THE CONCUSSION REPAIR MANUAL

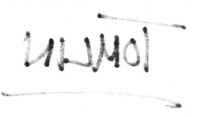

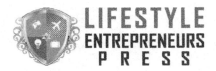

Publisher: Jesse Krieger
Write to Jesse@LifestyleEntrepreneursPress.com if you are interested in publishing through Lifestyle Entrepreneurs Press.

Publications or foreign rights acquisitions of our catalogue books.

Learn More: www.LifestyleEntrepreneursPress.com

Maryanska, Julia. "Dr. Dan Engle / Author Photograph." 2017.

ISBN: 978-1-946697-34-9

THE CONCUSSION REPAIR MANUAL

Visit ConcussionRepairManual.com,
FullSpectrumMedicine.com and
DrDanEngle.com for more information.

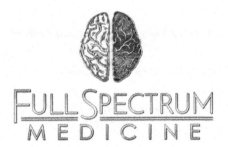

To all fellow voyagers along the path of Concussion Repair,

May your path to healing be a fulfilling journey of self discovery.

To all my teachers, mentors, and guides along this one precious life,

Thank you for your dedication to the healing arts and your willingness

to venture outside the box.

If you want to awaken all of humanity, then awaken all of yourself.
If you want to eliminate the suffering in the World, then eliminate all that is
dark and negative in yourself. Truly, the greatest gift you have to give is that
of your own self-transformation.

— *Lao Tzu*

SOME PRAISE FOR THE CONCUSSION REPAIR MANUAL

PHYSICIANS AND CLINICIANS

"A Game Changer. This book is the most useful piece of literature I have ever read on concussions. It gives patients all the tools, techniques and treatments they can use to heal themselves, as well as providing a workbook that lets them track their progress. It's also useful to doctors as the most comprehensive look at brain injury and all of the modalities currently available to treat it. In its class, it is the best book on the market."

~ *Matt Cook, MD* Founder, BioReset Medical

"The conventional model of concussion recovery is broken. Finally, there is a book that codifies what I truly believe; that there is another, more comprehensive and integrative approach that can vastly improve the lives of patients. Dan's CRM is required reading for concussion patients, their caregivers, and all allied healthcare practitioners who care for these patients. There is a better way and this is it."

~ *Scott Sherr, MD* Founder, Integrative HBOT,
Head of Protocol and Innovation at Hyperbaric Medical Solutions,
@hmsHBOT

"*Medice, cura te ipsum, Physician heal thyself.* Dr. Dan Engle has put together something truly valuable for those suffering from Trauamatic Brain Injuries. Dr. Dan's personal TBI recovery, as demanded by a cracking of his own "cosmic egg", opens the door for many warriors to recover from such an insidious ailment. This book takes deep cuts into understanding TBI's, and details approachable, effective treatments. Soldiers, football players, and physicians alike will benefit from studying its content in an ideal way."

~ *Jason McNeil, NMD* President,
North Valley Medical Center

"The real title of this book is "The Brain Health Optimization Manual." Whether or not you have had a concussion, read this book and follow the strategies used by biohackers like me to achieve optimal brain function: clarity, focus, memory, attention, cognition, concentration, learning, mood, stress adaptation, tranquility of thought, stillness of emotion, and "eye of the storm" equanimity. Except for injecting stem cells directly into my brain, I have used all the modalities laid out clearly by Dan, and they do work, especially if customized as a N=1 self-research protocol. The big secret that Dan is not telling you is that when you optimize your brain health, you optimize your entire body's health. And that is the biggest bonus of this book!"

~ *Dr. Ted Achacoso*, Founding Pioneer,
Health Optimization Medicine and Practice (HOMe/HOPe),
Interventional Endocrinology / Nutrient Therapy,
European Board Certified in Anti-Aging Medicine,
European Board Certified in Nutritional Medicine

"There are few topics in healthcare today receiving more attention than the long term damage from traumatic brain injury. Dr. Dan Engle has delivered the definitive resource that weaves together cutting edge technologies with traditional practices to provide both clinician and patient with the necessary tools to heal the injured brain. Whether you are a young athlete, military veteran, or an aging adult, *The Concussion Repair Manual*, is an invaluable guide to assist you on your path to recovery."

~ **Harry McIlroy, MD** Integrative Physician

ATHLETES AND ADVOCATES

"I've never read such a comprehensive manual for treating TBI's and concussions using the most cutting-edge protocols that exist - protocols that combine ancient wisdom and modern science in an informed, educational and easy-to-understand way. What I especially like about *The Concussion Repair Manual* is that the book can also be used as a simple tool to get smarter and think better, even if you haven't had a concussion. Whether you are a physician, a patient or simply an optimal health seeker, this book is a must-have for your personal health library."

> ~ *Ben Greenfield,* Human Performance Consultant,
> BenGreenfieldFitness.com

"When a problem has as wide a scope as traumatic brain injury, you need someone to tackle it from as many angles as possible, and Dr. Engle is exactly that guy."

> ~ *Aubrey Marcus,* Founder and CEO of Onnit

"No one plans for a brain injury and no-one knows what to do when they or their loved one is faced with the effects of one. Researching the safest and most effective treatments and modalities becomes a full time job with numerous twist, turns, and toll booths along the way. With today's bombardment of conflicting information, it is near impossible to sift through the contradictions and sales pitches to find the tools that are going to be effective to optimize brain function and repair.

This is not the kind of information that you will hear from your standard medical doctor. *The Concussion Repair Manual* provides an immensely useful guide to navigate **the turbulent waters of recovery by weighing the risks and unknowns to the possible benefits of** particular therapies.

For patients, practitioners, and loved ones, Dr. Daniel Engle, MD brings an invaluable resource."

> ~ *Cavin Balaster,* Author of How to Feed a Brain,
> Creator and CEO of FeedaBrain.com and
> AdventuresinTBI.com

"Dr. Dan Engle is simply magnificent. With his experience and knowledge transcending cultural, historical, and global medicine protocols- western clinical medicine, tribal technologies, eastern practices and much more it's safe to say the lens by which Dr. Dan evaluates and treats brain injuries is uniquely profound. As a TBI and Post Concussion syndrome sufferer myself, his insight has provided significant healing I could not find elsewhere. If you are suffering or know someone who is, stop what you are doing, and pick up this book immediately."

~ Guenter Bergmann, Entrepreneur and Adventurist, CEO,
High Five Digital, LLC

"The Concussion Repair Manual sheds light on many of the alternative health care modalities that are often over looked in the medical field. Many of these modalities have helped me tremendously in my own recovery, and my hope is that this book finds its way into the hands of those who are in need of these treatment options. It's never too late for your brain to heal"

~ Amy Zellmer, Faces of TBI,
Advocacy Platform and Podcast

"People and head injuries are like snowflakes in that no two are ever the same. They are uniquely individual. Likewise, the path of healing needs to be individualized based on each person's needs. Dr. Dan can talk the talk because he has walked the walk. *The Concussion Repair* Manual gives us the information, tools, and strategies needed to put together our own unique recovery plan. You can recover from head trauma to live and perform at elite levels. Dr. Dan and I are living proof. Let the CRM serve as your guide."

~ Andrew Marr, U.S. Army Special Forces (RET.),
Co-founder of Warrior Angels Foundation, Co-host of the Warrior Soul
Podcast, *Tales From The Blast Factory: A Special Forces Green Beret's Journey Back
From The Brink* (2017)

"Dr. Dan Engle is the one person I turn to when my brain isn't functioning at its full capacity. His wisdom and compassion are palpable, and through his experience both in and outside of academia, he shepherds those in need towards better brain health."

~ Jonathan Levi, Founder Becoming SuperHuman

TABLE OF CONTENTS

CRACKING MY COSMIC EGG

Not till we are lost. . . do we begin to find ourselves.
— Henry David Thoreau

IT'S SAFE TO say my worldview is a bit wider than that of the average doc—but by no means did it start out that way.

I'm board-certified in adult psychiatry and neurology, and I've completed psychiatric fellowships in child, adolescent, and forensic psychiatry. Still, I've come to realize there are many paths to healing. After deep and gradual exploration of transpersonal psychology, allopathic (i.e. Western medical approach) psychiatry, functional medicine, and many other alternative and integrated medicine practices, I've cultivated a mindset that appreciates and honors all aspects of wellness.

Author Joseph Chilton Pearce describes the "cosmic egg" in his contemporary classic, *The Crack in the Cosmic Egg*, as the way one's mind sees—and, as a result, the way one *experiences*—the world. He explains, "This circular trap of how we perceive reality is our cosmic egg, a shell of mind that both defines our world and helps shape it, just as that world, so shaped, defines the nature of our mind and experience." Furthermore, this bidirectional, interactive relationship between each of us and the world around us is fluid and evolutionary. As we grow and evolve so does the way we experience the world, and as the cultural identity of the external world around us grows and morphs over time, so it too affects our own sense of self and personal identity.

Pearce also notes, "There are experiences in which a crack forms in this egg, when non-ordinary things are possible, or non-ordinary solutions occur to the mind." These cracks in our cosmic eggs can be keys to new modes of thinking. Case in point, in some Amazonian cultures, when the medicine keeper of the tribe identifies a potential successor or apprentice, he will club that person on the crown of the head with a mallet. This figuratively (and frequently literally) cracks open the apprentice's cosmic egg, opening him up to receive the medicine keeper's teachings. At the very least this also tests the willingness and resolve of a would-be-student to actually go down the path of apprenticeship.

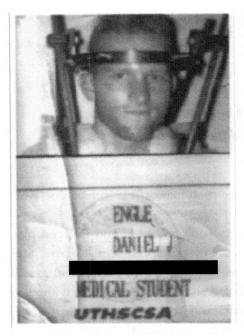

My own cosmic egg was cracked very wide open when I was 21. It happened just two weeks before I started medical school, and I had just arrived at my favorite fishing spot in Texas on the Gulf of Mexico. I was hot and tired after the long summer drive and had recently returned from celebrating college graduation with cliff diving in the tropics. Needless to say that sense of aerial freedom in flight was still programmed into my subconscious when I dove from 20 feet headfirst off of a pier into knee high water. This abrupt landing on a sandbar, which felt like getting blindsided by a dump truck, resulted in a compression fracture of my C5 vertebra and a newly acquired vulnerability. What also resulted was a healthy respect for the beauty and depth of life. My newly-liberated cosmic egg (disguised as a diving "accident") also catalyzed the beginning of an unexpected journey—one that would lead me to see myself and the entire field of medicine in a completely new way and eventually stimulate the deep investigation of brain trauma and the writing of this *Concussion Repair Manual*.

A brief backstory will paint more of the picture. Long before my deep dive into shallow water, I was an incredibly driven scholar and athlete. I grew up with an uber serious "Type A" personality focused on being the best at whatever I did, a natural asset to competitive sports. I played just about every sport in school and on club teams, which included me playing on the US Olympic development team in soccer and a club soccer team that won the gold medal in the Junior Olympics of 1989. At St. Edward's University, I was Academic All American, graduated Summa Cum Laude with a double major in Chemistry and Biology, and, as team captain, I didn't hesitate to lay into my teammates or drive them off the squad if they didn't perform. By the time I had graduated college, my level of intensity was at a fever pitch, and my broken neck associated TBI (traumatic brain injury) was only one in a series of major sports-related concussions. As anyone who's ever had a major dinger (i.e. concussion) will attest, there's nothing quite like the experience of not knowing who you are, where you are, and why you're there. Initially I thought breaking my neck was just another injury to overcome... and then reality and humility set in.

To immobilize my head and broken neck, I wore a halo device for three months and one day. Titanium screws in my skull connected a metal ring around my head to a plastic back plate and a chest plate. For the first time in my life, I felt quite immobile and surprisingly vulnerable. Needless to say, metal bolts screwed into your skull affects your concentration, and with the phone-book levels of information to memorize piling up in the first months of med school, my grades slipped a bit. Frustrated and finally forced to slow down, I reflected on my life. I had gained a wealth of early success and confidence in my life up to that point... and very little happiness. The previous level of drive had drawn me to the fast-paced fields in medicine of surgery and emergency medical care, but after the accident it all shifted. Psychiatry seemed like a much better fit, and, for the most part, it was—except for two little major hurdles. The first was Pessimism—not mine but the entire field of psychiatry and neurology, and the second was narcolepsy.

During my medical training (and pretty widely spread across the training programs throughout the country), many of the conditions assessed in the field of neurology and psychiatry were believed to have no known cure. The field itself is amazingly sophisticated in diagnosis and assessment, and yet quite limited in regards to resolution of the symptoms involved. Brain scanning machines, cerebrospinal assays, and biochemical blood markers were (and still are) only a few tools of the trade. We as physicians are very good at telling someone what is wrong symptomatically and pointing to the complex array of potential neurological areas affected, however, we are not historically very good at understanding the underlying mechanisms of causation and prescribing an effective intervention for resolution. Today, this is particularly relevant in the fields of autistic spectrum disorders, severe and chronic depression or anxiety, addictions, traumatic brain injury, and narcolepsy, to name just a few.

As mentioned before, I also previously experienced symptoms of narcolepsy, and it's my belief in hindsight that these were compounded by Post-Concussive Syndrome after multiple previous sports related concussions. I was formally diagnosed with narcolepsy in my third year of medical school by an MSLT (multi-sleep latency test) in the sleep lab of our medical school hospital, although the symptoms had certainly started much earlier. Essentially the core symptom of narcolepsy is consistent uncontrollable experience of falling asleep in situations where it is socially detrimental and physically dangerous. These issues came to a head in my third year of medical school when I fell asleep while driving home every day after an all-night call shift in the Labor and Delivery unit during my OB/GYN rotation. Even though I lived only 5 minutes away, I still couldn't't help falling asleep while driving, and the last time I woke up in oncoming traffic I knew I had to get it formally evaluated.

The MSLT is the diagnostic tool for narcolepsy, and I scored high marks in this test, too. My prize was being prescribed a very effective and heavy-duty pharmaceutical cousin of Ritalin called Cylert. My doctor told me that I would simply have to take it for the rest of my life to manage my condition and that there was no known cure. Not thinking much at the time about the "life sentence" to medication, I took it regularly—and well, it *really* worked. *There's a reason most people love stimulants.* From the US military to peak performance entrepreneurs, from high achieving students to long distance truck drivers, tons of people have been turned on to the pills. Just one pop of pill that neuro-chemically juices your brain like cocaine will most definitely get your attention… and for many hours. This certainly became quite advantageous through medical school and the rest of my psychiatric training. It was only after my medical training completed that I realized I was hooked to these pills with no end in sight, and furthermore, I couldn't help but notice that we psychiatrists were essentially doing the same thing to most of our psychiatric patients—getting them hooked with no plan or end point in sight. I had been taught first and foremost to prescribe meds to treat patients' symptoms, rather than start with the mindset of using medications only when necessary and while using a thorough plan to assess the underlying root causes for their problems. There had to be another way—maybe *many* other ways—to treat myself, not to mention my patients.

For the next several years, I studied the myriad branches of alternative medicine, training with chiropractors, naturopaths, homeopaths, Ayurvedic practitioners (focused on holistic, energy-based healing), acupuncturists, herbalists, Reiki healers, martial artists, and just about anyone else with a fascinating skill set in a formalized healing modality that had experience working with any mental health issue and was willing to teach me. When I couldn't find a living and willing teacher to work with, I dove into the available research and practiced on myself. I decided to put *myself* in the laboratory, because at the end of the day my own personal experience was the best barometer to assess the appropriateness of each modality. How else would I understand the nuances of so many paths to healing? How did each work? Why did they work? How did each one complement the other modalities I was or had been using?

I became a relentless detective. I analyzed everything I could think of that might have been a contributing factor. I overhauled my diet, regulated my sleep cycle, looked at my stress levels, and evaluated my hormone balance. I experimented with supplementation and used just about every technology and therapeutic device available to me for healing the brain (most of which are in this Manual), and each apparently blind alley opened up to a new wealth of information. When I exhausted all my known local resources, I moved to the Amazon rain forest to study herbal medicine and traditional healing techniques. What had been a relentless drive for perfection in the classroom and on the field during my childhood had gradually turned into a mission for developing the best strategies for optimal healing of the brain and mind.

This became a pilgrimage of personal development, and along the way I came to realize that the journey of healing *any* condition is a potential road to becoming one's best self. With experimentation in the reparative strategies making up this Manual, due diligence in my own healing protocols, and the grace of time, the symptoms of head trauma have almost fully abated, the experience of narcolepsy has completely resolved, and I'm off all prescription medications. Like many who have experienced multiple, significant concussions, I do still technically meet criteria for Post Concussive Syndrome, although my relationship to it now is vastly different than before. Now I use it as an ally and a tool. It works as a barometer constantly giving me feedback for how well I'm following my optimal lifestyle program, and how actively engaged I am in my own personal life's mission. The entire experience has become a form of Resistance Training, not so much for the body as much as for the mind. As such, the massive benefits of mindfulness, true presence, and simplicity and consistency in my daily routines have become paramount, and channeling this renewed passion toward the exciting new and growing field of holistic, integrative psychiatry and functional medicine has led to a whole new toolkit presented here in this Manual.

In this one precious life everyone has their own unique form of the Hero's/Heroine's Journey. Mine just happened to be initiated through a series of traumatic brain injuries. Through the fog, fatigue and helplessness of debilitating concussions, I found the modalities that worked and developed a way to not just recover but to thrive. I exceeded all expectations of the doctors treating me at the time, graduated from medical school, received board certification in psychiatry and neurology and became one of the leading clinician physicians in the field of neuroscience and cognitive restoration.

My passion and mission are to help guide, support, teach and treat patients and families on the journey of concussion recovery. I have worked with thousands of patients in healing their neurological conditions using all the strategies mentioned in this book. In some cases we used many tools, in others we used a "less is more" approach. With the appropriate therapies at the appropriate times, more and more patients will not only experience their own recovery, they too will exceed expectations and perform what they once believed was not possible. As the saying goes, "the journey of 1000 miles begins with one step." Let us begin......

HEADS UP!

The Concussion Repair Manual is not intended for acute patients who are currently on life support or those who have not yet been fully stabilized in a medical environment.

This manual is intended for traumatic brain injury survivors who already have been medically evaluated and stabilized and are now in transition, gradually healing and returning to their lives, their relationships, and their day-to-day activities.

The Concussion Repair Manual should be used with the awareness, support and supervision of a local physician or primary care provider

HOW TO USE THIS BOOK

Nothing has such power to broaden the mind as the ability to investigate
systematically and truly all that comes under thy observation in life.
— *Marcus Aurelius*

THERE REALLY ISN'T a wrong way to use *The Concussion Repair Manual,* but there is an *ideal* way to interact with this book.

First, bring your curiosity, patience, and an open mind. *The Concussion Repair Manual* is partly a guidebook, which will help you to understand what processes naturally happen inside healthy brains, how traumatic brain injury derails these natural processes, and what that means for you. It is also an overview of the most current, comprehensive TBI treatment tools and techniques that holistic and integrative medicine has to offer.

Some of these therapies come from the newest frontiers in neuroscience. Others are rooted in ancient medicinal and natural healing traditions. To really get to know the TBI condition and its treatment options, read through each of these chapters at least once.

Next, grab a pen and plan to really get to know *yourself* by using the worksheets included in the back of this *Concussion Repair Manual.* You will pay close attention to your symptoms, establish a symptom severity baseline, and systematically track your recovery progress. In the very last chapter of this book, you'll learn how to weave the various therapies together to create a personalized treatment protocol that works best for you.

The old adage "everyone is unique" will be reiterated many times throughout the Manual and really cannot be said enough. It's tempting to judge resolution of these chronically held and often frustrating symptoms by expectations of "speed of cure" or "because that person got so much better so much faster than me." This Manual is not about curing anything. It is about working towards recovery in the best way for each person and assisting in tracking that progress. As such, many factors contribute to symptom expression and recovery, and this Manual is aimed at taking a multi-pronged, holistic, and integrative approach to contribute to a return of optimal physical, neurological, and personal function. Hopefully, the road ahead for you in Re-becoming your best self is met with as much ease, effectiveness, acceptance, and inspiration as possible.

QUICK TIP Throughout this book, definitions of technical terms, quick tips, and really important notes are highlighted inside special boxes like this one.

Also, the beginning of every chapter includes a brief description of what that chapter is about and how you can get the most out of it. Notably, in regards to definitions for this Manual, the terms concussion and mild traumatic brain injury (TBI) are essentially interchangeable and will often be utilized as such.

INTRODUCTION – HISTORY OF TREATMENT AND CURRENT TRENDS

THE BIG PICTURE OF TRAUMATIC BRAIN INJURY – PAST AND PRESENT

AS A FAMILY of humanity and the species of Man, like it or not, we are collectively in the throes of an unprecedented evolution of global technology and digital information. Never before in our history has it been possible for this many people on the planet to share so much information so quickly. Every season, previous physical performance records are smashed, and every day more people are connected to the world-wide-web. Our individual and global human potential seems to know no bounds.

A perfect example of this degree of growth and technological expansion is in the field of Regenerative Brain Medicine. It is accelerating through an exciting time of unprecedented development in the research areas of neuro-diagnostics and reparative technologies for both healing the brain from disease and promoting its ability to achieve peak performance. This present day trend has largely been driven by three distinct forces: the aging Baby Boomer generation's growing prevalence of neurodegenerative conditions (predominantly Alzheimer's Dementia), the present day consumer concern over the effects of of Traumatic Brain Injury and the neuro-hacker contingency of cognitive performers looking to up-level their game.

Articles are written almost daily about the public concern over head injury and its potentially serious progression—from concussion to PCS (post-concussive syndrome), to PTSD (post-traumatic stress disorder) to the newest term for most people CTE (chronic traumatic encephalopathy), a form of accelerated dementia resulting from chronic head injuries. As a result, the paradigm of Concussion Care is actively shifting from one of relative acceptance of head injury in sports to one of mandating preventative measures be taken (especially for youth sports) and effective diagnosis and treatment be provided when it occurs. When I was in medical training, we knew traumatic brain injury occurred, but we really had no idea how to treat it when it didn't resolve on its own. Now the research field is revealing excellent new technologies and treatments for the injured brain, most of which are covered in this Manual.

If you've suffered a traumatic brain injury, you're certainly not alone. An estimated 3.17 million Americans are living with long-term disabilities related to TBI,[1] although that number is actually thought to be on the low side. In fact, in 2009 alone, nearly 3.5 million patients received medical attention—either hospitalization or treatment from an emergency department, outpatient center or physician's office—for the condition.[2] But even *that* number doesn't accurately reflect just how many people were affected in 2009, because it doesn't account for people who went unrecognized or untreated. It also doesn't include injured military personnel.

Quantifying the total number of TBI cases has been tricky, but, in general, the combined rates for TBI-related deaths, hospitalizations, and trips to the ER have risen by nearly 60 percent between 2001 and 2010.[3] There could be many reasons for that increase. Sure, it's possible that it's just bad news and many more people are sustaining traumatic brain injuries overall. But it's also possible that a larger portion of the injured population is finally taking even mild head trauma more seriously—seriously enough to seek medical care. That would be good news.

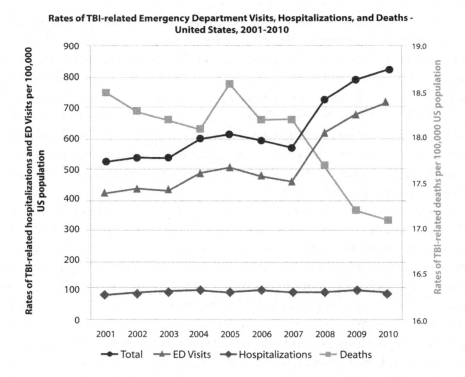

Rates of TBI-related Emergency Department Visits, Hospitalizations, and Deaths - United States, 2001-2010

Source: 2001 – 2010 U.S. data as reported by the Centers for Disease Control and Prevention office of the National Center for Injury Prevention and Control

LEADING CAUSES OF TBI

TBI-related emergency department visits, hospitalizations and deaths per 100,000 U.S. population

	ED Visits	Hospitalizations	Deaths	Total
2001	420.6	82.7	18.5	521.0
2002	433.9	85.6	18.3	537.2
2003	423.3	94.6	18.2	535.4
2004	486.3	97.6	18.1	601.3
2005	505.0	92.0	10.0?	615.2
2006	478.9	98.7	18.2	595.1
2007	457.5	91.7	18.2	566.2
2008	616.4	95.5	17.7	728.9
2009	677.4	98.0	17.2	791.9
2010	715.7	91.7	17.1	823.7

Falls, traffic accidents, sports injuries and active-duty military service are among the top causes of traumatic brain injury. On average, unintentional falls accounted for nearly half of the TBI-related ER visits and half of all TBI-related hospitalizations in the U.S. between 2006 and 2010.[4]

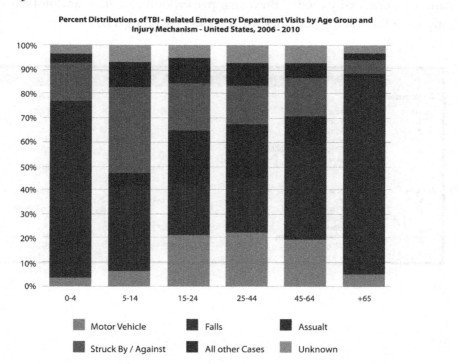

Percent Distributions of TBI - Related Emergency Department Visits by Age Group and Injury Mechanism - United States, 2006 - 2010

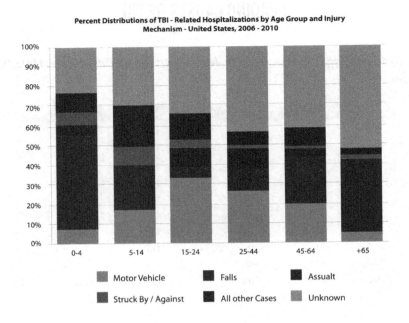

Percent Distributions of TBI - Related Hospitalizations by Age Group and Injury Mechanism - United States, 2006 - 2010

Researchers analyzed sports and recreation-related injuries treated in U.S. emergency departments between 2001 and 2012 and found that 7% of all of these were TBIs. Bicycling, football, and basketball were the leading activities among male TBI patients. Bicycling, playground activities, and horseback riding were the leading activities for females sustaining TBIs.[5]

Rank order by sex	Treated and released SRAs	%	Hospitalized/transferred As	%	Total* As	%
Male	N = 2 107 008		N = 216 368		N = 2 368 405	
1	Football	18.5	Bicycling	33.3	Bicycling	19.2
2	Bicycling	17.7	ATV	16.2[b]	Football	17.3
3	Basketball	8.1	Moped[c]	7.7	Basketball	7.6
4	Playground activities	6.2	Football	6.1	Playground activities	5.8
5	Baseball	5.9	Snow sports[b]	6.0[b]	Baseball	5.5
	All other SRAs	43.6	All other SRAs	30.7	All other SRAs	44.6
Female	N = 953 206		N = 77 385		N = 1 048 864	
1	Bicycling	12.7	Horseback riding	23.2[b]	Bicycling	13.3
2	Playground activities	10.5	Bicycling	19.8[b]	Playground activities	10.1
3	Soccer	8.6	ATV	16.5[b]	Horseback riding	8.3
4	Basketball	8.3	Snow sports[d]	5.4[b]	Soccer	8.1
5	Horseback riding	7.1	Exercise[e]	4.4[b]	Basketball	7.8
	All other SRAs	52.8	All other SRAs	30.7	All other SRAs	52.4

Interestingly, over time, soccer accounted for increasing numbers of TBI cases among both males and females.[6] It's worth noting that each time a player "heads" the ball—especially at high velocity—his or her brain may sustain some degree of trauma. Even mild headers can add up. For my part, I started playing soccer when I was just four and continued until I was 20—that's 16 years' worth of low-grade brain trauma!

Traumatic brain injury also has become increasingly common in some branches of the U.S. military. More than four percent of the total 5.6 million people serving in the Army, Air Force, Navy and Marine Corps between 2000 and 2011 were diagnosed with a TBI.[7]

[handwritten margin note: Soccer heading]

Estimated Overall Annual Incidence Rates of TBI among Active-Duty U.S. Military Service Members by Service Branch, 2000–2011

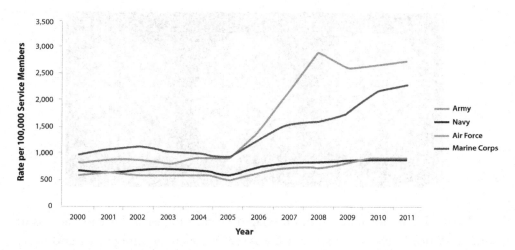

Source: Defense and Veterans Brain Injury Center (via 2013 Report to Congress on Traumatic Brain Injury in the United States)

During the period studied, the largest increases in the incidence of TBIs were among active-duty segments of the Army and Marine Corps. By 2011, the TBI rate was 3.3 times higher than it had been in 2000 for active-duty Army personnel. As for active-duty Marines, by 2011, the TBI rate was 2.4 times higher than it had been in 2000.[8]

LONG-TERM EFFECTS OF TBI

Fortunately, most mild TBIs heal spontaneously with rest and recovery. However, with more significant trauma, symptoms often persist, lasting even months to years, nagging and limiting personal function and life enjoyment. As a result of your own TBI, you may have problems with your thinking and memory, trouble communicating with others, issues with your vision, hearing or other senses, mood swings, sleep problems, and a whole lot much more.[9] While this can be challenging at the present moment, your injury's impact in later life can be even more deleterious. That's why getting proper treatment as soon as possible is absolutely critical. (So is avoiding repeat TBIs if you've been injured!)

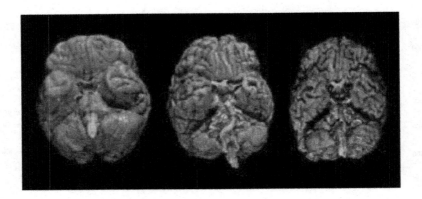

Partly due to advances in brain imaging technologies and greater access to injured donor brains for further study, researchers are learning more and more about TBIs' long-term effects and are finding significant correlations between traumatic brain injury and early onset dementia. If you've had a moderate brain injury, your risk for developing Alzheimer's disease is more than double. And, if you've had a severe brain injury? Your Alzheimer's risk is four and a half times higher.[10] (We will talk more about the genetics of Alzheimer's as it relates to TBI later on in this chapter.)

Researchers have also found associations between TBI and Parkinson's, chronic traumatic encephalopathy (a neurodegenerative condition often linked to boxing and other long-term, high-impact sports like football) and even premature death.[11] (See the section on Repeat TBI for more detail on chronic traumatic encephalopathy.)

The *financial* ramifications for individuals and society as a whole are massive as well. Looking back at TBI cases occurring in the U.S. civilian population during the year 2000, researchers have estimated the associated economic costs to be more than $221 billion (in 2009 dollars.) That amount included $14.6 billion for medical costs, $69.2 billion for work loss costs, and $137 billion for the value of lost quality of life.[12,13] What's more, unemployment rates for TBI patients of working age have been shown to be much higher than the U.S. national average. Between 2003 and 2012, the unemployment rate for patients who had completed inpatient rehabilitation for TBI between 2001 and 2010 was 60.4%. (The average unemployment rate for the U.S. population during the same period was just 9%.)[14]

So, what does all of this mean for your own long-term outcome? Well, that depends on multiple factors like the severity of your injury, how old and how healthy you were at the time of your injury, and your genetic makeup. Although you can't control those particular factors, the good news is there are plenty of others factors that you *can* control, which can be leveraged to help you recover and optimize your brain function.

As you'll see, there are more TBI therapy options available than ever before, and TBI survival rates and treatment outcomes have improved dramatically.

JUST HOW FAR HAVE WE COME?

Necessity is the mother of invention.
– *Plato*

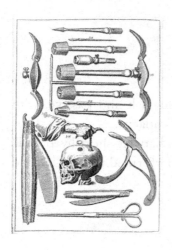

Up until recent history, medical practitioners didn't clearly understand the link between brain injury and psychological symptoms. Brain injury can give rise to virtually any type of psychiatric symptomology including depression, mania, psychosis, obsessive-compulsive disorder, psychosis, substance abuse, apathy, aggression, and personality changes.[15] These consequences are pervasive and identified in virtually all patients with moderate to severe injuries for an initial period up to about three months, with a smaller percentage exhibiting persistent symptoms for months to years.[16]

Take a moment to imagine that you'd sustained a TBI back in the Stone Age. Fossil records suggest that some of the earliest human civilizations treated severe brain injuries by scraping, cutting or drilling into a live patient's damaged skull with sharpened stones. (At least, by the end of the Neolithic period, surgeons graduated to surgical instruments made of bronze.)[17] The practice was known as "trepanation" (from the Greek *trypanon*, meaning "auger" or "borer"[18]) and was widely practiced well up until the Civil War era.[19]

Used by Hippocrates and his ancient colleagues, "bloodletting" was another popular technique used to treat brain injuries (and myriad other medical conditions, for that matter.) It was thought that, by intentionally withdrawing a patient's blood, the natural balance between the body's four main fluids—yellow bile, black bile, blood and phlegm, according to Hippocrates—would be restored or maintained. Physicians would continue the practice of "bleeding" their patients for the next 2,000 years.[20]

> **Down-regulation**—the process by which function is limited, decreased or entirely suppressed by external factors.

Or suppose that you experienced your head injury sometime during the 1800s or even the early 1900s. Let's say you survived the initial treatment for your wound, but as a result of the TBI you suffer ongoing depression, mood swings, anger, agitation and so on. At that time, long-term confinement to asylums for the mentally ill was pretty common—so common that they became overcrowded.[21]

Partly to solve that overcrowding problem plus the lack of other obviously effective treatment options, frontal lobotomy was developed in the 1930s. The most common approach was for surgeons to disconnect and literally "scramble" the prefrontal lobe of the brain—sometimes by injecting alcohol into this tissue or cutting into it with various instruments. As a result, and *not at all surprising*, lobotomized patients often became sluggish and passive, with noticeably blunted emotional ranges and intellectual capacity.

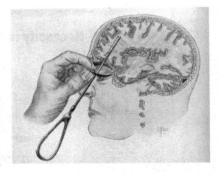

The practice was controversial and, fortunately, relatively short-lived. Still, it's estimated that 60,000 frontal lobotomies were performed in the U.S. and Europe between 1936 and 1956.[22]

HOW HEALTHY BRAINS ARE SUPPOSED TO WORK

Brain researchers have learned SO much about the entire nervous system and the human brain within the last few years. (To say it is a complicated organ is an understatement.) So, what follows here is a window into the basics for understanding how healthy brains ideally function, how an injury disrupts some of the brain's natural processes, and how those disruptions can create a seemingly endless cascade of problems.

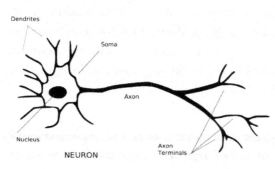

But first, a rundown of some essential anatomy. (The technical terms that are going to come up again in the context of traumatic brain injury are highlighted in bold.)

On the outside, the brain and spinal cord are enclosed within protective membranes called the **meninges**.

On the inside, the average human brain contains billions of **neurons** (nerve cells) and **glial cells.** Neurons transmit electrochemical signals to and from the brain. A neuron is made up of a cell body (which contains DNA), branching dendrites (which receive signals) and a slender nerve fiber projection called an **axon** (which conducts signals.) Glial cells support the work of neurons in many ways, such as providing nutrients and oxygen and removing harmful debris.

Although there are different subtypes of these supporting glial cells, we're only going to focus on two of them for now: the **microglia** and the **astrocytes**. Microglia are the brain's primary immune cells, and astrocytes (making up about half of the brain's volume) perform many functions, including producing energy and helping to form the blood-brain barrier. The **blood-brain barrier (BBB)** is a semi-permeable, protective shield of cells, which separates the brain from the circulating bloodstream.

Got all that? Before we see how all of this fits together, here are a few other concepts to keep in mind.

- Your neurons contain **tau proteins**. In healthy brains, these proteins serve as a kind of support scaffolding for the axons. Tau proteins transport fats, glucose, and other important cargo along a neuron's axonal fibers to the end of the axon. Moving this cargo to that spot is essential for the transmission of signals between neurons. And this transmission of signals, called neurotransmission, is essential to normal brain function.

- When our cells metabolize oxygen, free radicals called **reactive oxygen species (ROS)** are naturally released. Because they have unpaired electrons, these molecules are highly unstable and chemically reactive. While they do serve some important roles in the brain, reactive oxygen species can also cause damage. In healthy brains, there are super important mechanisms at work to keep the amounts of ROS in check.

- Just as the rest of the body has a lymphatic system to help rid itself of toxins and bacteria, the brain has a **glymphatic system** with a similar function. These brain specific lymphatic vessels surround the neurons and astrocytes and are responsible for removing waste and debris that build up in the brain.

HEADS UP! *Be careful to avoid repeat injury while recovering from TBI!*

This is probably the single most important recommendation in the whole Manual, and will be repeated often to make the point. Exposure of the initial injury to subsequent, large amounts of ROS and neuro-inflammation will cause already weakened cells to be increasingly susceptible to cell death. Thus, sustaining additional blows to the head can push already-stressed cells to their limits.

THE INJURED BRAIN

So, just what happens when you sustain a head injury? Well, there are essentially 3 areas of associated symptoms:

- Neuro-biological
- Neuro-psychiatric
- Neuro-cognitive

In looking at the **neuro-biological** ramifications, the type, severity, and frequency of the injury dictates how much tissue damage occurs. With major brain trauma, the connective tissue of the meninges tears, and the damaged tissues release reactive oxygen species (ROS) in such massive amounts that cells—including astrocytes making up the blood-brain barrier—begin to die. As these cells die, the BBB becomes weakened, and the metabolic cascade continues. Potassium, chloride and sodium begin to leak through the compromised barrier and into the brain, causing the brain to swell, the synaptic junction becomes paralyzed and loss of consciousness can occur.

Incidentally, with loss of consciousness upon injury, there can be even more cell death due to oxygen deprivation. Normally, astrocytes produce energy through a process called glycolysis. During **glycolysis**, astrocytes break down glucose and make lactate as a byproduct. When lactate combines with oxygen, energy is created. But, if the brain is oxygen-deprived, oxygen is unavailable to the lactate. Instead of combining with oxygen to convert to energy the neurons can use, the lactate levels build up, causing even more cell death.

Now your brain's immune response is triggered, and your microglia swing into action, trying to clean up the dead cell debris and shore up weaknesses in the blood-brain barrier. This is the same reactive process that occurs elsewhere in the body, when proteases and cytokines are sent in for tissue repair, and is seen as the four classic signs of injury—redness, heat, swelling, and tenderness. The excitatory neurotransmitter glutamate is then released and **excitotoxicity** ensues, leading to further neuronal cell death.

As mentioned before, with consistent rest after injury, the brain usually heals itself, and this is through the release of BDNF (brain-derived neurotrophic factor). However, if another injury occurs before the brain can start to heal, the immunological response is stuck in "action mode," the excitotoxic cascade continues and neuronal damage mounts. This is essentially the biggest risk for accumulated brain trauma—the brain cell damage accruing over time while the reparative mechanisms are sidelined.

Activating the immune system also causes deposits of **amyloid beta plaques** to accumulate outside of neurons and in between glial cells. These plaques disrupt glycolysis and cause even more reactive oxygen species to be released. Their presence also activates additional microglia, which will try to remove the amyloid beta plaques—sending more pro-inflammatory signals in the process.

The accumulation of *amyloid beta plaques* and *tau tangles* are two hallmark features in the brains of patients with **Alzheimer's disease**. It's true that these plaques and tangles gradually accumulate in all brains as part of the natural aging process, and we've also just described how head injuries can markedly speed up this process. Other conditions associated with brain trauma are CTE and BIN. **Chronic traumatic encephalopathy**—CTE—is a condition of accelerated dementia resulting from successive head injuries. There is still growing research into its full etiology and what predisposes one to its effects.

Lastly, the term BIN—**Blast Induced Neurotrauma**—is a separate and quite unique condition described by the military where a soldier is exposed to a high frequency and high velocity explosive blast, and a result the brain experiences multiple small ricochet traumas as it bounces rapidly and repeatedly inside the skull. This extraordinarily high impact exposure may account for the high prevalence rate, on the order of 20 percent, of all soldiers returning home from service abroad having TBI and its often-associated post-traumatic stress disorder—PTSD.

In looking at the **neuro-psychiatric** ramifications of TBI, post-traumatic stress disorder (PTSD) is the one classically discussed. However, we learned before, brain injury can give rise a host of psychiatric symptoms. Depression is one of the most common psychiatric outcomes in TBI survivors and is prevalent among 20 – 60% of individuals. Depression following TBI is associated with reduced levels of serotonin and disruptions in brain circuitry in the prefrontal cortex, amygdala, hippocampus, and basal ganglia.[23] Individuals with TBI are also at increased risk for developing addiction. A recent population-based study indicated 1 to 3 years after injury, individuals with TBI are almost twice as likely to report binge drinking,[24] and in my clinical experience this is a conservative estimate.

TBI is a complicated picture involving many different clinically symptomatic pictures and personal life experiences, and the clinical association of such a broad spectrum of neurological issues can be challenging to fully assess and resolve. The most frequent neurologic symptoms associated with TBI include: headache, light and sound sensitivity, dizziness/nausea, fatigue/lethargy, and insomnia. Headaches can manifest as cluster type, tension type, and migraine, and the chronicity of these neurologic symptoms may persist for decades depending on the nature of the injury.[25] To complicate matters further, neurological symptoms can also arise months and even years after an initial injury, making identification of the primary insult challenging, and about 15 percent of people will experience chronic symptoms lingering for months or even years in a condition known as Post Concussive Syndrome.[26]

Neuro-cognitive deficits are common after TBI and vary based upon the location, type, and severity of injury. Impairments following TBI can arise in attention, working memory, executive functioning, information processing speed, and long-term memory. Impairments in cognition can be due to many of the aforementioned underlying neurobiological such as diffuse axonal injury, inflammation, and mitochondrial dysfunction. Neurocognitive deficits may be some of the most devastating consequences of TBI as individuals experience limitations accomplishing pre-injury tasks that may have been automatic and previously required little cognitive effort. Tasks such as sustaining attention while reading, planning a daily schedule, finding the correct words in conversation, remembering people's names or organizing personal items may be extraordinarily difficult, and frustration over one's cognitive limitations only exacerbates co-occurring psychiatric symptoms. Typically these cognitive difficulties resolve (or at least significantly improve) over time, but many will persist indefinitely and continue to hinder the functional experience and quality of one's life.[27]

GENETICS AND THE ALZHEIMER'S LINK

With further advances in research the relationship between Alzheimer's Dementia and TBI is clarifying, and it's currently estimated that your risk of Alzheimer's more than doubles if you've had a moderate brain injury, and it's even higher if your injury was characterized as severe.[28]

As it happens, there is one other factor—your genetic makeup—that increases your Alzheimer's risk even further.

To understand how, you first need to know a little about apolipoproteins. These are special proteins in the brain, which are crucial for healthy function. There are several different kinds of apolipoproteins, and the one that's most relevant here is called Apolipoprotein E. Abbreviated as Apo-E (pronounced

AY-POE-EE), this particular protein transports cholesterol and fatty acids to neurons and helps facilitate the growth of new synapses in your brain. Apo-E also assists with the removal of amyloid beta plaques and other debris.

Apo-E is genetically polymorphic, which means there can be slight variations in the sequence of its DNA. In the human population Apo-E has three variations known as ApoE2, ApoE3, and ApoE4, with each of these variations having a somewhat unique structure and function.

In review of basic genetics, each one of us gets one copy of every gene we have from our mother and another copy from our father. In terms of apolipoprotein E, that means we each have two chances to get one of the three variations of Apo-E. The majority of people carry the Apo-E3 variation, which typically functions well. The problem arises however, with the subtype Apo-E4, because unfortunately, amyloid beta plaques aren't as easily discarded in brains with ApoE4. This factor is implicated in the estimated correlation between Alzheimer's and carrying the Apo-E subtyped at approximately 40 to 80 percent. [29] [30] Notably, about one in every four people have at least one copy of ApoE4, and worse still, approximately two percent of the population is unlucky enough to have *two* copies of ApoE4.[31]

All of this boils down to the summary research finding that has tentatively concluded people who carry one or more copies of ApoE4 and have had a traumatic brain injury have a *tenfold risk* of developing Alzheimer's disease.[32]

The green highlighted areas in this positron emission tomography (PET) scan indicate tau tangles which have built up in the brain. The patient on the left carries the ApoE4 variation and appears to have more of this debris than the ApoE4-negative patient on the right.

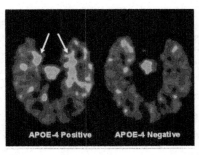

And remember those tau proteins? Well, in the case of TBI and in response to the activation of microglia, what were once essential cargo transporters become clumped together in messy **tau tangles**. Like a derailed train, these proteins can no longer deliver the goods. The downstream end result of all of this (and partly due to the compromised glymphatic system) is the piling up of the tau tangles, amyloid beta plaques and cellular debris, the breakdown of neurotransmission, the death of neural connections, the shrinkage and scarring of the affected brain area, and overall severe functional impairment.

During this cascading response to the initial injury, each of these negative effects compound, and this underlying process can go on for weeks, months, or even years. Meanwhile, on the surface, the symptomatic experience of this cascade is an assortment of problem areas, including short-term memory, communication, thinking, metabolic function, and so much more. All the energy the brain has is thus diverted from normal function to mounting a response to the insult and attempting to marshal repair.

Fortunately, there are tests (like the 23 and me) that can determine a person's genetic status. This can be particularly helpful in the event that someone is having a challenge recovering from a TBI. When treatment resistance occurs, especially when there is a positive test for the ApoE4, it becomes much more important to increase the recovery protocol intensity to match the increased neurological need.

THE LIMITS OF CONVENTIONAL TBI TREATMENT

A multitude of standard medical strategies exist for treating TBI, and while they exceed in stabilizing acute trauma, they are also limited in several essential ways. The current mainstream medical treatments for TBI are essentially the same ones taught to me in medical training 20 years ago and include surgery, behavioral and functional rehabilitation, physical therapy, and nutritional recommendations. These approaches are primarily designed to minimize complications of the initial injury and rehabilitate lost functional abilities, though they are frequently lacking in their power to mitigate the inflammatory cascade and foster neurogenesis and repair. While emergency and rehabilitation medicine are good on the "battle field" and are equipped to deal with acute brain injury, there is a significant lack of efficacious treatments for secondary and degenerative effects. We are just now stepping into a golden age in regenerative medicine in which we are finding strategies to truly restore brain function.

Fortunately, effective, cutting-edge medical strategies demonstrating early evidence of regenerative neurological effects are *definitely* on the rise and comprise the bulk of the material discussed here in the Manual. Many of these "new kids on the block" are still considered novel by the general medical field as they are still garnering more of the formal, large scale research data that is the standard process of becoming more widely accepted. However, the growing acknowledgment of TBI and concussion related catastrophic health impacts along with the epidemic of rising neurodegenerative conditions is outpacing standard research science investigation and stimulating the rise of new technologies. Examples of these include: hyperbaric oxygen,[33] stem cell therapy,[34] hypothermic therapy,[35] virtual reality,[36] and near-infrared laser photo-therapy.[37] As a result of the newness of the methods and research, most have yet to be widely utilized or supported by the medical industry and often fall outside the realm of third-party insurance companies.[38] Hence, the personal expense can be significant when engaging in a recovery program that uses novel approaches, especially when doing so without a guided plan supported by a knowledgeable clinician specialized in concussion care. All these factors are coming together to create a ripening field of scientific exploration and clinical growth, as the current crisis in brain illness and its related psychological epidemic warrants treatment solutions that are not merely palliative in nature, but have the capacity to heal, regenerate, and truly restore neurological health and function.

DIAGNOSIS AND CLASSIFICATION OF TBI

As we discussed previously, when brain trauma occurs, physical forces compress and sheer brain tissue, leading to a series of events from axonal injury and inflammation to neuronal degradation and cell death. This "neu-ro-metabolic cascade," as described by Giza and Honva, is a vastly com-plex cellular and neuro-vascular storm carrying with it a further windfall of pathophysiology effects that includes ionic shifts, abnormal energy me-tabolism, diminished cerebral blood flow and impaired neurotransmission. Symptomatically, what can be seen immediately as a result of a TBI can range from transient and self-limiting to catastrophic, including irreversible dysfunction and even death.[39] According to CDC guidelines in conjunction with the Department of Defense (DoD) and Veterans Affairs (VA), TBI is classified as mild, moderate, or severe based on three criteria: the duration of unconsciousness, the lowest Glasgow coma scale score within the first 24 hours of the inciting event, and the duration of post- traumatic amnesia.

GLASGOW COMA SCALE

Eyes Open		
	Spontaneously	4
	To speech	3
	To pain	2
	Never	1
Best verbal response		
	Oriented	5
	Confused	4
	Inappropriate words	3
	In comprehensible sounds	2
	None	1
Best Motor response		
	Obeys commands	6
	Localized pain	5
Flexion to pain		
	Withdrawal	4
	Abnormal	3
	Extention to pain	2
	None	1
	Total	**3-15**

Coma scale.

The term concussion is often used interchangeably with mild TBI (mTBI) in medical literature, and we will also use these terms synonymously in the Manual. Multiple classifications systems exist, and generally the concussion grading guidelines by Cantu (2001), which correlate severity with the longer-term consideration of post-concussive symptoms (see TBI effects) are a hallmark system in the field.

Whatever the extent of severity of TBI one experiences, it remains clear that early assessment and recognition of the injury is associated with significantly better health outcomes. On presentation, the assessment includes a thorough history of the inciting event, physical exam, mental status exam, cognitive screen, post-concussive assessment, and a review of mental health.

The vast majority of sports related concussions typically fall on the benign end of mild TBI, and notably, about 90 percent of diagnosed concussion do not include a loss of consciousness. That being said, even the mild types deserve serious attention and warrant appropriate treatment. The variety of **possible signs and symptoms of mild TBI/Concussion include:** headache, confusion, poor coordination, abnormal behavior, light sensitivity, nausea/vomiting, slurred speech, any tingling or numbness, visual changes (blurring, double vision), and problems with concentration or memory (particularly of the event causing the injury).

WHEN IS NEUROIMAGING NECESSARY?

The need for neuroimaging has historically been determined by the Canadian Head CT rule to assess for lesions requiring neurosurgical intervention, such as hemorrhage. This takes into account the severity of head injury, how it occurred, the age of the person, extent and duration of any alteration in consciousness and obvious physical exam signs of skull fracture. It has the benefit of carrying a high degree of specificity and sensitivity for assessing a significant injury's need for a head CT scan to discern further neuro-surgical intervention. There are also novel imaging tools for assessment being explored on the field of play and battle for use when rapid and timely diagnosis is critical. (For example, a portable hand held device called the Infrascanner uses near infra-red light to detect pooled blood in and around the brain) The on-site portability of such units greatly assists in the acute evaluation and triage process, leading to more appropriate early treatment measures and better overall outcomes. *** We delve into this all further in the Assessment Tools for Concussion in Chapter 8. ***

The majority of TBIs are classified as mild, and, fortunately, most will spontaneously resolve with care and rest. In the event that further assessment in a medical facility is warranted, the following criteria are used for safe discharge to home observation following the period of initial assessment within the medical arena:

- No mental status changes with clinically improving post-concussive symptoms, at least four hours post-injury
- Normal head CT scan or no clinical risk factors requiring the need for CT head scanning

-   - No clinical indicators for prolonged observation including: clinical deterioration, focal neurological deficits, changes in mental status, known coagulopathy, presence of drug or alcohol intoxication, concurrent medical problems, or age greater than 65.

Classification Criteria Of Tbi

	Duration of Unconsciousness	Glasgow Coma Scale (lowest score)	Post-Traumatic Amnesia
Mild	<30 Minutes	13-15	<24 hours
Moderate	30 minutes to 24 hours	9-12	1-7 days
Severe	>24 hours	3-8	>7 days

While most outcomes for mild TBI resolve fully to the level of previous function, the outcomes still remain unpredictable and heterogeneous, depending on a variety of pre-existing risk factors, social support utilized, and treatments explored. There is often a period of reduced cognitive function within the first few days of injury, which is expected to resolve to the pre-injury level within a period of a few days to a few months. Ideally clients and family are well-educated by trained clinicians on what to expect in the acute healing phase, as well as strategies to maximize outcomes. The goals of treatment are to facilitate the return to full pre-injury function as quickly as possible, and when significant symptoms persist for longer than two to three months, more comprehensive assessment in a specialized brain care center is warranted.

The hallmark diagnosis for continued symptoms is **Post Concussion Syndrome—PCS**. So often it goes recognized and untreated, mostly because of its very vague nature and nonspecific symptomatology. While no single explanatory model exists to elucidate the wide range of symptoms and unpredictable recovery course of TBI, it likely involves a complex array of pre-injury health, nutrigenomic profiles involving methylation pathways (which we get deeper into in the Section on Foods for Recovery), constitutional recovery mechanisms, co-existing inflammatory conditions, ongoing environmental toxic exposures, psychological make-up and attitudinal styles, social supports, sleep hygiene, lifestyle influences and other untold forces.

Diagnosis of PCS requires the development of at least three psychomotor symptoms within four weeks of the head trauma and lasting for 3 months or longer. These generalized neuro-psychiatric symptoms include: headaches, fatigue, dizziness, irritability, anxiety, insomnia, light/noise sensitivity, and poor concentration/focus. Notably, it does not require a loss of consciousness. *(DSM V – Manual of Psychiatry)*

The potential association of such wide-ranging, fairly vague symptoms leads to a high potential for misdiagnosis, making a clinical differential diagnoses looking at other underlying causes ever more important. Interestingly enough, and typically going against one's expectation, the diagnosis of PCS does not require a loss of consciousness and also does not seem to correlate with the severity of the injury. When persistent TBI related symptoms are suspected, clinically validated tools (such as the Post Concussion Symptoms Questionnaire) can be utilized to support the accurate diagnosis of PCS, further encouraging a treatment protocol based on target symptoms and working towards functional and psychological recovery.

THE KEYS TO EFFECTIVE TREATMENTS

The therapies you'll learn about in the next chapters help heal the brain in one (or more!) of the following ways. They may work through:

- Nerve Growth & Repair
- Decreasing Inflammation & Oxidation
- Increasing Circulation & Oxygenation
- Removing Scarring, Proteins & Tangles
- Improving Cell Signaling & Function

You can think of these as the five main keys to effective TBI treatment. You'll come to understand the mechanics of each of these keys as you learn how healthy brains are supposed to function (in the next section) and as you read more about the individual TBI therapies themselves.

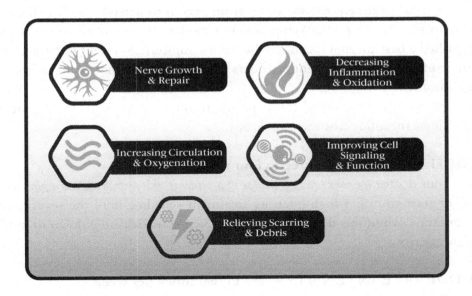

QUICK TIP As you explore individual TBI therapies throughout The Concussion Repair Manual, look for these icons to see which of the five keys to effective treatment each therapy represents.

LEVELS OF ENGAGEMENT OF THE TREATMENTS OFFERED

As a scientist and a physician, I evaluate available treatments based on their potential efficacy, their risk-benefit ratios, and their track records. I also consider their practicality, availability, cost of use, ease of intervention, and likelihood of "playing well" with other interventions. As a result, each of the individual sections is led with the therapies I've personally observed to be the most effective for the largest numbers of people or those therapies that appear to have been especially effective within a short period of time.

Because every case is unique, some people may have better results with certain therapies than others. I encourage you to see your doctor and investigate many different treatments to determine how well you tolerate each of them and which ones work best for *you*.

Optimal treatment *intensity* varies from person to person, too. You'll learn how to start tracking your symptoms in Chapter 10, and, once you have established a baseline and identified the main symptoms you want to target, you can work with your treatment providers to devise an ideal therapeutic schedule and protocol.

Unless otherwise noted for a specific technology, here are some general guidelines regarding treatment intensity.

HIGH INTENSITY—three to four times per week

Your doctor (*or your primary treatment provider if this provider is not a physician*) might start you on a high-intensity treatment schedule until the severity of your target symptoms decreases by 50%. Then you could step down to moderate intensity.

MODERATE INTENSITY—one to two times per week

When your target symptoms have become mild and/or you've noticed another 50 to 75% reduction in the severity of the symptoms you've been working to improve, your doctor might switch you to a low-intensity treatment schedule.

LOW INTENSITY—once or twice per month

You and your doctor may decide to continue with a low-intensity treatment schedule for maintenance and ongoing symptom relief as needed.

CHAPTER 1

PRIMARY TECHNOLOGIES

In This Section

You'll learn about these therapy types:

- Floatation therapy—REST (Restricted Environmental Stimulation Technique)
- Low-level laser (light) therapy (LLLT)
- Hyperbaric oxygen therapy (HBOT)
- Pulsed electromagnetic fields (PEMF)
- Transcranial magnetic stimulation (TMS)
- Transcranial direct current stimulation (tDCS)

PEMF and floatation (REST) can be particularly effective, they are safe and they easily complement other treatment strategies, so, if you're not quite sure where to start, start by investigating these.

Don't let what you cannot do interfere with what you can do.
— John Wooden

CASE REPORT

CODY, A 24-YEAR-OLD Iraqi War veteran presented with severe chronic lower back pain, ongoing anxiety, trouble focusing and being in large, stimulating environments, fatigue, headaches, insomnia, and PTSD after "getting blown up twice" while stationed abroad four years prior. He experienced these two significant events with concussions that included loss of consciousness both times, each one spaced about one month apart. The first one happened when his Hum-V hit an IED, the second happened in a rocket attack. The latter incident led to a fusion at lumbar vertebrae L3-5, intermittent shooting pain down both legs, and, as a result, he was on the following prescriptions daily: two different opiate pain relievers, one anti-anxiety medication, and one sleeping pill. His symptoms remained constant and worsened with stress, and he had unsuccessfully attempted several times to wean off his meds.

He chose to try floatation therapy at the suggestion of a fellow veteran, and upon emerging from the tank the first time reported, "that was the best and worst thing that could have ever happened." He relived both explosions in vivid detail, with full physical re-experiencing, although was a bit emotionally separated from it, observing it "like it was happening right next to me." It left him with noticeably improved anxiety for the next day or two while his physical pain essentially remained unchanged.

Over the following 3 weeks, he floated a total of seven times and noticed a considerable improvement in his sleep, pain, anxiety, and headaches. With these gains he was motivated to start a slow exercise regimen again, made an effort to socialize with friends and family more, and restarted a reading hobby. Gradually over another 6 months, he continued floatation twice a month and chose to lessen his pain medications, sleeping pill, and benzodiazepine. Eventually, he came off three of four of his medications and continued one pain reliever intermittently as needed at about one-quarter the previous dose. Currently, he is pain free due to floating regularly, maintaining sobriety, managing stress effectively, and sticking to a regular sleep schedule.

Cody's case is a great example of floatation therapy's effectiveness, though this may not be the degree of everyone's success in using it. What it highlights in general is that when pain, sleep, and anxiety are relieved, even just a little bit, it can spark more optimism and motivation to re-engage life in a healthier way. He was very motivated to continue the progress made, even though he was initially quite skeptical and only tried it at the recommendation of a friend.

Often times, early gains can be leveraged over time, and with perseverance can really pay off.

PRIMARY TECHNOLOGIES OVERVIEW

"Primary" technologies are therapies based on the building blocks of life. These building blocks are essential to our well-being, to our long-term development, and to our survival. I've divided the following therapies into four primary categories—Water, Light, Oxygen, and Frequency.

Note: The fifth of these primary therapies—Food—is covered later in a chapter all to itself, and Light is further covered in the section on Nature's Medicine.

HEADS UP! The information in this section is not intended to replace an individual consultation with a licensed healthcare professional. Consult your doctor or primary treatment provider before incorporating any of the primary technologies into your treatment plan.

WATER: FLOATATION THERAPY

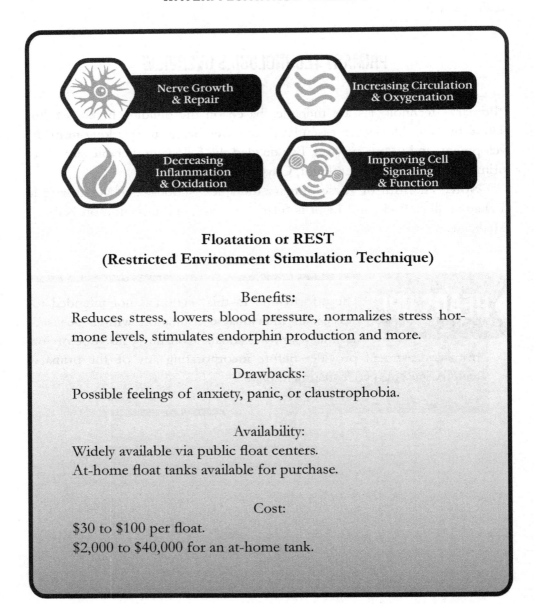

Nerve Growth & Repair

Increasing Circulation & Oxygenation

Decreasing Inflammation & Oxidation

Improving Cell Signaling & Function

**Floatation or REST
(Restricted Environment Stimulation Technique)**

Benefits:
Reduces stress, lowers blood pressure, normalizes stress hormone levels, stimulates endorphin production and more.

Drawbacks:
Possible feelings of anxiety, panic, or claustrophobia.

Availability:
Widely available via public float centers.
At-home float tanks available for purchase.

Cost:
$30 to $100 per float.
$2,000 to $40,000 for an at-home tank.

You may not have heard of "Floatation or REST (Restricted Environment Stimulation Technique) therapy" before, but odds are, you *are* familiar with the concept of the sensory deprivation tank. (You may also have heard these called "isolation tanks" or "sensory attenuation tanks.") Designed to eliminate—or at least greatly restrict—external stimuli like sounds, light, and temperature, these darkened, sound-insulated pods or chambers are filled with about 10 inches of a warm water solution of magnesium sulfate (Epsom salts).

During a floatation therapy session, you are completely enclosed inside the warm, dark tank. About 1,200 pounds of salts are typically used, and, because the salt solution is so highly concentrated, it is naturally buoyant, causing you to float effortlessly within it. As you experience weightlessness, there is no need for you to actively support your body, and muscle tension is gradually released.

Also, because the tank's liquid is held to the temperature of human skin, there is little need for your brain to concern itself with temperature regulation. In fact, since the usual auditory, visual, cognitive, gravitational, electromagnetic and other types of sensory input have been removed from the environment, many regions of your brain get a much-needed rest. It's essentially the first time since conception that one has the pleasure of being without sensory experience from the environment, thus enabling the mind-body connection to recalibrate in several ways. (See "Benefits" section for details.)

HISTORY

Floatation therapy has its roots in the sensory deprivation research of Dr. John C. Lilly, a neuroscientist who invented the first sensory deprivation tank in 1954. Dr. Lilly was a true pioneer and **psychonaut**. Studying at the National Institute for Mental Health, he explored sensory deprivation as a means to understand the origins of consciousness.

> Psychonaut - One who explores altered states of consciousness through meditation, spiritual practices, the use of psychoactive substances and other methods to heighten awareness and better understand the human condition.

In subsequent years, the National Aeronautics and Space Administration also used flotation tanks to study the effects of weightlessness on astronauts. Despite floatation research's early start and positive findings, many people still haven't been introduced to floatation therapy. There are a few reasons for this. One of the most notable is the quite trippy movie *Altered States*, which dramatically portrayed sensory deprivation tanks as dangerous. Released in 1980, the sci-fi flick was (very) loosely based on Dr. Lilly and his work. As the original movie poster exclaims, "In the basement of a medical school Dr. Jessup floats naked in total darkness. The most terrifying experiment in the history of science is out of control... and the subject is himself."

It's true that Dr. Lilly was a famously colorful character, and wearing a Davy Crockett style raccoon pelt hat on a 1980s nationally syndicated television interview didn't easily engender identification with the masses. He was known for spending many years experimenting with psychoactive drugs (mostly Ketamine), studying interspecies communication between humans and dolphins, and rather than considering sensory deprivation tanks to be tools for healing the body, he viewed them in more self-exploration or psychedelic terms.

This challenge in connecting with the lead man of the sensory deprivation movement plus the AIDS scare of the 1980s were major setbacks to the widespread use of flotation tanks. The public was unclear about how HIV/AIDS could be transmitted, and it led to a chilling effect on the use of public float centers that had begun to spring up nationwide.

Fortunately, we're now in the midst of a renaissance in floatation therapy. There has been a huge influx of new research, as well as improvements— such as UV and ozone filtration systems—to the flotation tanks themselves. Currently, floatation therapy is being used to combat psychiatric issues, cardiovascular conditions, and skeletal muscle inflammation, to name just a few treatment areas. It is easily one of the cornerstones of frontier medicine, addressing many of the top reasons people see their primary care physicians— for pain management, stress management, weight management, and the desire to get off of psychiatric or pain medications.

BENEFITS

In a meta-analysis of 27 different studies that were conducted between 1983 and 2002, researchers looked at floatation REST therapy's physiological effects and its influence on well-being and performance in a total sample of 449 people. Compared to biofeedback and other stress-reduction techniques, flotation therapy appeared to be more effective. The researchers also noted that the effects of floatation therapy appear to become stronger through repeated exposures (thus offering an additive effect over time towards a threshold saturation point) and that flotation therapy could be of particular use for chronic fatigue.[40]

Just how does floatation therapy work to reduce stress in the body? Well, the short answer is similar to many modalities that work directly with the psychology and mental arena—we're still studying it. From a physiological brain perspective, while in the sensory-deprived environment of a floatation tank, there is less stimulation to your brain's reticular activating system. Located at the base of your brain, this system continually scans all incoming sensory data (like sights, sounds and physical sensations) and looks for information that may be important. Less stimulation to your reticular activating system results in reduced neural firing to the sympathetic nervous system—responsible for fight-or-flight mode. This, in turn, lowers your levels of circulating stress hormones like cortisol. High cortisol levels can interfere with healthy metabolism, immune system function and other important processes.

Researchers studied the effects of floatation therapy on blood plasma levels of cortisol and found a 20% decrease in the stress hormone within just one 35-minute session. (They also noticed a decrease in the levels of ACTH—a hormone which stimulates the release or cortisol.) Overall, repeated floatation sessions were associated with a significant decrease in plasma cortisol levels, as compared to the control group. Furthermore, the cortisol levels of the flotation REST study group remained low even at four to five days after treatment.[41]

Lowering the levels of stress hormones like cortisol, ACTH, norepinephrine, and epinephrine helps to normalize the nervous system and shift your body from sympathetic overdrive to a more relaxed, parasympathetic state. (Your parasympathetic nervous system governs the basics of healing—think digestion and waste elimination—while your body is at rest.) You can essentially think of this as working towards a healthy reset of the neuro (brain and spinal cord)–endocrine (hormonal) systems.

Floatation therapy also has been shown to relax the brain into a theta state.[42] Theta brainwaves are present during light sleep. You may also fall into a theta state during deep meditation, but it is usually accessible only in the brief moments before falling asleep. During theta, your body's pain-reducing endorphins are naturally released. This level of consciousness also provides access to the right hemisphere of brain, which is associated with concentration, creativity and learning. The brain can more easily retain information while in the theta state.

All of this redirected energy from sympathetic overdrive to a more restful and meditative state also encourages a significant degree of deeper self-reflection and personal introspection. As in the above example of Cody shared above, the continued use of floatation therapy was massive for healing the psychological trauma of intense war related experiences, while supporting the body to release the physiologic tension and chronic pain associated with the Post-Traumatic Stress.

AVAILABILITY AND COST

The number of dedicated, public float centers is again on the rise. (Visit http://floatationlocations.com to find a float center near you.) Floatation tanks can also be found in chiropractic offices, fitness and sports therapy centers, and spas. Floating in these settings is relatively inexpensive, but prices vary, depending on your location. On average, you can expect to pay between $30 and $100 per individual float. (Sometimes you can purchase multiple floats in advance to end up with a better per-float rate.)

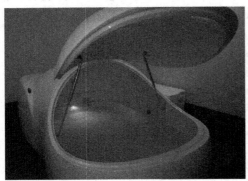

When choosing a Float Center, depending on personal tastes and availability, you might prefer a Float Pod style (like the ones manufactured by True Rest) or a float room style (like those manufactured by Zero Gravity Institute). I'm personally familiar with both systems, and they are truly state-of-the-art. Each is a fiberglass unit with internal lighting and many other upgradeable features, the difference essentially being the space involved. The pod you slide into and is a huge tube with a couple of feet of head room. The float room has a side door you step into and has about eight feet of headroom. My own individual preference is the float pod style because I like the experience of being held close while in the tank. The price point varies depending on upgrades and is generally under $20,000 for the commercial pod and under $40,000 for the commercial grade room.

Both of the above systems are available for at home use, and at the other end of the at-home spectrum, marketed as "the world's first affordable isolation tank," is the Zen Float Tent. It began as a Kickstarter project in 2014, and now the pyramid-shaped flexible structure isolation tanks are available from the Zen Float Company for under $2,000 each. Think of it as a waterbed

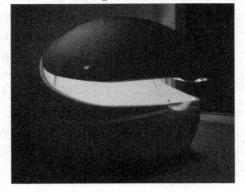

with the top cut out, sitting in a sturdy tent of the same sized footprint.

RISKS

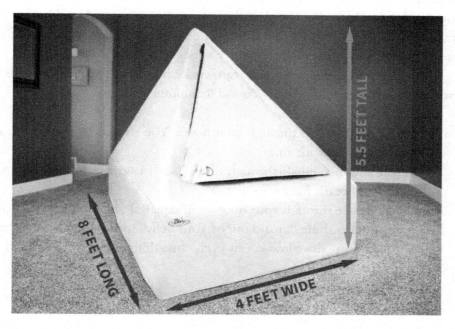

Overall, the benefit-to-risk ratio for flotation therapy is *exceedingly* weighted toward benefit, as there is minimal risk involved. This is one of the reasons I like floatation therapy SO much. Essentially, just about anybody can float and will receive benefit. Though, for the sake of thoroughness, let's go ahead and look at the risks.

Repeat these steps two to three times or until you feel more relaxed.

Give it a little time, and your mind and body will relax. Little by little, you can use the isolation tank itself to help unravel any fear cycle, and, as you start to reestablish balance in the neuroendocrine system, your brain's fear center will start to quiet its level of over activity. And as mentioned before, the benefit of a quieter fear center can significantly persist even when you are outside of the tank, gradually working toward an overall better experience of ease and flow in your every day.

As for other potential risks? Technically, it is possible to get saltwater in your eyes, and speaking from experience it's a buzz kill, so try and avoid it. Also, if you have a cut or an area of broken skin, you'll want to apply a little petroleum jelly to prevent the sting of saltwater. That's it. Too bad all therapeutic modalities don't come with similar risk-benefit ratios!

For most people, their first time in a floatation tank is also the first time they've been without sensory input. This can be a very relaxing experience, but it is possible to feel some anxiety or even panic. Some people may also feel claustrophobic in the confined space. Should this arise, an easy remedy is to prop the door open with a towel, and once you become comfortable, you can remove the towel. Notably, many clients and friends of mine have cured their claustrophobia and panic disorder with a series of float sessions.

If you begin to feel anxious, you can work on your self-regulation skills by practicing deep breathing. Here's a good technique to try:

1. Take a deep breath through your nose. (You should be filling your diaphragm/belly with air.)
2. Exhale and then inhale through your nose to a slow count of 4 seconds.
3. Hold that breath for four seconds.
4. Slowly exhale through your nose to an equal, slow count of 4 seconds.
5. Focus on breathing "in and out of your belly" more so than your chest.
6. Aim to repeat this slow count cyclic breathing pattern for at least 10 minutes.

LIGHT: LLLT (AKA COLD LASER THERAPY)

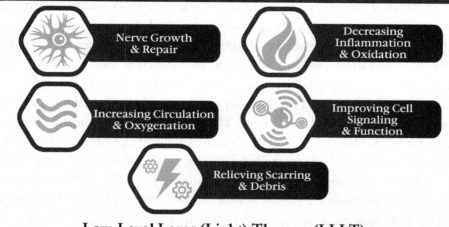

Nerve Growth & Repair

Decreasing Inflammation & Oxidation

Increasing Circulation & Oxygenation

Improving Cell Signaling & Function

Relieving Scarring & Debris

Low-Level Laser (Light) Therapy (LLLT)

Benefits:
Controls pain, reduces inflammation, increases blood flow and has been shown to stimulate nerve tissue growth and to improve memory and focus

Drawbacks:
Potentially damaging to eyes and skin, if not properly used

Availability:
Found in physicians' offices, head trauma clinics and Rehabilitation Medicine Centers. At-home systems available for purchase

Cost:
Vary widely depending on the frequency spectrums and intensity levels, preprogrammed settings and number of lights per unit. $500 to $15,000 to buy a new, at-home system

We encounter lasers every day. We use them to play our CDs and DVDs, to print high-quality documents, to check out our library books, and to scan groceries and other merchandise. Lasers are also frequently used in medicine. With many surgical applications, high-powered, medical-grade lasers are routinely used to cut through or remove certain types of tissue and to cauterize wounds. And, emitting light at lower energy levels, other medical-grade lasers are used in low-level laser (light) therapy (LLLT) to control pain, reduce inflammation and increase blood flow to damaged tissues.

Sometimes referred to as "cold lasers," the low-level lasers used in LLLT do not generate heat like high-powered lasers do. Lasers used for LLLT typically operate in the range of one to 1,000 milliwatts (mW) at wavelengths from 632 to 1,064 nanometers (nm).[43] (Additionally, in lieu of low-level lasers, some clinicians are now using light emitting diodes (LEDs) with success.)

During LLLT, the part of the body to be treated is exposed directly to low levels of red and near-infrared light. This stimulates a biological response on a cellular level. Here's how: our cells contain chromophores—light-sensitive groups of atoms—which react to the photon energy in light. This photon energy stimulates electrons and kicks off important tasks like cellular respiration and ATP production for energy synthesis. You can think of ATP being the "energy currency" that runs cellular function.

Now, if you remember, in the section called "The Injured Brain," you learned what happens on a cellular level when you sustain a head injury. In short, you may have tissue damage, the release of harmful free radicals, lactate build-up and lots of cell death. This can weaken the protective blood-brain barrier and touch off an immune response leading to an ongoing cascade of serious issues. By triggering basic cell functioning, low-level laser light therapy can help the brain to reverse these processes.

BENEFITS AND RISKS

LLLT has been the subject of much study and is thought to have many clinical applications. It is commonly used in sports medicine to relieve pain, reduce swelling and increase healing rates. Also, some military branches have had positive results when using LLLT for symptomatic improvement in the field. In one instance, Navy SEALS with chronic, non-healing leg injuries were treated with an array of LEDs with wavelengths of 670, 720, and 880 nanometers combined in a single unit. Including range of motion, pain intensity, and other factors, their musculoskeletal injuries improved overall by more than 40 percent. And, in a separate naval crew, lacerations treated with a similar LED array were shown to heal 50 percent faster than those of an untreated control group.[44]

But what about the effects of LLLT on traumatic brain injury? In studying mice with TBI, researchers have shown that the treatment can stimulate the growth of new nerve tissue. Spatial memory and learning also improved with treatment.[45]

They also suggest that—again, in brain-injured mice—LLLT may "significantly improve neural function, decrease lesion volume, augment cell proliferation and even protect the brain against neuronal damage to some degree."[46]

There are also case studies of LLLT used to treat human patients with TBI, and the treatment outcomes have been largely favorable. Interestingly, however, in some cases, patients have reported the need to continue weekly LED treatments, in order to maintain relief from their symptoms.[47] For example, one patient who had sustained a TBI in a car accident seven years earlier, was unable to focus her attention for long periods. Pre-treatment, she could work on her computer for no more than 20 minutes at a time. After eight weekly LLLT treatments, her focus improved, enabling her to work on her computer for three hours at a time. According to the case report, "The patient performs nightly home treatments (five years); if she stops treating for more than two weeks, she regresses."[48]

With a history of multiple TBIs, a second patient had been on medical disability for 5 months. After 4 months of nightly LLLT treatments, she was able to return to work full-time. What's more, after 9 months of LLLT treatment, neuropsychological testing revealed improvements in executive function and memory and reduced PTSD symptoms. But, as with the previous patient, her condition regresses if she does not maintain a regular treatment schedule.[49] These positive treatment reports and pilot studies have stimulated larger trials for efficacy now ongoing in many centers around the country.

There are some caveats associated with LLLT. Because lasers can be damaging to your eyes, both you and your clinician should wear laser-protective safety glasses when lasers are in use. Also, if you have dark skin or are heavily tattooed, you may feel some heat in treated tissues.

Lasers should not be used on cancerous or suspicious skin lesions or positioned over your thyroid. Finally, if you are pregnant, you should avoid laser contact with your abdomen.

AVAILABILITY AND COST

If you do a quick Internet search for "laser therapy clinics" or "laser therapists," you'll likely turn up lots of results, but not necessarily the *right* results for you. Laser therapy is currently available in multiple settings, including chiropractic practices, dermatology clinics, spas and, even dedicated "hair re-growth" centers, but not all laser treatment is alike.

Low-level lasers are used in many different ways, depending on the wavelength of light delivered, the power density of the device, duration of treatment and other factors. That's why it's important to seek out practitioners who have experience treating traumatic brain injury with LLLT. They are more likely to have the best equipment for the job and they should be familiar with the treatment parameters most optimal for use in TBI patients. You can expect the average LLLT treatment to cost between $500 - $5,000 for an at home unit.

If you try LLLT and have good results, you might want to consider purchasing a low-level laser or LED light therapy system for at-home use. To make this task a little easier, make note of the type of LLLT system your healthcare provider uses—including its available wavelengths and power levels—before you start shopping for yourself. Although you might not be able to afford an identical model, knowing its specifications will help you as you wade through the many choices on the market.

The FDA groups lasers into four major classes, according to hazard level. (Class I products are least harmful, and Class IV devices are most harmful.) Most medical-grade lasers fall into Class III or Class IV—some Class III lasers can cause immediate eye damage upon exposure, and Class IV lasers can cause eye damage and skin burns.[50] In order to purchase a Class III or Class IV device for at-home use, you must have a prescription from a healthcare provider.

For best results, choose a device which has officially been "cleared" for use by the FDA. (Look for the word "cleared," rather than "registered" or "listed.")[51] You can expect to pay between $5,000 and $15,000 for a new class III or IV laser. It is also possible to find used laser therapy systems. A used class III, medical-grade laser may start at $1,000, while a more powerful class IV laser can go for $5,000 or more. (Visit http://www.coldlasers.org for more information about choosing a laser for at-home use or see Resources for more options.)

QUICK TIP   Before you spend big money on a device for at-home use, try it a few times in a clinician's office first to make sure it's right for you.

OXYGEN: HBOT

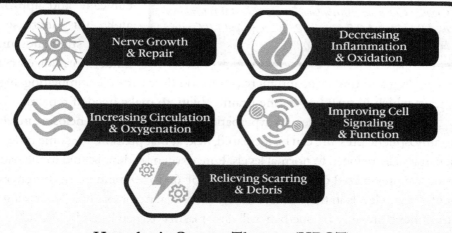

Nerve Growth & Repair

Decreasing Inflammation & Oxidation

Increasing Circulation & Oxygenation

Improving Cell Signaling & Function

Relieving Scarring & Debris

Hyperbaric Oxygen Therapy (HBOT)

Benefits:

Improved brain and tissue oxygenation; shows promise for relief of many TBI-related symptoms.

Drawbacks:

Claustrophobia, mild pain in ears, sinuses or joints, potential oxygen poisoning, damage to the ears or lungs.

Availability:

Widely available in hospitals, outpatient centers and private clinics. At-home hyperbaric chambers available for rent or purchase

Cost:

$108 to $250 per hour (private clinics); $1,000+ per hour (hospitals). $4,000 to $20,000 to buy a portable, at-home unit

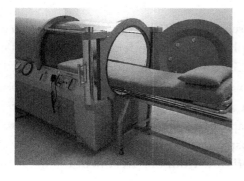

Our brains must have oxygen in order to generate the energy needed to function. Because it stimulates fundamental processes like cell production and growth, oxygen is also critical for healing damaged tissue. By using hyperbaric oxygen therapy (HBOT), it's possible to increase the level of oxygen

that is available to the brain. When applied clinically and appropriately, this increase in oxygen stimulates nitric oxide, normalizes cellular signaling and function, and increases blood flow through stimulating angiogenesis, which in turn boosts the brain's ability to make needed repairs.

HBOT requires the use of a hyperbaric chamber—a special enclosure in which the atmospheric pressure can be increased, held at that pressure for some time, and then gradually reduced to normal levels. Pure oxygen is administered to the patient inside the pressurized chamber for a period of 60 to 90 minutes. In this environment, oxygen levels in the blood increase dramatically. For example, increasing the atmospheric pressure by one-half will raise plasma oxygen levels by 700%.[52]

HBOT is routinely used to treat decompression sickness, carbon monoxide poisoning, and thermal burns. (The FDA has officially cleared HBOT to treat these conditions and 13 others, in fact.)[53] Although there is some controversy surrounding common "off-label" uses of HBOT, there is a growing body of evidence to support its use for a variety of conditions, including autism. In one study, for example, after receiving 40 hourly HBOT sessions, 33 autistic children showed "significant improvements in overall functioning, receptive language, social interaction, eye contact, and sensory/cognitive awareness" compared to 29 children in a control group, which did not undergo HBOT.[54]

BENEFITS AND RISKS

But is HBOT an effective treatment for traumatic brain injury? There is a mountain of anecdotal evidence, including patient video testimonials and case stories suggesting TBI survivors, particularly those with moderate-to-severe injuries, are seeing amazing benefits.

As for relevant quantitative research, a 2012 *Journal of Neurotrauma* study followed 16 U.S. servicemen who had mild to moderate blast-induced post-concussion syndrome (PCS) or PCS with post-traumatic stress disorder over a 29-day treatment course. The subjects were treated with HBOT at 1.5 atmospheres twice a day for five days per week. HBOT sessions lasted for one hour each and were at least three hours apart to make sure individual patients had adequate rest time at normal atmospheric pressure.[55] The figure below shows the increased global cerebral blood flow from one treatment to 40.

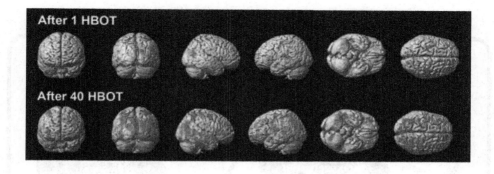

After 1 HBOT

After 40 HBOT

TABLE 3. SYMPTOM CHANGES (15 SUBJECTS)

Symptom	Better (%)	No change (%)	Worse (%)
Headache	87 (13/15)	13 (2/15)	0
Sleep disruption	75 (9/12)	25 (3/12)	0
Short-term memory	92 (11/12)	8 (1/12)	0
Cognition	93 (14/15)	7 (1/15)	0
Energy level	87 (13/15)	13 (2/15)	0
Post-traumatic stress disorder symptoms (P), or nightmares (N)	50 (2/5) P (2/3) N	50 (3/5) P (1/3) N	0
Short temper/irritability	82 (9/11)	18 (2/11)	0
Mood swings	87 (13/15)	13 (2/15)	0
Imbalance	55 (6/11)	45 (5/11)	0
Fine motor incoordination	75 (3/4)	25 (1/4)	0
Decreased hearing	20 (2/10)	80 (8/10)	0
Tinnitus	37 (3/8)	63 (5/8)	0
Depression	93 (13/14)	7 (1/14)	0
Arthralgias	0	100 (5/5)	0
Photophobia	44 (4/9)	44 (4/9)	11 (1/9)

Combined symptoms from subjects' prioritized symptom list and primary author's standard questionnaire.

Out of 15 subjects—one subject withdrew from the study before its completion—12 reported improvements in most of their targeted symptoms after HBOT. "Headache, sleep disruption, short-term memory loss, cognitive problems, decreased energy, self-characterized PTSD symptoms or nightmares...short temper/irritability, mood swings, imbalance, photophobia, and depression, which were present in a majority of subjects, were improved in 44 – 93% of the subjects." The subjects also experienced an average 14.8-point increase in IQ scores and noted significant increases in their cognitive, physical, and emotional function after treatment.[56]

HBOT does have its risks. Some patients may experience claustrophobia or mild pain in their ears, sinuses or joints. More serious risks can include oxygen poisoning and damage to the ears or lungs.

AVAILABILITY AND COST

Hyperbaric chambers can be found in hospitals, outpatient centers, and private clinics, but you'll need a prescription from your doctor to access this therapy. On average, the cost for a single, hour-long treatment ranges from $108 to $250 in private clinics and may exceed $1,000 per treatment in hospital settings.[57]

Again, with a prescription, you can also rent or purchase hyperbaric chambers for at-home use. These portable, soft-sided HBOT systems typically operate at lower pressures than the more durable chambers found in most hospitals and private clinics. Used hyperbaric chambers sell for about $3,000. New HBOT systems may cost between $4,000 and $20,000.

PULSED ELECTRO-MAGNETIC FIELDS (PEMF)

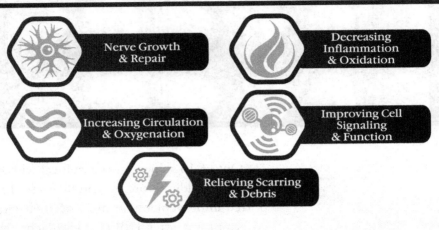

Nerve Growth & Repair

Decreasing Inflammation & Oxidation

Increasing Circulation & Oxygenation

Improving Cell Signaling & Function

Relieving Scarring & Debris

Benefits:
Stimulates cellular processes, has been shown to boost neuronal cell growth and may reduce the brain's post-traumatic inflammatory response.

Drawbacks:
Potential side effects include temporary drop in blood pressure, light headedness or fainting.
May interfere with battery-powered medical device implants.
May aggravate some pre-existing medical conditions.

Availability:
Found in chiropractic clinics and sport medicine centers.
At-home systems available to rent or purchase.

Cost:
$350 to $5,000 for an at-home PEMF system.

We've long known that biological organisms, including humans, respond to certain frequencies of electromagnetic fields. Many researchers regard the EM fields as the fifth element in health, behind water, light, food, and oxygen. Some of these EM fields occur naturally, others are man-made and we are continually surrounded by them. It was in the mid-1970s that three different groups of researchers, working independent of one another, suggested essentially that "during evolution Mother Nature created preferable levels of recognition of the signals from (external) magnetic fields."[58]

While this makes intuitive sense, what does it mean for treatment? There are specific "biological windows" or ranges on the electromagnetic spectrum that can induce certain biological effects, and researchers have discovered that, within these biological windows, the parameters of a signal—like the shape and length of electromagnetic waves and the number of waves per second—produce different biological responses.

PULSED ELECTROMAGNETIC FIELDS (PEMF)

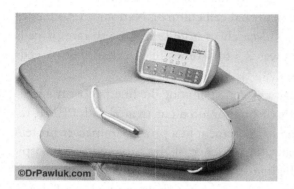

On a cellular level, weak electromagnetic fields can stimulate the transport of energy, information and other materials in living tissues,[59] so it should come as no surprise that physicians have been treating patients with pulsed electromagnetic fields (PEMF) for many years. During PEMF therapy, intermittent bursts of electromagnetic waves are directed at the area of the body to be treated.

Although the FDA originally approved the use of PEMF to stimulate bone growth, this therapy is routinely used "off-label." Many scientific and clinical studies have shown the treatment can reduce pain and swelling, increase blood circulation, and stimulate the immune and endocrine systems. It also has been used to help accelerate the healing of skin ulcers, surgical wounds and burns.[60]

I was first introduced to PEMF therapy as a patient with an acute injury, although it was for a rib and not my brain. While learning to surf I cracked a rib, and as a result couldn't lift my arm above my head or breathe very deeply without being in a ton of pain. Sleeping was next to impossible. Amazingly enough, within the first 15 minutes of my first PEMF treatment, I felt about 60 to 70 percent better. Unfortunately, as is the case with most treatments for structural damage and inflammation, the initial benefit dropped (to about 30 percent by the next day for my rib) and more treatments were warranted. After two more sessions that week and two more over the following month, I was essentially pain free and back to full function. Undoubtedly, the PEMF treatments sped up my recovery time and it massively sparked my ongoing interest in pulsed wave therapies.

BENEFITS AND RISKS

PEMF therapy appears to have real potential for the treatment of TBI. In studying the effects of PEMF on neuronal cell cultures, National Aeronautics and Space Administration (NASA) researchers noted the growth rate of cells exposed to electromagnetic waves was 2.5 to 4 times higher than that of cells that had not been similarly exposed.[61]

The therapy may also have a major effect on limiting the brain's post-traumatic inflammatory response. In a study of brain-injured rats treated with PEMF, researchers reported reductions of up to 90 percent in a pro-inflammatory protein called interleukin-1beta.[62] (In humans, the presence of this protein in cerebrospinal fluid has been correlated with high intracranial pressure and poor outcomes.[63] And, in other animal studies, injections of interleukin-1beta resulted in cell death, fluid buildup, swelling[64] and further breakdown of the blood-brain barrier.)[65][66]

One of the main therapeutic effects of pulsed E-M fields is through stimulating vasomotion - the oscillatory contraction within the microcirculation. Notably, 75% of all the blood vessels in the body are in this microscopic network, and enhancing function here can have a myriad of benefits, like improved oxygen delivery, nutrient utilization, nitric oxide and ATP production.

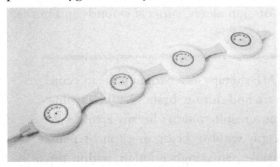

If you are pregnant or have a history of seizures, you should consult your doctor before trying PEMF therapy. Side effects associated with PEMF therapy may include a temporary decrease in blood pressure, which can cause lightheadedness or fainting. Also, if you have an implanted pacemaker, insulin pump, or other battery-powered medical device, strong electromagnetic pulses may interfere with their operation.[67]

In part, other potential health risks depend on how often you undergo PEMF therapy and which portions of your body make contact with the PEMF system. (There are small PEMF units designed for use on very localized areas and larger systems to target your whole body. See "Availability and Cost" section for details.) As an example, let's say you have a pre-existing, overactive thyroid. Frequent exposure to electromagnetic fields at high intensities might aggravate that condition.[68]

Women who are on their periods and have PEMF therapy targeted at their pelvic regions may temporarily experience heavier menstrual flows. And people undergoing PEMF treatment who have active bleeding—from hemorrhoids or a stomach ulcer, for instance—may have trouble clotting.[69]

AVAILABILITY AND COST

Many chiropractic clinics and sports medicine centers offer in-office PEMF therapy. The average session lasts 10 – 30 minutes and may cost around $50 – 100 per treatment. At least initially, you may find that frequent treatments over a period of weeks or months are beneficially compounded over time.

There are scores of PEMF therapy devices on the market for at-home use. Some are large mats meant to be reclined upon for full-body PEMF exposure. Others are much smaller pillows, belts, patches or wands intended to direct electromagnetic fields to a specific part of the body. The main differences between the available devices on the market are two fold—the frequency range and the intensity of the pulsed waves delivered. These differences essentially dictate the effect of the waves on the target area and usually the cost of treatment for a unit session. While inexpensive systems start at about $350, more sophisticated (wider range frequency and higher maximum intensity level) models may cost up to $5,000. As you investigate, you'll find PEMF therapy devices of all sorts offering these various, multi-wave shaped, wide range frequency and intensity options. Some also have pre-programmed settings for specific applications. (For a further overview resource, visit http://drpawluk. com/resources/buyers-guide for a good primer on choosing a PEMF system and see Resources section.)

QUICK TIP It is sometimes possible to rent PEMF systems for short-term, at-home use. This can be a good way to try a few different systems for yourself, before you buy your own.

TRANSCRANIAL MAGNETIC STIMULATION (TMS)

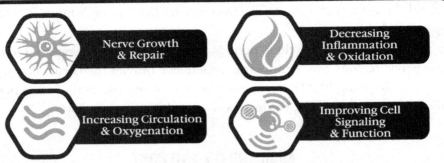

Nerve Growth & Repair

Decreasing Inflammation & Oxidation

Increasing Circulation & Oxygenation

Improving Cell Signaling & Function

Transcranial Magnetic Stimulation (TMS)

Benefits:

Stimulates activity in the brain. Has been shown to reduce post-concussion symptoms and neuropathic pain. Can localize treatment to specific areas of injury or low function.

Drawbacks:

Potential side effects include headache, scalp numbness, light headedness and facial twitching, temporary hearing loss, mania and seizures are rare but also possible.

Availability:

Found in physicians' offices, head trauma clinics and rehabilitation centers

Cost:

Typically around $150 per treatment, done in a series of 10 – 20 sessions.

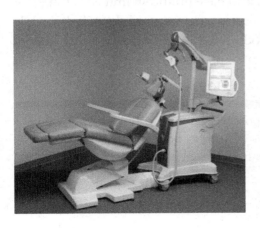

Transcranial magnetic stimulation or TMS is another type of electromagnetic therapy, but, unlike PEMF therapy, TMS cannot be performed at home. You can think of TMS as a more powerful brain specific PEMF unit. The equipment required for TMS treatment delivers electric current to a magnetic field generator that is positioned close to the patient's skull. Up to 20,000 times stronger than the Earth's own magnetic field, the magnetic field generated by the device passes through the scalp and is converted to electrochemical energy that excites neurons and stimulates activity in the brain.[70][71]

The FDA has cleared transcranial magnetic stimulation for use in patients with treatment-resistant depression, but TMS is also being used "off-label" to treat many other conditions, such as PTSD, schizophrenia, migraines, stroke, and TBI.

BENEFITS AND RISKS

Several case studies detailing the use of TMS to treat mild to severe traumatic brain injury have been published, with largely positive results. But researchers are still working to determine how changes in certain treatment variables—like the number of electromagnetic pulses per second and the length and number of sessions—may affect outcomes for different patient populations.[72]

In a recent study of 15 patients with mild TBI and persistent post-concussion symptoms, participants were treated with TMS five days per week over a four-week period. (12 of the participants completed all 20 treatment sessions. Three other patients withdrew from the study.) When comparing the severity of each patient's post-concussion symptoms before and after completion of all TMS sessions, researchers noted severity scores declined by an average of 14.6 points. There was a statistically reliable decrease in symptom ratings for headaches, and the researchers also saw decreases in severity scores for fatigue, trouble falling asleep and difficulty remembering, among others.[73]

There are potential side effects associated with TMS, including mild headache, tingling or numbness of the scalp, lightheadedness, and facial twitching. Because the magnetic pulses that are generated make loud, clicking sounds, ear protection is worn during TMS therapy, but temporary hearing loss is possible. Although much rarer, mania and seizures are other possible side effects. Also, if you have any metal fragments in your body or certain implanted medical devices, you may not be a good candidate for TMS.

TMS VS PEMF

A natural question arises in comparing TMS to PEMF to see which is better for TBI. While both have a history of clinical efficacy for the brain in a variety of conditions, there have not been comparison studies (at least that I am aware of) assessing the superiority of one over the other. Notably, there is a wide array of PEMF units on the market, most of which generate a much lower level of intensity than with TMS. TMS is head/brain specific, while larger PEMF pads can generate pulses to a larger section of the body, and theoretically covering more area can offer more effect globally, though this doesn't necessarily translate to better brain outcomes.

Given all this, if the only obvious target indication for treatment is the post traumatized brain, there is an available TMS provider in the area, the financial means are available for a treatment course and with your own further research it feels like a good fit, then go with TMS first. In cases where there are other areas of the body experiencing chronic pain or inflammation, and after your own further investigation PEMF seems like the better fit, then go with it. In either case, ask any prospective clinicians providing treatment about their experience with using pulsed magnetic field therapies for TBI and make an educated choice. For both therapies, the risk benefit ratio is relatively good, and in the care of a trained professional their use warrants a trial.

AVAILABILITY AND COST

Transcranial magnetic stimulation therapy must be administered in a clinical setting by a healthcare provider. The average TMS session may last between 40 minutes to an hour, and multiple treatments over a period of weeks or months may be necessary. Treatments cost between around $150 – $200 per session and a typical course is 10 – 20 sessions.

TRANSCRANIAL DIRECT CURRENT STIMULATION (TDCS)

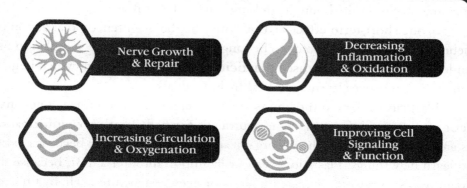

Nerve Growth & Repair

Decreasing Inflammation & Oxidation

Increasing Circulation & Oxygenation

Improving Cell Signaling & Function

Transcranial Direct Current Stimulation (tDCS)

Benefits:
Wide ranging from improved attention and concentration, to support with depression, insomnia and potentially pain management.

Drawbacks:
Can cause localized skin irritation in susceptible individuals. Some units require a physician's prescription

Availability:
Widely available online and in some rehabilitation clinics.

Cost:
Variable and typically around $150 – $300 for a hand held unit.

Transcranial Direct Current Stimulation, or tDCS, is a type of Direct Current Stimulation that refers to the application of low currents to the scalp for improved brain function. Many studies in healthy individuals have shown that tDCS improves attention, learning, and memory.[74] Research has not yet unified an understanding as to *why* tDCS has this effect, but it may be related to the increased polarizability of neurons near the tDCS wires.

When two ends of an object are different from one another—like the two ends of a magnet, for example—scientists refer to the object as being "polarized." With differing salt concentrations inside and outside their membranes, neurons are polarized, too. The neurons' polarization enables them to transmit signals in the brain via pulsing waves of salt flow.

So, one short-term effect of tDCS may be the heightened polarization of neurons, but there also seems to be long-term benefit *after* the stimulation has ended. Neurons have increased **plasticity** after a tDCS session, which may be why tDCS improves learning in healthy individuals.

"Plasticity" refers to the brain's ability to change. As you learn, a new pattern of connections among your neurons is formed. That's how information is stored in the brain. When reorganization is made easier, it becomes easier to learn new things. Plasticity is especially important after a TBI, because the brain needs to reform damaged regions or even restructure itself by utilizing healthy tissue to perform the tasks previously handled by regions which may have become irreparably damaged.

In prior studies, only brain regions near the tDCS anode wire show improved function. For instance, when tDCS was used to help patients recover their ability to speak after a stroke, the anode wire was placed over the right Wernicke's area,[75] a brain region involved in speech. When tDCS was used to help patients recover motor function in their hands after a stroke, the anode wire was placed over the presumed hand region of the damaged hemisphere.[76] In a more contemporary similar fashion using brain scanning devices, transcranial direct current stimulation studies in laboratories are targeted to the precise regions of the brain implicated in the recovery of lost physical or cognitive function.

BENEFITS AND RISKS

To date, there have not been published studies on the use of tDCS for TBI patients immediately after an injury. Although the side effects of tDCS are typically very mild in healthy patients, including headaches and scalp tingling, we don't yet know whether tDCS will be equally safe for patients to use *immediately after* a TBI.

There have been several studies of tDCS used for patients suffering from the *chronic* stages of traumatic brain injury. The researchers were testing whether the benefits to learning, working memory, and attentiveness seen in healthy patients might translate to similar benefits for those suffering from the lingering malaise of a prior TBI. The results of these studies have been mixed.[77]

Not all TBI patients showed improvement in the measures under study in the tDCS trials. But, some TBI patients treated with tDCS saw a temporary increase in attentiveness as measured by reaction time.[78] Further experiments will be needed to determine for which type of patients, and for what types of recovery, tDCS is most helpful.

AVAILABILITY AND COST

Most Transcranial direct current stimulation devices can be purchased for home use and cost between $150 and $300. There are newer more sophisticated versions out there like the Focus that include a cell phone app interface.

CHAPTER 2

INTERVENTIONAL THERAPEUTICS

In This Section

You'll learn about these therapy types:

- Hormone replacement therapy (HRT)
- Cognitive rehabilitation devices
- Neurofeedback
- Acupuncture
- Stem cell therapy
- Pharmaceutical nootropics

To get the most out of this section, read through it and see which ones are most interesting, available and doable. When in doubt, hormone testing can at least give you an idea if HRT is warranted, cognitive rehabilitation is helpful for most, and acupuncture is high in potential benefit while being very low in potential risk.

Be faithful in small things because it is in them that your strength lies.

~ Mother Teresa

CASE REPORT

Roy, a 42-year-old, married accountant presented at the request of his wife, also a client, who noticed him over the previous several years to be gradually "tired but wired," emotionally distant, grumpy, self-absorbed and short-tempered. When they had first married ten years previously his disposition was much lighter and buoyant, and she attributed his change in mood to a climbing accident where he fell from about 20 feet and broke his lower leg. When questioned alone he tended to minimize any symptoms including overt pain or depression, although acknowledged he hadn't been as active as he had been previously and he did desire to get back into some of his previous hobbies like hiking and skiing. When interviewed together and presented more directly with his wife's concerns, he reluctantly acknowledged them and also added frustration at a lack of libido, decreased erectile function, feeling "foggy" throughout most days, and worsening short term memory.

Upon exam, he had good global physical and cognitive function, walked normally, had a slightly irritated tone, and did not appear to be in any pain. When asked about his history of hobbies and any accidents, he noted several minor ones and the broken leg several years prior. With further questioning, he also elaborated on the fall and described hitting the front of his head hard on the side of the wall, without losing consciousness. And, while his head did hurt after the fall (for several days afterwards), it was overshadowed by the greater pain of his broken tibia and fibula.

We did a routine hormone panel, and he was borderline low normal in testosterone, notably low in cortisol levels throughout the day, and low in DHEA-S and 25-OH-Vitamin D. Additionally, several of his inflammatory markers were elevated and thyroid function profile was normal. He was willing to start a trial of hormone support with low dose testosterone and vitamin D. He also started fish oil, melatonin, and rhodiola (an adaptogen known to support energy levels), as well as trying acupuncture once every couple of weeks given the convenience of its close proximity to his office.

After 2 months, his symptoms were significantly improved. Both he and his wife noticed he had more energy and sex drive, he was more engaged with her, he had restarted hiking on the weekends, he seemed like he had less brain fog, and he was sleeping better. Lab reports showed improved testosterone and vitamin D had both moved to the mid-normal range. He continued the supplements and phased out the acupuncture with ongoing improvement.

This is an example of a multi-armed approach to addressing concerns that Roy himself did not even initially come in complaining about, namely using HRT, acupuncture, and targeted supplementation. It also highlights the common experience that many partners and friends/family have about their loved ones post-TBI, namely the often-present lack of personal awareness to present "disconnection" from others and life in general, plus the limited motivation to change the situation. While these are certainly generalized symptoms that could be simply called "depression" by a general practitioner or psychiatrist and treated with medication, it is a case where a possible frontal head concussion in the setting of lifestyle changes from an accident and thus, worsening probable age-related trending down of androgens (testosterone) all contributing to some symptoms of Post-Concussive Disorder. In this case, the presenting symptoms were addressed using an integrative medical approach and treated with methodologies that more effectively corrected the core imbalances present.

THERAPEUTICS OVERVIEW

While you could pursue most of the therapies in Chapter 1 by yourself, you'll need the assistance of skilled professionals to access most of the technologies in this section. From ancient art to state-of-the-art, the "Interventional Therapeutics" presented here are carried out by a wide range of experts who step in to help guide your recovery. They may include general practitioners, endocrinologists, neurofeedback specialists, and acupuncturists, among others.

As you learn about these therapies—and as you seek out experts to deliver them—you'll be better prepared to ask the right questions and be your own advocate along the way. And note too, the practitioner supported therapies included here are by no means the only ones available or potentially beneficial. Others such as neurological chiropractic, physiotherapy and craniosacral therapy, to name a few, do have a following of supporters. Ultimately, do your research, and if there is a technology or treatment not included in the Manual that "speaks to you" then try it out.

HORMONE REPLACEMENT THERAPY (HRT)

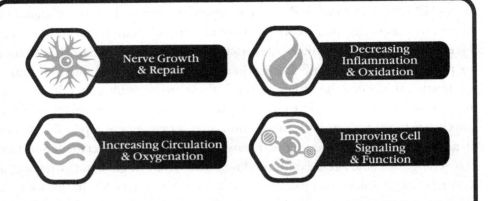

Hormone Replacement Therapy (HRT)

Benefits:
Dependent upon which hormonal deficiencies are corrected. Has been shown to improve cognition, verbal memory and mental speed.
May influence neuronal survival and repair

Drawbacks:
Dependent upon type of HRT supplement, delivery method and frequency

Availability:
More and more providers nationwide.

Cost:
Testing profiles are typically $200 – $500, depending on those tested. Treatment costs vary according to providers, route of treatment and the duration of care.

Immediately after an injury is sustained—and even many years later—traumatic brain injury can wreak havoc on your endocrine system. *** It is *easily* one of the **most overlooked issues** for people in post-concussion care, and because SO many people experience hormonal dysregulation after a head injury, we are going to go deeper into this discussion than most other areas in the Manual. ***

Made up of several hormone-secreting glands, this is your body's master control center or master switch. It uses a sophisticated stew of chemical signals to regulate our sleep cycles, metabolism, sexual arousal, reproductive processes, and many other physiological essentials.

Located inside the brain, three important parts of the endocrine system are the hypothalamus, the pituitary gland, and

> **Down-regulation** - the process by which function is limited, decreased or entirely suppressed by external factors.

the pineal gland. This master gland triad is particularly susceptible to damage by the sheering and impact forces of traumatic brain injury and its aftereffects, and when this occurs their function is noticeably reduced (over time this can be dramatically decreased), in a process known as **down-regulation**. When this happens, the gland's functional output is reduced as a result of external factors, and, as a result, the brain begins to have major difficulty in governing the rest of the bodily functions. (Some examples of these external factors, as they relate to TBI, include exposure to harmful free radicals, toxins or pro-inflammatory proteins.)

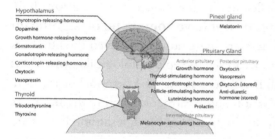

To see how and why their down-regulation is a problem, you must first understand what roles the hypothalamus and the pituitary and pineal glands play. About the size of an almond, the **hypothalamus** is a small but mighty powerhouse. Some of its most important tasks include regulating body temperature, sleep cycles, hunger, thirst, and the body's response to stress. The hypothalamus secretes different hormones to trigger or suppress the release of other hormones from the pituitary gland. For its part, the **pituitary gland** controls the body's growth and development as well as certain reproductive processes. The pituitary secretes hormones which help govern the thyroid, adrenal glands, and gonadal glands (testes or ovaries.) Lastly, shaped like a tiny pinecone and historically in spiritual cultures described as the "third eye" and the "seat of the soul," the **pineal gland** secretes melatonin, a hormone which helps to regulate reproductive hormones and sleep-wake cycles.

In addition to down-regulation, your endocrine system may also be affected by what many practitioners with an understanding of integrative medicine call "interference fields." An **interference field** is a blockage or impediment to the natural flow of energy through nerve, lymphatic, and other pathways in the body. To give you a picture of this, imagine turning on a garden hose and watching water flow freely through it. Now imagine that in parking a car in the driveway the tire comes to rest on the hose, pinching of the free flow of water through it. Under those circumstances, it's much harder—if not impossible—for water to flow through the hose. Likewise, physical scars in the brain can act as interference fields, decreasing the flow of energy and impairing function.

Hormonal deficiencies and imbalances are very common in TBI patients. Unfortunately, they frequently go undiagnosed and untreated. Some numbers to consider: after studying 78 TBI patients and 38 healthy control subjects, researchers found that *more than half* of the TBI patient population showed hormonal disturbances three months after sustaining their head injuries. Checking in a year after the initial injuries took place, researchers found hormonal disturbances in one-third of the TBI patients studied.[79] Another set of researchers studied the prevalence of pituitary dysfunction in 50 TBI patients over a five-year period. Within four or five years, a whopping 54% of the study's subjects had developed pituitary dysfunction. Pituitary dysfunction occurred in 38% of patients with mild TBI, in 57% of those with moderate TBI, and in 59% of people with severe TBI.[80]

Summary statement for these smaller studies mentioned here — **about half of all people with a major head injury will have some type of significant hormonal imbalance as a result**. These are huge numbers! Given the numbers of people with TBI in the US alone, one can see the epidemiological implications of TBI on overall vitality and general health as a result of hormonal disruption, hence its primary importance in evaluation and treatment. Even if the numbers were only one quarter affected (noted in the following study examined), you are still looking at massive cultural, societal, and personal ramifications that worsen over time, as hormone productivity tends to wane over the years even in healthy people as a natural process of aging. Thus, for most people a significant, untreated TBI will likely lead to noticeable and significantly accelerated aging.

Looking at a much larger sample size, a separate group of researchers pooled and analyzed data from 19 past studies including 809 patients with TBI. The pituitary glands in nearly 28 percent of these patients were significantly under producing (or failing to produce) certain hormones. (See chart for details.)[81]

Table 4. Frequencies of Anterior Hypopituitarism in Adults in the Chronic Phase After Traumatic Brain Injury (TBI) or Subarachnoid Hemorrhage (SAH)[a]

Source	No. of Adults	No. (%) [95% CI]					
		Growth Hormone	LH/FSH	Adrenocorticotropic Hormone	TSH	Hypopituitarism	Multiple Deficiencies
TBI alone	809	100 (12.4) [10.2-14.8]	101 (12.5) [10.2-14.8]	66 (8.2) [6.5-10.3]	33 (4.1) [2.9-5.7]	209 (27.5) [22.8-28.9]	60 (7.7) [5.6-9.2]

Abbreviations: FSH, follicle-stimulating hormone; LH, luteinizing hormone; TSH, thyroid-stimulating hormone.
[a] Defined as at least 5 mo.
[b] Significant compared with TBI.

Out of 809 TBI patients:
12.4% exhibited deficiencies in growth hormone
12.5% exhibited deficiencies in LH/FSH (gonadal...)
8.2% exhibited deficiencies in adrenocorticotropic (ACTH)
4.1% exhibited deficiencies in thyroid-stimulating hormone (TSH)
7.7% had multiple hormonal deficiencies

For instance, 4.1% of the TBI patients were deficient in thyroid-stimulating hormone.[82] This hormone, in turn, triggers the thyroid gland to produce other hormones, which have been shown to be vital to the maturation of neural cells and for learning, memory and general cognitive performance.[83 84 85] Having levels of these hormones that are too low has been associated with reduced executive function in the brain.[86 87]

Researchers have determined that many different hormones affect brain function. Thyroid hormones, gonadal hormones (such as estrogen and testosterone), and adrenal hormones all "participate in the birth, differentiation and survival of neurons and/or glial cells." Additionally, progesterone is another hormone that appears to influence the repair and survival of neurons.[88] Even growth hormone plays some part in attention, memory and executive function.[89 90]

RESETTING THE MASTER SWITCH

Fortunately, it is possible to reboot or reset the body's master switch by correcting hormonal deficiencies with targeted hormone replacement therapy (HRT). Identifying any deficiencies you might have is the first step. To start, your primary care provider, hormone specialist or endocrinologist would likely order extensive blood work, including a complete metabolic workup with hormone levels. Once you have the results, you can work together to supplement what's missing in your system. As you undergo HRT, your doctor should order additional blood work periodically. Using your original blood work as a baseline, you will be able to track your progress and see whether the supplementation is working.

BENEFITS AND RISKS

In part, specific treatment benefits will depend on *what hormones* are being supplemented. A deficiency in growth hormone, for example? There have been a few small studies—each randomized and placebo-controlled—which showed

TBI patients treated with replacement growth hormone resulted in significant improvements in overall mental speed,[91] verbal memory, [92] and general improvement in cognition.[93] Or, say you have low levels of luteinizing hormone (LH) or follicle-stimulating hormone (FSH), both secreted by the pituitary gland. Because deficits in these can cause low libido and sexual dysfunction, supplementing your LH and FSH may help improve these conditions.

Depending on the *type of supplement* and *how it is administered*, the risks associated with HRT can vary. Supplemental hormones come in many forms. They may be injected, taken orally, delivered through transdermal creams or patches worn on the skin, or even delivered through small HRT "seeds," which are implanted underneath the skin. Hormones may be continually released or their delivery may be "pulsed" to mimic the body's natural cycles.

Pulsed or intermittent delivery of HRT is often preferable over continuous use. However, this varies depending on a person's age, relative production of an ideal hormone pattern, current level of symptomatology, and desired schedule of hormone use. Because our bodies do not produce hormones continuously under normal circumstances, problems can arise when supplemental hormones are delivered continuously. On a pulsed or intermittent HRT schedule, you might take supplemental hormones for a few weeks and then discontinue them for another week, cycling on and off, according to your prescriber's instructions.

While some hormone supplements are completely synthetic, it is possible to find hormone preparations that come from natural, plant- or animal-based sources. And, taking "natural" to the next level, some doctors treat patients using "bioidentical" hormones. **Bioidentical hormones** have been specially prepared to precisely match the molecular structure of the hormones produced naturally in your body.

The safety of bioidentical hormones is another hot topic area of discussion amongst the medical communities. Overall their safety and efficacy can vary depending on how they

> **Bioidentical hormones** - supplemental hormones which come from plant - or animal-based sources and have been specially processed to precisely match the molecular structure of hormones found in the human body.

are compounded, and some medical organizations (like the FDA and AMA) take the standpoint that the evidence does not show greater safety and side effect profiles than for non-bioidentical counterparts. It's outside of the scope of this Manual to go deeply into all the relevant science and present debate, as there is exhaustive data to support both sides of the discussion. (Please see the Reference section for more resources on the matter). However, because it's such a relevant topic to proper care in the post-TBI setting, we will go further into the reasons for the larger debate in this growing field of HRT medicine.

DIFFERENCES OF OPINION

There are a ton of different clinical opinions on how best to address hormonal disruptions, and the discussion between different treatment providers often gets quite passionate and even inflammatory. Generally, the differences of opinions among the medical community boil down to four areas: **when to prescribe, what to prescribe, who to prescribe to, and how to deliver it.** Currently there are inconsistent Standards of Care regarding HRT. Manuals, reference guides, and medical conferences seem to be always updating the protocols and encouraging advancement in the delivery of what many see as a "research science." State Medical Boards have often chimed in on doctor's prescribing habits, filing investigations, and even leveling significant reprimands for what other clinicians in the industry would see as appropriate health care practice. In the end, it has to be a personal choice if and when to pursue HRT, ideally done with a knowledgeable practitioner aware of the latest science and offering safe, effective, affordable options.

On the first point of **when to prescribe**... Now in reality this question is part of a much larger discussion, and its implications are significant for anyone in the U.S. involved in medical care, either as a prescriber or as a patient. Many hold the view (as do I in my practice) that the Reference Laboratory Values in a routine lab report dictate "normal" and "abnormal" results frequently based on the minimum values to avoid overt illness and disease. While it is most certainly helpful to identify a crisis situation and know when it is necessary to intervene to correct a severe problem, it is equally helpful to practice a system based on the understanding of optimal function and ideal physiology. The "abnormal" values in standard lab reports are generally placed at 2 standard deviations of what would be considered "normal." This means that only 5% of the results will be "abnormal," and as a result worthy of treatment (2.5% will be considered too high and 2.5% will be considered too low). Unfortunately, in the age of increasing obesity, inflammation, and chronic disease, the reference range for normal is getting pushed further and further away from optimal. Waiting until the numbers are outside the reference range and a crisis is (potentially) at hand, is akin to waiting to plant crops until 95% of people's food rations are threatened. At this point it's SO much more difficult to easily intervene and make substantive change.

The other three points of **what, who,** and **how,** these factors are often practitioner specific according to latest trends in the research and literature. **What to prescribe** can be related to bio-identical vs. non-bio-identical hormones and herbal vs. glandular (as discussed above), as well as what the entire HRT cocktail is to be given. Ideally not just one hormone is prescribed without taking a look at all the other hormones potentially involved, as they are all a part of one Endocrine Orchestra. This also brings in to discussion safety profiles of the prospective hormones, and when the data is meticulously investigated, it is usually quite good in safety profiles for those who are candidates (for example testosterone in men who are depleted and estrogen/progesterone in women who are low).

Notably for competitive athletes, because most of the hormones addressed for brain repair typically accelerate the performance of the rest of the body, they are not allowed by professional athletics organizations and would be considered "doping."

This brings us to the **who**. As mentioned before it is ideally the personal choice of a client to receive HRT, based on the recommendation of a skilled practitioner using the most recent, accurate, un-biased data. Furthermore, the decision to use HRT by a prescriber is ideally directed to the client's primary symptoms and not only laboratory data. As I was taught in medicine, "treat the patient, not the labs." This means if someone presents with all the symptoms of low thyroid while the lab values are "normal," ideally that person is seen and examined to evaluate any possible underlying cause and treated as soon as possible, not waiting (while the patient suffers) until the numbers become "abnormal" and it is more difficult to intervene.

Lastly, **how to treat** with HRT is also practitioner specific. We discussed this above regarding different options in the method of delivery (ex. transdermal vs oral vs injection) and different treatment courses (intermittent vs continuous). A second part of the how discussion is **how to test**, which typically involves saliva vs. blood vs. urine. Holding true to the trend, it too is provider specific.

LAB TESTING PROFILES

General tests to look for regarding the hormone status of the ones we have overviewed here include:

- **thyroid profiles**: TSH, free T3 and T4, reverse T3, and, if signs of clinical hypothyroid is present, then check thyroid antibodies. (Notably, signs and symptoms of low thyroid include lowered core body temperature, cold hands and feet, constipation, tiredness, dry skin, loss of lateral third of the eyebrows, thin hair, slow heart rate, inability to lose weight, and carpel tunnel syndrome)

- **adrenal profiles**: adrenal stress index with 24-hour cortisol, DHEA-S

- **gonadal sex hormone profiles**: testosterone, estrone, estradiol, estriol, 17-hyroxyprogesterone

- **other**: 25-OH-Vitamin D (this is a hormone produced by the skin), SHBG (sex hormone binding globulin, produced mostly by the liver and affects sex hormone availability and function)

Additionally, brain specific hormone and neurotransmitter profiles can also be used in the full assessment of TBI related impairment:

- **brain hormone profiles**: melatonin, ACTH, ADH, TSH, GH, LH, FSH, and oxytocin

- **neurotransmitter profiles**: testing urine metabolites of major neurotransmitters is possible, and even though there is some debate about the accuracy and reliability of these testing methodologies it may serve as a baseline marker of function to be able to assess progress of HRT or TAAT (targeted amino acid therapy) over time, especially if there are significant psychological symptoms associated with TBI and its recovery phase.

AVAILABILITY AND COST

There is a growing arena of practitioners in HRT worldwide, especially in the U.S. Every year there are more and more conferences and academic HRT training programs for physicians and other curious medical practitioners. As a result, there should be relatively easy access to trained HRT practitioners, however the field of HRT related to TBI is somewhat specific, so you may inquire about the prospective provider's history of working with TBI related clients.

Cost is variable. Testing profiles can run between $200 – $500. The types of HRT recommended vary even more widely, depending on all the hormones requiring support, their route of administration, and total time course for therapy.

LEARNING: COGNITIVE REHABILITATION DEVICES

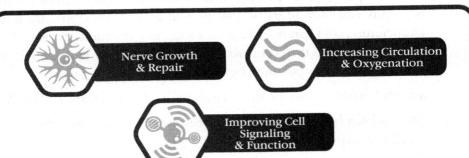

Nerve Growth & Repair

Increasing Circulation & Oxygenation

Improving Cell Signaling & Function

Cognitive Rehabilitation Devices

Benefits:
Growing new neural pathways. Improved cognitive function. And with accelerated improvement, contributing to self-confidence and even relearning previously held physical function.

Drawbacks:
Very low side effect profile. Cognitive fatigue may dictate treatment levels of intensity.

Availability:
Personal units are widely available in the U.S.

Growing number of practitioners are also available depending on which methods are used.

Cost:
Typically around $300 – $400 depending on the home unit.

Strength and resistance training are common components in the recovery of most types of physical injury. Just as you might use free weights and resistance bands to rehab torn ligaments or broken bones, a similar kind of strength training for your brain can be utilized.

After a traumatic brain injury, the ability to process certain kinds of visual information may become impaired. Distinguishing between similar-looking letters can make reading more difficult, or you might have problems with depth perception or visual-spatial navigation, making you more accident-prone. You could also find it difficult to focus your thoughts or concentrate on a specific task.

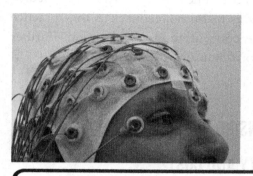

EEG Recording Cap" by Chris Hope. Licensed under CC BY 2.0. (Wikimedia Commons)

Wearable neurofeedback monitors, virtual reality technology, and visual-motor reaction boards are a few different types of cognitive rehabilitation devices that have been found to be able to help in recovery from TBI. We're going to focus on three specific examples of these technologies—the Muse Brain Sensing Headband, Oculus Rift, and Dynavision D2, respectively. (See Resources section for a more complete list of available products.)

WEARABLE NEUROFEEDBACK MONITORS

If you've ever been the subject of a sleep study, then you already may be familiar with electroencephalography (EEG). During a non-invasive EEG, many small sensors are placed on the outside of your scalp to measure your brain's electrical activity. At one time, only hospitals and researchers could afford the technology required to record the brain's wave patterns in this way, but, because EEG sensor technology has become more affordable and widespread, that's no longer the case.

Today, there are a handful of wearable neurofeedback monitors on the market—and still more coming along all the time. Intended for *at-home use*, they don't include

> **Neurofeedback** - a type of biofeedback focused on the use of real-time information specific to brain activity. Individuals monitor this real-time feedback as they practice controlling certain brain functions like concentration or relaxation.

nearly as many sensors as medical-grade EEG systems do, but, ranging from $80 to $500, they are relatively inexpensive and work fairly well.

These devices enable *at-home* users to see and monitor their own brainwaves and are especially useful for the practice of **neurofeedback—NF**. In traditional biofeedback therapy, many different kinds of monitors are used to display real-time, physiological information like heart rate and muscle tension. Patients use this real-time feedback as they practice deep breathing and other stress-management techniques. Neurofeedback (or neurobiofeedback) is similar; however, its focus is solely on real-time *brain* activity. During neurofeedback therapy, individuals monitor this real-time feedback as they practice controlling certain brain functions like concentration or relaxation. Further in the discussion, we will talk about more clinically driven and intensive EEG directed NF therapy.

MUSE BRAIN SENSING HEADBAND

AVAILABILITY AND COST

One of the more popular wearable neurofeedback monitors being used as a personal training device is InteraXon's Muse, which retails for just under $300. The device analyzes the balance of alpha, beta, theta, gamma, and delta waves in your brain and how these change over time. Muse is intended to be Bluetooth-connected to your smartphone or tablet and used in conjunction with the company's "Muse Calm" mobile app to help learn how to calm and relax your mind.

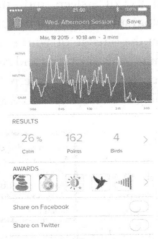

Within the app, relaxation sessions can last from 3 to 20 minutes, and you're required to perform a one-minute device calibration exercise before every session. During sessions, you close your eyes and try to calm your thoughts.

When your mind is relaxed and focused, you hear the sounds of ocean waves. If you become distracted, the wave sounds grow louder—your cue to try to refocus. When you mind is calmest, you'll hear birds chirping. When sessions end, you can view graphs of your mental state.

Muse works with seven EEG sensors that are distributed across its "brain sensing" headband. Capable of reading four channels of data, there are individual sensors positioned at the left and right sides of the forehead and along the tops of the left and right ears. The three remaining sensors run across the front of the forehead.[94] (Check out the "Developer Kit" section at www.choosemuse.com for more complete technical specs and documentation.)

It's important to note that, although the Muse picks up on your brain's alpha, beta, theta, gamma, and delta waves, the Muse Calm app does not display the raw data for these. Instead, brain wave activity is expressed as either "calm," "neutral" or "active." If you would like access to that raw data, you can purchase a separate, user-made app called "Muse Monitor."

BENEFITS AND RISKS

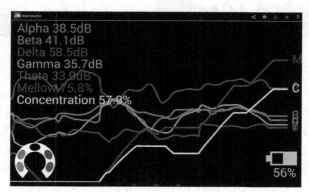

Screen captures from "Muse Calm" app (top right) and "Muse Monitor" app.

Because most of the NF devices on the market are still so new, there is a lack of scientific, peer-reviewed research about specific benefits they may provide. That being said, in my clinical experience and in examining the anecdotal evidence available, there is strong support to suggest these technologies have helped many users learn over time to improve their ability to focus, calm, and center their mind and achieve a great overall sense of well-being.

Currently, there are no known health risks associated with the use of wearable neurofeedback monitors like Muse. However, when it comes to ease of use, functionality, and customer service, user reviews of *all* available devices and their accompanying apps have been mixed. Regarding the Muse Brain Sensing Headband, in particular, some users have expressed frustration about the time required for setup. They have had trouble getting the headband and sensors correctly positioned, and, sometimes, they have ongoing difficulty keeping the sensors in position during use.

VIRTUAL REALITY (VR) TECHNOLOGY

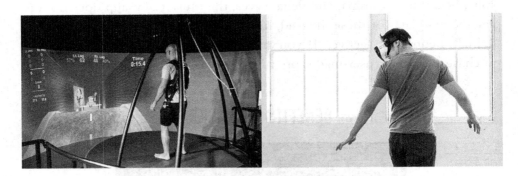

Virtual reality technology is used to help rehabilitate a serviceman at Walter Reed Army Medical Center.

Pairing specialty computer hardware and software to create a VR (Virtual Reality) experience isn't exactly new. Technically, VR was used as early as the 1960s when new pilots—with their feet planted firmly on the ground—trained on high-tech flight simulators. Since then, head-mounted displays, elaborate motion-capture video systems and other advances in virtual reality (VR) technology have enabled users to interact with increasingly lifelike, computer-generated environments.

VR is commonly employed for military training and in gaming, but it happens to have therapeutic uses as well. Made by GestureTek, the Interactive Rehabilitation and Exercise System (IREX) is one of the more elaborate virtual reality devices used in hospitals and sports rehab facilities. Typically installed in a permanent location, IREX uses immersive video gesture control technology and a green screen to "place patients into virtual sport or gaming environments where they are guided through clinician prescribed therapeutic exercise regimes."[95]

We will get into some of the more user-friendly, inexpensive models currently available for at home use down below.

BENEFITS AND RISKS

VR technology is used in medical settings to help assess the treatment needs of patients having difficulty processing sensory information. It has been shown to improve general cognitive abilities, memory, auditory and visual learning, and speed of information processing.[96]

And, in a small study of post-stroke patients, participants being rehabilitated with virtual reality technology showed significant improvements in visual attention and short-term visuospatial memory.[97] VR training also has been shown to help some post-stroke patients physically, by increasing the range of motion in their knees and ankles.[98]

Virtual reality can have its drawbacks though. With symptoms ranging from a slight headache to occasional nausea and vomiting, some people experience "cybersickness," a form of motion sickness, after immersion in virtual environments. On the more severe side of the spectrum, the aftereffects of cybersickness, such as disorientation, problems with balance, and reduced eye-hand coordination, can last up to several hours after a VR experience.[99] [100] If you're significantly prone to motion sickness, you may also be more likely to experience "cybersickness" and therefore, start with more brief exposure and gradually work your way up in length of time used and intensity level of programs experienced.

AVAILABILITY AND COST

Showing players and their body movements in real-time, scaled-down versions of systems similar to the IREX are now available for at-home use. (For instance, used with Sony's PlayStation 4, the PlayStation Camera and PlayStation Move gaming controller are equipped with motion sensors to show players on-screen.) But VR technology is becoming more portable and compact.

There are now many inexpensive, "head-mount" products out which enable users to convert their smartphones into wearable, stereoscopic headsets suitable for 3D gaming and watching 3D movies. And, at the other end of the spectrum, there are much more sophisticated VR headsets like the Rift by Oculus VR.

Oculus Rift features two visual displays running at a total resolution of 2160 x 1200 pixels, and users experience a 360-degree field of view. The Rift also has an audio component and "Adjacent Reality Tracker," including a magnetometer, a gyroscope, and an accelerometer for smoother tracking across three-dimensional space.[101] As of early 2017 Oculus' Rift sells for around $500.

DYNAVISION BOARDS

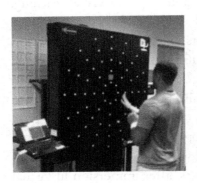

The Dynavision device was originally developed to help athletes work on their visual-motor skills (and it is still used that way), but it has since been adapted to help patients with brain injuries to improve many aspects of visual attention and processing.

The large board features more than 60 target buttons arranged in five concentric circles. Each button contains a colored light, and individual buttons randomly light up. (Sound is also sometimes incorporated into the exercise.) When training, you focus your eyes on the center of the board and use your peripheral vision to notice when different buttons illuminate. If you see a button light up, you press it as quickly as you can. There are many variations on this activity, depending on the visual attention skills being tested.

The Dynavision board can be used as a diagnostic tool to help determine what kinds of visual attention deficits you may have developed after your injury. And, because your responses are carefully recorded as you train, performance baselines are easily established. These are used to track your progress during recovery.

BENEFITS AND RISKS

Working with a Dynavision board has shown to improve eye-hand coordination, visual-motor reaction time, peripheral visual awareness, concentration, simple cognitive processing, and physical endurance.[102] One small study of post-stroke patients found significant improvements in visual attention after six weeks of Dynavision training. The study subjects were between the ages of 45 and 80, and all made progress in their overall endurance, speed and visual reaction times.[103]

There are no serious health risks associated with the use of Dynavision boards.

AVAILABILITY AND COST

Due to its hefty size and cost, the Dynavision board isn't necessarily as well-suited for at-home use as the other cognitive rehabilitation devices mentioned here. Mostly in hospitals and sports training and rehabilitation facilities, more than 1,000 units are currently in use worldwide. The company's original model, the Dynavision 2000, can be found in 36 countries and in more than 500 hospitals across North America.[104] (Visit http://dynavisioninternational. com and click on the "Client Map" tab to see which treatment centers near you might have a Dynavision board.)

Curious about buying your own Dynavision board? The newer Dynavision D2 model retails for about $16,000, and it's sometimes possible to find a used Dynavision 2000 for sale for about $7,000.

BRAIN TRAINING MOBILE APPS

While not cognitive rehab devices per se, there are quite a few brain-training mobile apps that add state of the art gamification quality to the basic rigors of mental tests and tasks, which are then tracked over time to assess progress. These can therefore be stacked on any concussion repair strategy to aid in determining if a given protocol is helping and in what ways.

The big 5 in currently popularity are Lumosity, Peak, Elevate, Cognito and Fit Brains Trainer. These are free at a basic level with opt ins for ongoing monthly subscriptions to access the full features at a few bucks per month.

NEUROFEEDBACK

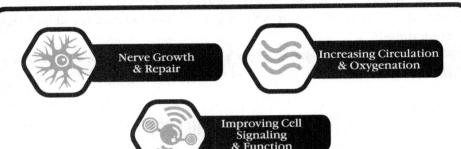

Neurofeedback

Benefits:
At-will access to alpha brainwaves that are conducive to healing. Preservation of alpha activity has been linked to neuronal survival and positive prognoses in brain-injured patients.

Drawbacks:
Currently no known health risks.

Availability:
EEG neurofeedback specialists widely available.
Alpha training immersion programs also available in some areas.

Cost:
$75 to $175 per hour for most EEG neurofeedback.
$5,000 to $15,000 to attend 10 day alpha training immersion programs.

We covered at-home neurofeedback devices a little bit in the last section, but now we're going to go into more detail about EEG neurofeedback—and alpha brain state training, in particular. Recall that, with traditional biofeedback therapy, patients use real-time feedback (provided by heart rate, muscle tension and other physiological monitors) as they practice stress-management techniques.

In neurofeedback therapy, individuals see and respond to real-time information about the electrical activity in their brains as they practice self-regulation of certain brain functions like concentration or relaxation.

I took the opportunity to experience this type of program a couple of years ago, and it is indeed rocket fuel for self-awareness. The EEG alpha brain state training developed by Dr. Jim Hardt is a very specialized type of neurofeedback therapy that facilitates speedy access to positive brainwave states performed by the Biocybernaut Institute. This program is by no means for the faint of heart as it involves approximately 12 hours of focused brain wave training per day for 7 days. The results are pretty phenomenal as a form of meditation on steroids. A pilot study of 17 subjects with no prior experience with yoga, meditation, or alpha training found that, after just seven alpha training sessions, it was possible to achieve the same brainwave patterns that some Zen meditation practitioners work 20 years or more to master.[105] The key for many in maintaining the gains (as it was for me) includes regular practice in continuing to access the alpha brain wave state at will, which can be facilitated even more robustly by 1 – 2-day "booster shot" programs at Biocybernaut every 6 – 12 months.

BENEFITS AND RISKS

We are most likely to register alpha brainwave activity when we are feeling simultaneously alert and focused but also relaxed. When in an alpha state, we shift out of sympathetic overdrive and into a calmer, parasympathetic mode that's more conducive to healing. It follows that the longer you are able to maintain an alpha state, the longer your system is primed for recovery. And, indeed, studies have linked the preservation of alpha activity to neuronal survival and positive prognoses in brain-injured patients.[106] [107] Researchers have also related alpha activity to "attention mechanisms, including maintaining an optimal cerebral arousal state."[108] [109]

During alpha brain state training, EEG sensors on your scalp enable you to see your brainwave activity in real-time. You'll learn what your brain's alpha activity looks like and which specific thoughts, feelings, memories, and ideas bring you closer to your ideal alpha state—and which ones take you farther away. Once you see which areas of focus contribute to your alpha activity, you can concentrate and build on those areas. With practice, you may become adept at producing and maintaining your own alpha state at will.

Currently, there are no known health risks associated with EEG alpha brain-wave state training.

AVAILABILITY AND COST

When checking out individual neurofeedback specialists, be sure you understand exactly how they work and what kind of training you can expect from them. (Many practitioners and available training methods utilize variations on the alpha training concept. For example, in one of the more common of these, the brainwaves of hundreds of healthy subjects are pooled and averaged to create an ideal or "norm." Rather than identify and achieve their own ideal alpha states, client trainees instead work to pattern their brainwaves as closely to the pooled "norm" as they can. While this can and has worked for many people, it too has drawbacks. It may be sensitive in working from a baseline toward a higher concentration of alpha states, however it may not be specific in assisting you to develop and maximize your own neuro-physiological alpha pattern signature).

Individual neurofeedback sessions in your area may cost between $75 and $175 per hour. (If you purchase multiple sessions in advance, you may be able get a discounted hourly rate.) And, ranging from about $5,000 for a couple of days to as much as $20,000 for a full week, alpha training immersion programs are also available. (See Resources section for details.)

STEM CELL THERAPY

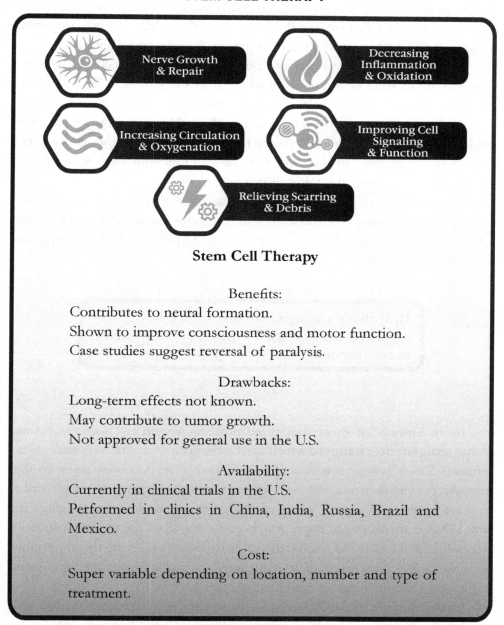

Stem Cell Therapy

Benefits:
Contributes to neural formation.
Shown to improve consciousness and motor function.
Case studies suggest reversal of paralysis.

Drawbacks:
Long-term effects not known.
May contribute to tumor growth.
Not approved for general use in the U.S.

Availability:
Currently in clinical trials in the U.S.
Performed in clinics in China, India, Russia, Brazil and Mexico.

Cost:
Super variable depending on location, number and type of treatment.

We have culturally been hearing about stem cell therapy for many years, however most treatments, with the exception of bone marrow/hematopoietic stem cell transplantation, still haven't been officially approved for treatment in the U.S. Elsewhere in the world, stem cells are used extensively, including for help in TBI-related patient injuries. To get around this barrier in the US, some practitioners offer them as an "experimental treatment procedure," and as with any new procedure that catches the curiosity of the culture, it's very important to know what the practitioner's background and success rates have been.

When stem cells are injected into a damaged brain, they become integrated into the pre-existing neural network where they are needed.[110] To understand how this process works, it helps to know some stem cell basics.

We have many types of cells in our bodies—like skin cells, muscle cells, and the neurons in our brains to name just a few. Now, even though these cell types are recognizably different and have distinct functions, they all started out in the same way. They all originated from stem cells.

You can think of stem cells as a kind of blank canvas in the body. Stem cells contain the same DNA as every other cell and the same basic set of proteins, but they're missing other more specialized proteins that give each cell type its unique identity.

> **Epigenetic changes** – changes in the way genetic sequences are expressed which result in variations in cell function.

In the absence of these specialized proteins, a stem cell does not yet undergo **epigenetic changes,** which affect the way a genetic sequence is expressed. DNA genetic sequences are modified to fit necessary roles, so that the *same* genetic sequence can have *different* functions in different people and in different cells. Additionally, some of those genetic modifications include the way DNA is *stored* not just expressed, because not all of the genetic material is accessible all the time. (In the last decade scientists are realizing the importance of epigenetics—not just genetic sequences—in making everyone unique and influencing health, longevity and life in general).

Stem cells were originally harvested from embryos. An embryo is the initial cluster of cells that forms after a sperm fertilizes an egg. Over time, this cluster of cells will divide to form an entire human being. Cells that have been extracted from an embryo have the ability to differentiate. That means they can adopt a specific function to fulfill a role that the body requires. Extracting cells from embryonic tissue as a practice has started to fall out of favor, both because of moral implications as well as the potentially uncontrollable genetically driven outcomes of using foreign donor cells in a separate host's body.

> **Pluripotency** – the capacity of a cell to adopt a specific function to fulfill a role that the body requires.

Usually, once a cell differentiates to take on a specific function, it loses its ability to fulfill any other roles in the body. However, scientists have recently found ways to cause some cell types to undergo **induced pluripotency**.[111, 112]

In other words, a cell that had previously differentiated is turned back into a stem cell. Epigenetic changes are erased,[113] and the cell is once again a blank canvas. This cellular blank canvas can be used to repair any damaged tissue in the body. For TBI repair, these stem cells are injected into the brain and can form new neurons[114] or whatever cell types the damaged brain needs.[115]

BENEFITS AND RISKS

According to anecdotal case reports, some patients with multiple sclerosis achieved full remission after undergoing stem cell therapy, and some TBI and stroke patients reported a reversal in paralysis. Quantitative studies also suggest introducing stem cells into the human brain is safe and effective. For instance, after injecting stem cells into the brains of 97 TBI patients, researchers found that 46% of patients who began the study trapped in persistent vegetative states showed improvements in consciousness. And, 37% of patients who began the study with disturbances in motor function showed improvements in this area.[116]

> **Autologous cells** – one's own cells which will later be reintroduced into his or her body.

Each of these patients had been treated with **autologous** cells—cells that had been harvested from their own bodies. Because it's now possible to cause differentiated cells to return to a "blank canvas" state, individuals can be treated with their own stem cells. (Cells to be reintroduced into a patient's brain typically come from that patient's own cerebral spinal fluid, fat tissue, or bone marrow.)

As with kidney donation, when new cells are introduced into a body, the immune system can negatively respond by attacking the foreign tissue material and causing it to be rejected. In kidney transplantation, that risk can be lowered by using a donor who shows genetic similarities to the recipient.[117] When autologous stem cells are used, the donor and recipient are the same person. This greatly reduces the likelihood of an immune response.

Still, even treatment with one's own stem cells carries some potential risk. One concern is that induced pluripotent stem cells could give rise to tumors.[118] Because these cells are manipulated to make them more able to divide and flourish, they might continue to do so—past the point at which we would want them to. So far, this risk has been most noticeable in animal studies. In humans, more long-term studies are needed, in order to better understand the balance between risks and benefits.

AVAILABILITY AND COST

Stem cell therapy is not approved for general use in the U.S., but there are ongoing clinical trials, some of which may be recruiting new patients. You can find these by searching for "stem cell traumatic brain injury" on the U.S. government-sponsored website www.clinicaltrials.gov. The major cost of enrollment would be relocating to the site of the study. Phase 2 clinical trial participants often receive free medical care.[119] Alternatively, there are clinics in the U.S. that offer treatments under an "experimental therapy" designation, allowing clients to choose to participate in a novel treatment that has not been fully legalized. Many of these treatments are for a variety of chronic pain and degenerative joint diseases, cosmetic uses and even brain/neurological recovery. Due diligence in investigating any treatment provider's stem cell specific training background is highly recommended before engaging in therapy.

Additionally, stem cell therapy *is* fully legal and available via clinics in other parts of the world, including Mexico,[120] where the regulatory environment is less restrictive.

Notably, the cost of stem cell therapy varies widely given the style of treatment and methodology used, the body location and number of treatments given and the facility location worldwide (for example treatments in Mexico are often a third to a fourth of the cost of treatments in the US).

ACUPUNCTURE — COAUTHORED BY DR. ANDY SWANSON

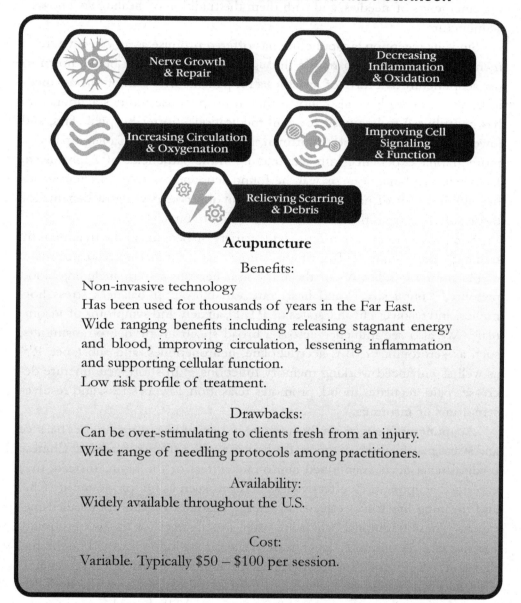

Nerve Growth & Repair

Decreasing Inflammation & Oxidation

Increasing Circulation & Oxygenation

Improving Cell Signaling & Function

Relieving Scarring & Debris

Acupuncture

Benefits:

Non-invasive technology

Has been used for thousands of years in the Far East.

Wide ranging benefits including releasing stagnant energy and blood, improving circulation, lessening inflammation and supporting cellular function.

Low risk profile of treatment.

Drawbacks:

Can be over-stimulating to clients fresh from an injury.

Wide range of needling protocols among practitioners.

Availability:

Widely available throughout the U.S.

Cost:

Variable. Typically $50 – $100 per session.

For many people, just the mention of needles conjures fear. Yet, acupuncture has been shown to be one of the most relaxing, therapeutic modalities for individuals who have suffered a recent traumatic incident. How is this possible that these small pointed objects can offer profound relief from trauma?

Let us travel back to the stone age, where we find human's earliest record of using sharpened stones as medicine. These so called Bian stones were used to drain abscesses.[121] With the discovery of bronze, silver, and gold, we see the emergence of needles, and with them the tradition of healing we know as acupuncture.

Since its inception, acupuncture has offered promise as an effective treatment for pain. Operating rooms throughout Asia have even been known to use acupuncture as a form of anesthesia for patients who cannot tolerate medications.[122] Studies have also shown that in hospital use settings acupuncture has contributed to less need for pain medication, shorter hospital stays, and lower medical costs. Robert Koffman, MD and U.S. Navy Captain, paints a more graphic experience with acupuncture in the battlefields of Afghanistan. In the starved limitations of war, he found acupuncture to offer clinical uses beyond the scope of pain relief. Dr. Koffman observed psychiatric benefits for those suffering from the most severe forms of trauma.[123]

Similarly, acupuncture offers a wide variety of benefits in the treatment of traumatic brain injury (TBI). Studies show that acupuncture regulates many of the common indicators of the autonomic nervous system, including blood pressure,[124] pupil size,[125] and heart rate variability.[126] It balances stress hormones, and resolves chronic states of PTSD, anxiety and symptoms of insomnia.[127] We also see influence across a broad spectrum of neurotransmitters, such as serotonin, GABA, acetylcholine, neuropeptides, and substance P,[128] as well as enhanced working memory functions.[115] In short, acupuncture decreases pain, regulates mood, promotes relaxation, lowers stress, and resolves symptoms of insomnia.

Acupuncture's effects on the nervous system and neurotransmitter balance and stress may be the best theory for how it works. Of course, ancient Chinese medical texts never mentioned neurotransmitters or the brain. Instead, they explained acupuncture's effectiveness in terms such as Qi (pronounced "Chi" and meaning life force) effects on energy channels of the body called meridians. These traditional beliefs are often too abstract for the western mind. For the sake of simplicity, lets return to the car analogy. Qi would be the fuel that converts to power when pumped through the cylinders of the engine. The meridians would be the fuel line. Unlike the car however, the body has many sources of power, such as water, oxygen, ATP, thyroid hormone, glucose, growth hormone, and testosterone. Qi would be that which drives the absorption, production, circulation, and utilization of all of these substances, and the meridians assist in guiding the Qi through the organs of the body. While Qi remains invisible to the eye, we are all aware of what Qi looks like in abundance when we see a vital, strong, healthy human being (think Michael Jordan in his prime).

When we move and enhance Qi in the body with acupuncture, we relieve pain and restore balance to all organ systems. Thus we see greater hormonal balance, neurological repair, increased neurotransmitter supply and regulation, and, ultimately, a brain that's able to heal.

A note to practitioners: Less is more. Acupuncturists experienced with treating clients with TBI know these individuals (more than most) require a tranquil environment. Those who have experienced a significant level of trauma have a sensory system that is operating on overtime. All sounds, smells, touch, and light will move them closer to the point of overwhelm. With acupuncture, and with most therapies involved in TBI care, less is often more, i.e. fewer needles, shorter treatments, and less stimulation. Dimmed lighting and a quiet setting are ideal. All sensory stimulation must be carefully selected, moving the patient towards a relaxed, parasympathetic experience. (Notably, there is similarity to the benefit of floatation therapy as a sensory deprivation, low stimulus environment). It's also a good idea for clients to have a snack before a treatment to avoid hypoglycemic episodes during a needling.

PHARMACEUTICAL NOOTROPICS

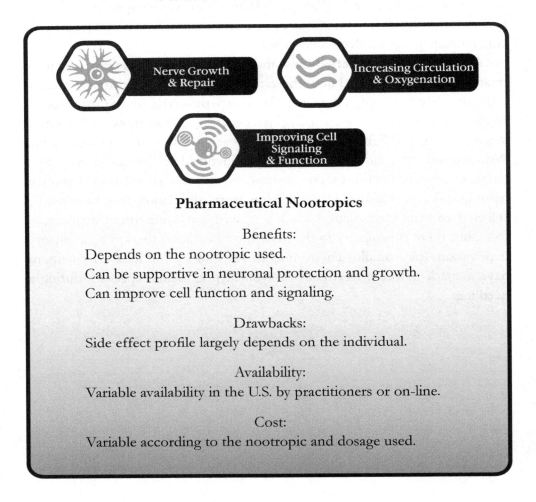

Nerve Growth & Repair

Increasing Circulation & Oxygenation

Improving Cell Signaling & Function

Pharmaceutical Nootropics

Benefits:
Depends on the nootropic used.
Can be supportive in neuronal protection and growth.
Can improve cell function and signaling.

Drawbacks:
Side effect profile largely depends on the individual.

Availability:
Variable availability in the U.S. by practitioners or on-line.

Cost:
Variable according to the nootropic and dosage used.

In my clinical practice, I tend to judiciously use pharmaceuticals when other modalities have failed and when there is an obvious direct benefit with low chance of side-effects. The biggest downside to pharmaceutical interventions is the long-term side effect profile in the setting of using something external to treat the symptom of a deeper underlying imbalance. When this happens, the body's signal of the imbalance becomes relieved, while the underlying issue typically worsens, in the end often causing a chronic, more nagging, and more difficult to treat issue.

That is not to say that medication therapy does not have a time and a place to use them. When in crisis at a severe level of symptomatology, medications often work very well to dampen down the symptoms. Ideally, they are used with a plan in mind that honors the client's desired goals in the least harmful and most effective way, while looking for the root cause of the symptoms in the first place. That being said, the pharmaceutical nootropics listed here tend to have a relative low risk of side-effects and have proven efficacy in supporting brain function and cognitive performance.

Nootropics are a class of "smart" drugs and supplements used to enhance brain function, and they represent many of the substances that people the world over have used for millenia to "get stuff done."

Imbibing in substances like caffeine, nicotine, and even cocaine to improve cognitive function is actually an ancient practice, but the term "nootropic" wasn't coined until the 1970s. It's based on the Greek roots "noos" for "mind" and "tropein" for "towards."[129, 130] It translates to "turning toward the mind", and through the use of nootropics, it's possible to turn the mind toward improved performance by increasing mental focus, stamina, and memory.

Although we'll cover many other more "natural" nootropics in detail in Chapter 3, in this section, we'll discuss four of the best-known *synthetic* nootropics: Cerebrolysin, Modafinil, Aniracetam, and Piraceram. With no naturally-occurring biological analogs, these nootropics must be chemically synthesized.

HEADS UP   Ask your doctor before adding pharmaceutical nootropics to your TBI treatment protocol.

CEREBROLYSIN

Memories are stored in the brain by the pattern of connections between neurons. However, these connections become disrupted in TBI by swelling and neuronal cell death, often leading to the experience of memory loss and other cognitive symptoms. Studied since the 1970s, Cerebrolysin is a pharmaceutical nootropic made up of porcine proteins derived from the brains of pigs. It has been used extensively to improve long-term memory in TBI patients.

Researchers have learned from animal studies that Cerebrolysin promotes neurogenesis. The drug works by boosting the production of new brain cells to replace those that had been damaged or destroyed.[131] Furthermore, Cerebrolysin halts dangerous blood brain barrier leakage[132] and speeds the recovery of cognitive and physical abilities.[133]

BENEFITS AND RISKS

Significant benefits have also been demonstrated in human subjects taking Cerebrolysin. One recent study tracked the recovery of patients suffering from TBI caused by concussive blows (typically the result of auto accidents). Recovering far more of their pre-injury capabilities within a 30-day period, the patients taking Cerebrolysin had markedly better outcomes than their control group peers.[134]

Although it's likely that patients taking Cerebrolysin soon after sustaining their TBIs will see the biggest benefits, it can help people who take it much later during their recovery. It has been used successfully for neuroprotection and neurorehabilitation in elderly patients and stroke victims,[135][136] suggesting that Cerebrolysin has a place in long-term treatment of chronic symptoms.

Cerebrolysin may even help *healthy* individuals to age more gracefully. The gradual accumulation of oxidative damage in the brain contributes to our gradual cognitive decline. In a study of Cerebrolysin used to treat brain cells from healthy human participants, the drug was shown to reduce oxidative stress-induced cell death.[137] A single dose of Cerebrolysin given to healthy elderly patients was shown to increase brain activity and improve performance on a memory test.[138]

Regarding the drawbacks associated with Cerebrolysin, some people initially experience mild side effects such as vertigo, agitation, and flushing, but these typically dissipate with continued use.[139] You should not use Cerebrolysin if you have kidney failure, epilepsy, or are pregnant. Also, antidepressant medications, including monoamine oxidase inhibitors, as well as some other nootropics may negatively interact with Cerebrolysin.[140]

AVAILABILITY AND COST

Approved as a nootropic supplement in only a handful of countries, Cerebrolysin is not available for sale in the U.S. However, it can be obtained through some online retailers. Currently, this pharmaceutical nootropic can only be administered via injection and is typically sold in 1-, 5-, and 10-milliliter vials. Depending on the quantities purchased, prices may range from two to five dollars per milliliter.

MODAFINIL

Modafinil was originally developed as an anti-narcolepsy drug, but it has many other well-tested applications. Since the 1990s, Modafinil has been used to fight fatigue in patients recovering from TBI.

Clinically proven to boost intelligence in healthy individuals,[141] Modafinil is also taken as a cognitive performance enhancer. Research professors have even reported taking the drug themselves to combat jet lag, increase mental energy, and tackle difficult intellectual challenges.[142] And, according to an informal *Nature* poll, Modafinil was the second most popular cognitive enhancer among survey respondents. (Methylphenidate, also known as Ritalin, came in first.)[143]

BENEFITS AND RISKS

Frequently used to treat excessive daytime sleepiness and attention deficits,[144] Modafinil has been shown to increase alertness and reduce fatigue in patients recovering from TBI.[145] When administered to 10 people with closed-head brain injuries, Modafinil markedly decreased excessive daytime sleepiness for 9 of the 10 patients. They reported experiencing normal nighttime sleep as well as "increased wakefulness and feelings of normality." Some also mentioned gaining cognitive benefits, such as improved focus.[146]

Although Modafinil has been approved for or is under investigation to treat a wide range of brain-related conditions, it is not entirely without risk. Some patients taking Modafinil have experienced insomnia, headache, nausea, rashes, nervousness, increased heart rate and increased blood pressure.[147]

AVAILABILITY AND COST

In the U.S., the U.K., Canada, and many other countries, this pharmaceutical nootropic is not available without a prescription.[148]

PIRACETAM

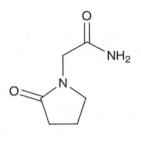

Piracetam

First approved in Europe in the early 1970s, Piracetam has long been used to treat vertigo and many age-related disorders.[149] The drug has been shown to be a neuroprotective agent, acting on the central nervous system in several ways, including stimulating synaptic transmission, influencing glucose metabolism, normalizing neuronal activity, and more.[150]

BENEFITS AND RISKS

Over the last four decades there have been many clinical trials of Piracetam in the context of neurological disorders. Seeking a big-picture view of the use of Piracetam for age-related mental impairments, researchers examined results from 19 different double-blinded, placebo-controlled trials that had been conducted between 1972 and 2001. In their resulting meta-analysis, they reported that, while only 32.5% of patients in the placebo groups showed improvement, improvement was seen in 60.9% of the Piracetam-treated patients. The study's authors concluded, "These results provide compelling evidence for the global clinical efficacy of Piracetam in a diverse group of older subjects with cognitive impairment."[151]

Piracetam's benefits have been demonstrated in younger subjects, too. In a study of 42 closed-head trauma patients between the ages of 12 and 18, researchers administered Piracetam to 20 subjects for one month. (The remaining 22 patients received no medications.) Those in the Piracetam treatment group showed significant improvements in the areas of visual, kinesthetic, and auditory-speech memory. The drug also provided "positive therapeutic effects on impairments to higher mental (memory, attention, executive) and motor (coordination) functions and on measures of the speeds of cognitive and motor operations."[152]

In a different study of patients being treated for concussions, the patients given Piracetam regained significantly more color vision than did the patients who were given a placebo. (Many people with traumatic brain injuries suffer from blurred vision, which can include a loss of the ability to see certain colors.) A comparison of pre- and post-treatment abilities in the Piracetam group revealed marked improvements in the perception of dim light. After treatment with Piracetam, patients were able to see colored light that was three to five times dimmer than the light they originally had been able to perceive.[153]

And, in patients undergoing coronary bypass surgery, Piracetam has been shown to protect against short-term memory loss after a temporary drop in oxygen flow to the brain.[154]

Piracetam appears to have anti-depressant properties as well. Researchers treated a pool of 70 patients who had "probable vascular dementia" due to stroke or chronic cerebral circulatory insufficiency with daily doses of Piracetam. Over the course of eight weeks, 30 patients were given 1,200 mg of Piracetam per day, and the remaining 40 patients were given daily Piracetam doses of 2,400 mg. Several statistically significant changes were noted, with the severity of stroke-related depression chief among them. Overall, the greatest clinical effects were seen in the group of patients taking the larger daily doses of Piracetam. The study's authors also observed, "Patients noted vivacity, increased levels of daily activity, with improvements in concentration, increased well-being, and self-confidence, the appearance of being at peace, and subjective improvements in mood. Patients evaluated their state and prognosis less pessimistically and became more positive with regard to further supportive treatment.[155]

People taking Piracetam sometimes do experience side effects like anxiety, agitation, insomnia and drowsiness, but these are often mild and temporary.[156]

AVAILABILITY AND COST

In the U.S., Piracetam is not approved for medical use and it may not be legally marketed as a dietary supplement. However, some U.S.-based suppliers do sell Piracetam in powder form for research purposes. (Depending on the quantities purchased, the cost of powdered Piracetam may range from 15 cents to as much as $1.25 per gram.) Largely used in Europe, Asia and South America, the drug is available via online retailers and may be imported for personal use in some other countries.[157] Piracetam is commonly sold in 800 mg capsules, and a bottle of 180 capsules costs about $40.

ANIRACETAM

Aniracetam is in the same general family of drugs as Piracetam, meaning they have comparable chemical structures and may affect brain cells in some of the same ways. Despite their similarities, Aniracetam seems to act more quickly on the brain than Piracetam. Soon after it is ingested, Aniracetam crosses the blood-brain barrier, reaching full concentration in just 20 to 30 minutes.[158]

Aniracetam

BENEFITS AND RISKS

As with Piracetam, Aniracetam boosts cognitive performance in animals and people. In one study, for example, after treating brain-injured rats with Aniracetam, researchers noted significant improvement in the rats' ability to solve a cognitive puzzle. Strikingly, some of the injured rats weren't given Aniracetam until 11 days after they had sustained their initial injuries, but even this group performed as well on the cognitive puzzle as healthy, uninjured rats.[159]

Aniracetam has also been shown to improve cognition in people with poor oxygen flow to their brains. In a study of patients with cerebral vasculature damage, those who were given 1,500 mg of Aniracetam daily performed better on a battery of cognitive tests than the patients who did not receive the drug.[160]

And, a separate study of 109 cognitively impaired patients between the ages of 65 and 80 showed similar results. Beginning at least six months before enrollment in the study, participants had exhibited signs of "gradual and progressive cognitive decline" and were thought to suffer from "probable dementia of the Alzheimer's type." Researchers split the participants into two groups. For six months, one group was treated with 1,500 mg of Aniracetam per day, while the other group received a placebo. Both groups were regularly tested in areas of perceptive and abstract reasoning, ability to focus attention, visual and spatial memory and verbal memory, among others. Although all patients performed comparably at first, by the study's end, the Aniracetam-treated group's average scores improved by more than 20 percent. Meanwhile, the placebo group deteriorated slightly in nearly every cognitive test area.[161]

Aniracetam affects the levels of several different neurotransmitters and may have antidepressant properties as well. The drug has been demonstrated to boost dopamine and serotonin transmission in rats.[162] Both dopamine and serotonin are intimately linked to pleasure and a sense of well-being.

When taking Aniracetam, some people have experienced headaches and gastrointestinal symptoms like diarrhea and nausea. Others have reported feelings of nervousness and anxiety. Generally, though, these side effects do not persist.

AVAILABILITY AND COST

Aniracetam is unregulated in many countries, including the U.S., the U.K., and Canada. It is widely available online and may legally be purchased without a prescription.[163] You can buy Aniracetam in capsules or as a powder. Aniracetam is commonly sold in 750 mg capsules, and a bottle of 100 capsules costs about $30. The cost of powdered Aniracetam can range from roughly 22 cents (for bulk discounts) to 75 cents per gram.

CHAPTER 3

BIOLOGIC NOOTROPICS

In this Section

You'll learn about many of the various Biologic Nootropics:

- Fish Oil – DHA/EPA
- Phosphatidylserine & Phosphatidylcholine
- Glutathione
- Vitamin C
- Lithium Orotate
- B12 – methylcobalamin
- Alpha Lipoic Acid
- Acetyl-L-Carnitine

Quick Tips:

- **The use of supplements in medicine is both a science and an art.**
- **When used at the right time, the right dose and for the right duration, most people will respond favorably.**
- **They can often be used in conjunction for a more robust effect.**
- **Professional line formulas tend to have more rigorous production standards, and are therefore, more trustworthy, leading to the adage "what you pay for is what you get."**

See other sections in the Manual for these nootropic supports:
- Melatonin see the section on Sleep.
- Vitamin D see the section on Sunlight.
- CBD/Cannabidiol see the section on Psychedelics.
- Turmeric/Curcumin see the section on Foods.
- Magnesium see the section on Sleep.

***

Note, the nootropics included here in the Manual are the ones typically used for TBI recovery, and there are still others with relevance and clinical data to support their usage. Those include – NAD+, astaxanthin, vitamin E, BCAA – Branched Chain Amino Acids, CBD oil (cannabidiol), DHEA, creatine and oxaloacetate to name a few.

When health is absent, wisdom cannot reveal itself, art cannot manifest, strength cannot fight, wealth becomes useless, and intelligence cannot be applied.

~ Herophilus

BIOLOGIC NOOTROPIC

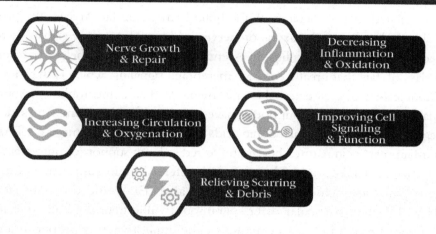

Biologic Nootropic –

Method of Action:
From 1 – 5 above, depends on its physiology.
Listed below for each.

Benefit:
Listed below for each.

Drawbacks:
Typically safe if used in dose range.
Do not use with conflicting medications.
Inform your treating provider you are taking to get their approval.

Availability:
Generally available over the counter.
Most brain treatment specialists will know about many of these.

Cost:
Variable depending on manufacturer, route of administration
and dose.

FISH OIL

It is estimated that 60 percent of the brain is made of fat. Myelin, the protective sheath that covers the axons of nerves, and preserves nerve signals, is composed of 70 – 85% fat. Fats high in essential fatty acids (EFAs) belong to a special sub-class of fats that greatly enhance membrane signaling, which is the way cells communicate with their external environment. As their name implies, they are essential to our diet because our bodies have no way of making them. EFAs include omega-3, omega-6, and arachidonic acid. Since omega-3 and omega-6 EFAs are anti-inflammatory in nature, they are preferred as brain supportive nutrients.

Omega-3 EFAs are highly prized as preferred brain supportive nutrients because they are rich in eicosapentaenoic acid (EPA) and docosahexaenoic (DHA). DHA in particular offers paramount value neurologically due to its high concentration in the grey matter of the brain, fostering proper functioning of the synapse, neurological repair, and membrane signaling.[164] In humans, between the last trimester of fetal development and the age of two, the brain expands dramatically. During this time, DHA is necessary for sensory, perceptual, cognitive, and motor development.[165] Likewise with TBI, its critical to rebuild the cell membrane to support the redox potential for neurons to heal and restore function, and DHA is an essential nutrient to help meet the demand.

Fish oil far exceeds any other dietary source as a combination of DHA and EPA omega-3s. While various forms of fish oil exist on the market, krill oil seems to be of the better options when we consider DHA concentration, purity, bioavailability, and sustainability of the environment.[166] Additionally, krill oil is lower on the food chain, giving it a reduced toxin load and is also a good source of astaxanthin, which is good for the eyes and skin and is beneficial to HDL cholesterol levels. The other major omega-3 EPA is particularly supportive in mood regulation as it lessens the inflammatory cascade of the brain and improves depression related to cytokine exposure and is more readily concentrated in fish oil. [167]

A note of caution to the consumer: please check that your fish oil has been sustainably harvested to assure we are preserving the health and diversity of our oceans. Also, the fish oil company should have a purification process in place that removes environmental contaminants. The oceans are no longer clean, and careful attention to the quality of your fish oil matters. When we supplement fish oil for brain health, it is essential that we are not adding contamination and toxicity to the equation.

The suggested dosage for brain support and repair is >2,000 mg per day of combined DHA and EPA, taken with meals.

PHOSPHATIDYLSERINE (PS) AND PHOSPHATIDYLCHOLINE (PC)

Every cell of the body wraps the inner environment of the cell in a protective outer coat comprised of phospholipids. Phosphatidylserine (PS) and Phosphatidylcholine (PC) are part of the family of phospholipids, and play an essential role in neuronal survival and recovery following injury. We find PS concentrated at key protein receptor docks on cell membranes. Proteins that land here communicate with the cell by activating chemical signals within. Survival of a neuron depends on these chemical messengers. These messengers are responsible for growth and regeneration of the neuron, in addition to function of the synapse. Recall that the synapse is where the neuron synthesizes and releases neurotransmitters. We find that higher concentrations of PS correlate with higher levels of neurotransmitters acetylcholine, norepinephrine, serotonin, and dopamine.[168]

Phosphatidylserine (PS) also helps the body adapt to stress by reducing cortisol output. Following TBI, many suffer from PTSD and chronic anxiety. The body and brain struggle with releasing trauma, and many TBI survivors suffer from a chronic state of stress. PS helps reduce the damaging effects of stress on the brain.[169] It also enhances our tolerance of stress, and reduces cortisol output by the adrenals.[170, 171] I consider PS an essential nutrient for repairing brain function and adrenal recovery following trauma.

Phosphatidylcholine (PC) serves as a phospholipid reserve that can be tapped when PS concentrations drop.[172] The process is metabolically demanding and requires a good supply of calcium and the amino acid serine. To reach the therapeutic doses required to optimize nerve function and healing, oral supplementation is highly recommended.

Also of interest, PS shows greater effectiveness when concentrations of DHA are high, which we acquire through fish oil. Other nutrients that enhance PS's cell membrane function include fat-soluble antioxidants, such as astaxanthin and other carotenoids, vitamin E, and coenzyme-Q-10.[173] Furthermore, Co-Q-10 not only supports cell membrane function, it also works as its own antioxidant and stimulates ATP production.

The suggested dose range for brain support and repair for PS is 500 – 1,000 mg taken at night before bed. The dosage range for PC is 800 – 2,400 mg per day.

GLUTATHIONE (GSH)

As the body's most abundant antioxidant, glutathione should be considered essential in any TBI treatment plan. Following injury to neurons, reactive oxygen species build up in the surrounding tissue. They are the natural result of the inflammatory cycle, however their existence slows healing and recovery over the long-term. Reactive oxygen species (ROS) include superoxide radical (O2-), hydrogen peroxide (H2O2) and hydroxyl radical (OH). As their name suggests, they are extremely reactive, and will do anything they can to achieve stability. In the process, they generate further damage by stealing electrons in their efforts to become a stable compound. This reactivity generates toxicity that damages molecules, such as lipids (causing lipid peroxidation and membrane damage), DNA (causing DNA breaks), and proteins (causing oxidation of amino acids and inactivation of essential enzymes).[174]

Beyond its role in easing oxidative stress, glutathione happens to be an important contributor to cell signaling and immune system defense. In the body, GSH is required for optimal immune function, supporting proliferation of T cells, and phagocytosis by dendritic cells.[175, 176] Dendritic cells serve a major role in antigen presentation. Through the process of phagocytosis, they consume the foreign body and then present it on their surface to signal for assistance and educate WBCs in the region. In fact, GSH deficiency has been shown to increase susceptibility to infections. Now let's consider how GSH works in the brain.

It was once taught that the brain functions without a resident immune system. Though we are only in the beginning stages of understanding the defense and regenerative faculties of the central nervous system, we can accurately say that the brain has a tightly regulated immune surveillance system that operates independently from that of the body. We know that dendritic cells function like they do in the body, recognizing foreign objects and damaged tissue, and notifying the surrounding region. Imagine Paul Revere shouting, "The British are coming!" Here, instead of a man on a horse, we have inflammatory cytokines that signal for assistance. The result is a series of inflammatory and regenerative agents designed to destroy any invaders, then clean up and repair tissue.

Astrocytes are called to duty by these cytokines, and the healing begins.[177] Glutathione is a necessary nutrient in this process. There is evidence that glutathione and its precursors, cysteine and glutamine, may be transported across the blood brain barrier. In addition, we know that there are ample stores of glutathione available in astrocytes. Astrocytes are essential cells of the central nervous system for many reasons, one being that they are more capable than neurons at scavenging reactive oxygen species (ROS). With astrocytes nearby carrying high concentrations of glutathione, neurons are more likely to survive in the toxic oxidative environment post-TBI.[178] In addition, dendritic cells and signaling systems all work better with glutathione present.

Glutathione is available *intravenously* and typically given at 500 – 1,000 mg per treatment. It can also be given *orally* by capsule or pill (although most of it gets chewed up by gastric juices and will not clear the digestive tract), *rectally* by suppository (with much better system whole body absorption), *transdermal cream* (which smells like a combination of eggs and dirty socks), and by *liposomal gel* for mucosal membrane absorption in the mouth (although still smelling and tasting horribly, there are a few manufacturers making a liposomal delivery with coconut oil or citrus flavor mixed in for much better taste) an acute TBI this may be the most effective delivery system as it's portable, can be used on-site as need, it's well absorbed and is easily tolerated.

Another less-utilized treatment approach that likely gets glutathione to the brain even more effectively than the others is to use it nebulized, where the liquid form is aerosolized (similar to treatments for asthma) and *inhaled into the nose* as opposed to the mouth. When inhaled through the mouth, the glutathione goes to the lungs, where it is often utilized as an effective treatment aid for asthma, allergies, bronchiectasis and other restrictive airway diseases. Nasal spray glutathione is also available, and it has the advantage over nebulization in ease of use. This is done by using either a traditional intranasal spray applicator or as an intranasal MAD (mucosal atomization device) applicator used at the tip of a 1 mL syringe. More often, the nasal spray is used for sinus conditions and is not quite as effective as the nebulizer, because the droplet size for the spray is larger, therefore it's not as well absorbed.

Whatever system is chosen, the *intranasal* administration has the advantage of a more direct delivery route into the brain via sinus cavity absorption, where it crosses the cribriform plate and goes through the blood brain barrier and into the brain. This mechanism bypasses the heart and liver (which consumes much of the IV glutathione) and the lungs (which utilize most of the orally delivered or inhaled glutathione). As a result, this is likely the most well delivered to-the-brain glutathione route of all the possibilities. The downsides to this approach include: the at-home set up can be a bit cumbersome, it takes 10 – 15 minutes of nebulization to get the full dosage, the liquid glutathione form needs to be made in a sterile compounding pharmacy with a prescribing provider involved, and unfortunately, there are relatively few practitioners nationwide that know of and utilize this approach. If you cannot find a provider offering IV or neb-ulized glutathione, consider using the liposomal glutathione or supplementing with its precursors N-acetyl cysteine (NAC) and glutamine.[179]

The target dosage for brain repair protocols with IV or liposomal glutathi-one is 500 mg. When using the intranasal spray or nebulizer the concentration of liquid glutathione is typically between 100 mg/mL to 200 mg/mL and used 1 – 2 mL per nostril per day in divided doses.

VITAMIN C (ASCORBIC ACID)

Vitamin C probably is probably the single most researched molecule for health in history. Entire volumes of its clinical data could easily fill a small library, and as with other areas of the Manual, our review of the research is specific to repair of the injured brain. Vitamin C is a sister molecule of glutathione. It serves as a very important antioxidant in the brain (the highest levels of ascorbate in the body are in the brain and neuro-endocrine tissues) and acts as a cofactor for the synthesis of several neurotransmitters.

Vitamin C reacts with oxidants directly and becomes a cofactor in recy-cling oxidized glutathione and vitamin E back to their antioxidant status.[180] Strong evidence supports the direct utilization of vitamin C by neurons of the brain, as well as storage in astrocytes. Further along the chain, neurons release oxidized vitamin C for uptake by astrocytes for recycling.[181] Lastly, consider using the liospheric form of vitamin C for improved bioavailability in the cells, the independent data of which is still growing; my own early experience with it has been positive.

The target dose range for vitamin C is 1,000 – 3,000 mg per day in divided doses.

LITHIUM OROTATE

"It takes the ouch out of the grouch," was a slogan used by entrepreneur Charles Leiper Grigg back in 1929 during the launch of his trademark soft drink, 7 Up. The name referenced the atomic weight of its active ingredient, elemental lithium.

The journey of this nutrient begins deep in the Earth, as a naturally oc-curring mineral that bubbles up in spring waters. Its use as a medicine was pioneered in the late 1800s by a London doctor, Alfred Baring Garrod, who discovered its effectiveness in the treatment of gout. Many years would pass before lithium emerged in 1949 as a psychiatric medication for manic depressive illness.[182]

Even today, psychiatrists consider lithium citrate and carbonate a first-line therapy for bipolar disorder. Standard of care guidelines suggest high doses of 300 to 900 mg for clinical effectiveness. At such high doses, the usefulness of this medication is limited by its extreme toxicity, particularly on the kidneys and thyroid[183] Fortunately, low dose options for lithium have emerged and clinical benefit has been seen at doses as low as 5 mg.[184] This is typically in the form of lithium orotate, as evidence suggests a much higher rate of absorption into the central nervous system of the orotate form over carbonate. (It should be noted that in cases of acute severe mania the target therapeutic lithium range is much higher than for neurological support post-concussion).

Despite its clinical use for over a century, we are only beginning to understand lithium's mechanism of action in the brain. It appears that lithium assists mood in two ways: repairing damaged neurons by stimulating neuronal growth and altering the neurochemical balance of dopamine, glutamate, and GABA. Additionally, lithium has shown to have a powerful influence on the expression of genes coding for histone modification and DNA methylation. This translates to influencing the expression of over 50 different genes, which support an environment that is both neuroprotective and neurorestorative.[185] And, at lower 5mg doses, there is little to no toxicity of this naturally occurring trace mineral, making it a favorable addition to any TBI treatment protocol, particularly given the high levels of associated post-TBI mood disorders such as depression, anxiety, and impulsivity.

Typical dose range is 5 – 10 mg per day in divided doses.

B12 (METHYLCOBALAMIN)

B12 exists in many forms. The three most common are cyano-cobalamin, hydroxy-cobalamin, and methyl-cobalamin. Of these, methylcobalamin is the only one in its activated state. The others must be methylated upon absorption into the body. When considering B12 for TBI treatment, methylcobalamin is the best form available. B12 has many functions throughout the body. Here we will focus on three main effects on the brain, and how these assist healing in the face of TBI.

First, methylcobalamin displays protective effects against glutamate-induced neurotoxicity.[186] Following brain injury, large concentrations of glutamate accumulate in the extracellular spaces.[187] Glutamate that has leaked out of damaged neurons over-stimulates neighboring neurons, generating a field of chaotic nerve signals, and studies suggest that part of methylcobalamin's detoxifying effect is through its mitigation of glutamate toxicity. While TBI is one cause of glutamate-induced neurotoxicity, another is dietary. Ingesting artificial sweeteners containing aspartame, and food additives like MSG, exposes the nervous system to high levels of glutamate. *** Notably, these foods are *highly discouraged* when recovering from TBI. ***

Second, methylcobalamin has a strong neuroregenerative property. Studies show it helps neurons remyelinate. Much like the coating on a wire, myelin wraps around the axon of a nerve, allowing for transmission of the electrical impulse.[188] Supplementation with methylcobalamin has been shown to enhance axonal recovery and myelination following injury.

Third, methylcobalamin is a coenzyme of methionine synthase, which assists the formation of methionine from homocysteine. These fancy words describe a biochemical process called methylation. Synthesis of DNA and neurotransmitters depends on optimal methylation, which requires an abundance of methylcobalamin.[189]

Dosage is typically 1,000 – 2,000mcg (1mg-2mg) sublingual daily in divided doses.

ALPHA LIPOIC ACID (ALA)

Alpha Lipoic Acid (ALA) has a unique quality: it's soluble in both fat and water, and therefore can travel through many substrates of the human body. For this reason, some call it "the universal antioxidant."[190] In 1959, Rosenberg and Culik first observed ALAs antioxidant properties. They noticed that ALA prevented deficiencies of vitamins E and C.[191] After further investigation, they found that ALA had a role in regenerating these two antioxidants.[192] Additionally, it likely increases intracellular glutathione[193] and restores supplies of coenzyme Q10, NADH, and NADPH, greatly improving mitochondrial production of ATP energy.[194] Given the wide range of importance of glutathione, vitamin E, and vitamin C for brain health, ALA is highly supportive for TBI recovery.

Oral dosages are typically up to 600 mg per day.

ACETYL-L-CARNITINE (ALC)

One of ALC's greatest offerings for TBI is capacity for it to expand dendritic networks.[195] While the study cited was considering ALC for Alzheimer's and age-related decline, the conclusion that dendritic networks recover and expand regardless of age offers a clinical pearl for TBI treatment. Long-term use of ALC shows increased areas of connection between neurons, which translates into better cognitive function.[196] In one double blind study, participants took ALC over a period of 40 days. They first noticed improved spatial recognition, judgment and mood stability. Soon after, they noticed better memory and social skills.[197]

Carnitine assists fatty acids across the mitochondrial membrane of cells, where they offer a non-carbohydrate energy source. The efficient use of fatty acids for energy prevents the toxic accumulation of fatty acids. When fatty acids linger, they become oxidative, damaging neurons in a process known as lipid peroxidation. Because they enhance the use of fatty acids, both carnitine and ACL are considered antioxidants.[198]

An important distinction exists between carnitine and acetyl-L-Carnitine (ACL). The acetyl group supplies the neuron with additional mitochondrial energy. Carnitine alone doesn't have this ability, and, in comparison studies, ALC shows improved effects on nerve regeneration.[199] For this reason, we recommend ALC as your primary carnitine supplement.

Dose range is typically 5,00mg – 1,000 mg twice daily.

CHAPTER 4

NATURE'S MEDICINE

In This Section

You'll learn about the five S's:

- Sleep
- Sun (heliotherapy)
- Sex
- Sound (music therapy)
- Skin (earthing technology)

If you're not recovering as quickly as you'd like, definitely start with the section on sleep!

The doctor of the future will give no medication, but will interest his patients in the care of the human frame, diet and in the cause and prevention of disease.

— Thomas Edison

The beauty of the big five S's—sleep, sound, sex, sun, and skin—is that they are all natural, widely available, and each is a foundational pillar among the building blocks of life. As with most of the therapies in *The Concussion Repair Manual*, each modality has solid, scientific clinical value in and of itself, and when used strategically in concert with one another (particularly exemplified with the big five of this section), the additive effect is often even stronger and more robust.

Although extensive research directly related to TBI hasn't been conducted for each of the five covered in this chapter, I've put them in order based on the amount of credible research available about them. In cases where formal, TBI-related research may be lacking, I've relied on my own experiences with patients, as well as others' case studies and anecdotal evidence.

Because sleep has been widely studied and shown to be critically important in healing both acute and chronic brain injuries, it leads the pack. I also encourage you to look into *all* of nature's medicines for yourself and try each on for size to see which combinations work best for you.

CASE REPORT

The story to share here regarding Nature's Medicine is not from one particular person. It's more of an overview of an approach to healing that is deep in the bones of being human, from the Earth and connected to the natural world. Historically, in many traditional cultures and societies, those coming back from war were encouraged if not mandated to spend time in nature and work with the land "to get right" before coming back home into normal community and family life. Today there is a resurgence of this approach, called **Horticultural Therapy**—HT—and it is quickly gaining popularity for TBI and PTSD.

HT, aka "gardening as therapy" has been formally recognized and encouraged in centers in and around Europe for decades, and it is now starting to *take root* here in the U.S. as a novel approach to assist in the rehabilitation of many brain impairments, from TBI and PTSD to stroke and dementia. It is particularly well-suited for war veterans returning from the battlefield given the challenges of reintegration after exposure to so much violence and death, the keyed up fight or flight mechanism hallmarking post-traumatic stress and a sense of disconnection from life and loved ones. For many, the flavor of PTSD and PCS (post-concussive syndrome) has a common theme in the inner subjective experience of distance between one's mind and emotions from the outer world around. It is this very nature of separation and disconnection that leads many to have low motivation in treatment, depressive tendencies, pessimism, further alienation and addiction.

We crave connection as social beings, and the field addiction medicine is rife with examples of how improving the social infrastructure leads to lower addiction rates across the board (see Johann Hari's book *Chasing the Scream*). And the same can be inferred in concussion repair, particularly when there is a strongly associated psychological component to the process of recovery, which is all too frequently the case. Connection is key, and HT can provide an avenue for many of the natural elements covered elsewhere in the Manual to come together in a healing synergy: exercise, coordinated movement, sensory stimulation, fresh air, sun, grounding, meditation, and social connection.

The clear upsides of high benefit rates with next to no risk and relative low cost of inclusion are stimulating more start-up organizations to join the movement. There are now agencies using HT in a variety of contexts for cognitive, psychological, and physical benefit because of the wide-reaching nature of its effects, as well as the ability to tailor to a given person's baseline functional status (Please see Resources section for more information). For any significantly injured person, reestablishing a direct, personal relationship to the land and nature plays a powerful way in healing at the core.

SLEEP

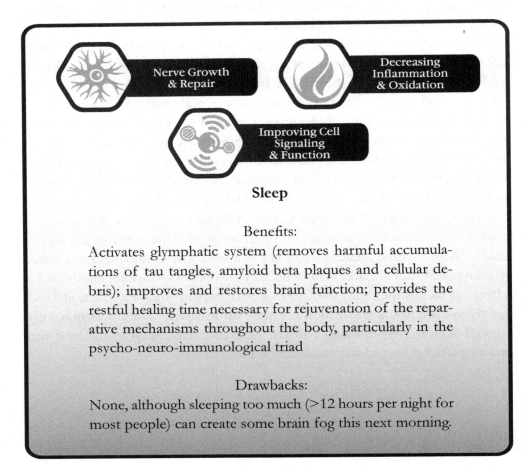

Sleep

Benefits:
Activates glymphatic system (removes harmful accumulations of tau tangles, amyloid beta plaques and cellular debris); improves and restores brain function; provides the restful healing time necessary for rejuvenation of the reparative mechanisms throughout the body, particularly in the psycho-neuro-immunological triad

Drawbacks:
None, although sleeping too much (>12 hours per night for most people) can create some brain fog this next morning.

We all know that getting enough sleep is important, and it's *extra* important if you're recovering from traumatic brain injury. When you're asleep—and particularly when you're in the deep REM stage of sleep—your glymphatic system gets to work, clearing away debris that can accumulate in the brain. (Remember, if tau tangles, amyloid beta plaques, and cellular debris are allowed to pile up, general brain function is impaired, neurotransmission breaks down, neuronal connections die, the brain shrinks, and a major negative cognitive cascade of poor short-term memory, communication, and thinking is set in motion. See "The Injured Brain" section for details.)

Paradoxically, even though TBI patients *need* their rest, they aren't always able to get it. Turns out, TBI patients are significantly more likely to experience sleep problems than the general population.[200] Approximately 40 to 65 percent of people with mild TBIs suffer from chronic insomnia.[201] [202] [203] This can be the result of a host of issues and vary from person to person, but generally include structural injury to the areas of the brain governing sleep architecture, inflammatory chemical messengers, hormonal dysregulation, and prescription medication side effects. Aside from trouble falling or staying asleep, sleep problems may include excessive time actually sleeping, changes in sleep patterns (such as less time spent in deep REM sleep), extreme daytime sleepiness, and difficulty not only in staying awake during the day but also in concentrating and focusing on the tasks at hand.

Not getting enough sleep can make symptoms of TBI worse. It can also limit or compromise your TBI recovery progress. Sleep, as dictated by the circadian rhythm, is vital for organizing all organ function based on the optimally timed function of the "body clock." This has been appreciated in Eastern Medicine for centuries and is gradually becoming more appreciated in Western medicine. Although western culture is still popularly exposed to late night technology (especially of the blue light spectrum that keeps the brain stimulated) and therefore, confusing the "body clock" about what time it actually is. Even people who *think* they've gotten over their TBIs may still be susceptible to the consequences, since sleep problems often become chronic, persisting up to five years or more after an injury is sustained![204] Worse still, long-term sleep disturbances have been linked to impaired immune function, increased health problems like cardiovascular disease, psychological issues including depression and anxiety, and an overall negative impact on greater lifestyle issues like poor work performance, fatigue, and a lousy sense of well-being.[205]

TOOLS AND TECHNIQUES

Most people do best when they aim for eight to nine continuous hours of sleep each night, with one or two brief naps (30 minutes or less) during the day as needed. Having trouble getting the sleep you need? First, take a look at your before-bed habits. Ideally, do not eat anything a minimum of two hours of going to sleep. You should also avoid vigorous exercise, bright lights or watching stimulating, aggressive movies within an hour before bedtime.

If you happen to wake up in the middle of the night, definitely try to avoid turning on the lights, as this will stimulate daytime brain function. If you find that you can't get back to sleep after 30 minutes, get out of bed while keeping any lights you *do* turn on at the lowest setting. Opt for a relaxing activity like stretching, journaling, reading, or meditation until you feel sleepy enough to return to bed.

Also, if you haven't already done so, start thinking about your sleep architecture—the structure and patterns of your sleep. How consistent is your sleep schedule? What time do you usually go to sleep? What time do you wake up? Do you wake up feeling refreshed? Make copies of the Sleep Architecture Log and begin using it to track the quality of your sleep each day for a couple of weeks. The data you collect during this time will serve as your baseline. Next, as you experiment with different therapies, continue to track your sleep each day, comparing your new scores with your baseline scores to determine whether a particular therapy is effective for you. This is invaluable information to help detect where the potential glitch is in your sleep system and therefore be able to effectively troubleshoot it.

There are entire clinics devoted to the study and treatment of sleep disorders and already plenty of books on insomnia and improving sleep quality, too. So, rather than reinvent the wheel here, I'll simply suggest a few things for you to investigate on your own. (See the Resources section for more information on these and other sleep aids.)

> **HEADS UP!** Some of the supplements included here can interact with antibiotics, birth control pills, and other medications. Consult your physician before incorporating supplements into your treatment plan.

- **Calming botanicals** – In lieu of sleeping pills (which can impair cognitive function and cause daytime drowsiness all by themselves), opt for calming botanicals to take before bed like valerian, chamomile, hops, passionflower, magnolia, lemon balm, and kava kava. You can find these in many forms, from teas and tinctures to powders and capsules.

- **Melatonin** – Secreted by the pineal gland, melatonin regulates our sleep-wake cycles. When given to TBI patients, melatonin has been shown to boost their daytime alertness, improve sleep quality and duration and help them fall asleep faster.[206] Most people know of it as a sleep hormone that's produced in the brain and helps circadian cycles, and it also an underappreciated hormone, brain and immune support agent for global health benefits. For the purpose of brain support post TBI, it serves as a neuro-protectant, anti-inflammatory and anti-oxidant support. Furthermore, when looking down the time line, sleep disturbances after head injury are predictive of more negative long term neurological outcomes, and since melatonin is supportive to establishing healthier sleep cycles and patterns, it makes good sense to support here as soon as injury occurs. Melatonin supplements are inexpensive and widely available. Sublingual forms are best and ideally taken at the same time each night 30 – 60 minutes before sleep time. [207] [208] [209]

- **Magnesium** – Although magnesium is prevalent in nuts, seeds, leafy greens, and chocolate, many people are deficient in this essential nutrient. Inexpensive and easy to find, supplemental magnesium is often used to relax muscles, reduce anxiety and help promote sleep. There are different forms of magnesium: chelate, glycinate, orotate, threonate, carbonate, chelate, citrate, chloride, sulfate and lactate. For our purposes the orotate form is important given its ability to create RNA and DNA, as well as its ability to penetrate the cell membrane to be delivered to the mitochondria and nucleus. Magnesium's **threonate** form is even more applicable for brain restoration given its unique up-leveled absorption into the brain and its enhanced ability to activate nerve channels involved in synaptic plasticity.

  It is known that magnesium has the effect of mitigating the action of the excitatory neurotransmitter glutamate. When a TBI occurs a couple of things happen relating to magnesium. Firstly, its levels are reduced in the brain and secondly, there's an influx of glutamate and calcium into the neuron, causing damage and likely leading to leading to cell death. So it stands to reason that supporting the brain with magnesium would help immediately after a concussion, however the majority of studies to date that have used magnesium *sulfate* did not show significant improvement. At present there are studies in the works for the use of the *threonate* form immediately post head injury, and still a strong case can be made for the use of the threonate form in the sub-acute recovery phase given vital role in proper nervous system, energy metabolism, cardiovascular health, protein synthesis and much more. [210] [211] [212]

- **Other thoughts** – The amino acids 5-HTP and tryptophan help build serotonin and assist in regulating healthy sleep cycles. Lastly, many people are significantly low in a variety of trace minerals and often benefit from using a quarter teaspoon of Himalayan crystal salt or sea salt in warm water before bed.

- **Inversion** – Before you go to bed, try this inversion position for 20 minutes. It's the easiest one for most people to do and requires no props. Lie on your back, positioning your butt against the wall while pointing your legs straight up the wall to form a 90-degree angle with your body. There are a host of other inversion poses and postures, including bridge pose in yoga, lying on an inversion table, and my personal favorite—going Batman style totally upside down with gravity boots hooked into a pull up bar. Whichever position you choose, gravity causes blood to pool into your cerebrovascular system, helping move you into a more relaxed, parasympathetic state.

HEADS UP! Inversion is not recommended for use in the first 48 hours after a concussion. Increased pressure can worsen existing headaches and cranial fluid congestion. Start inverting slowly and for brief periods, gradually increasing the inversion de-gree and slant according to your own tolerance. Check out Chapter 5 for more on Inversion Therapy.

- **Acupressure mats** – Akin to a bed of nails, acupressure mats like the ones from Heavenly and Spoonk also stimulate the parasympathetic nervous system. The hundreds of plastic spikes distributed across these mats can feel a little uncomfortable at first, although they should not puncture your skin. After lying on an acupressure mat for 20 to 30 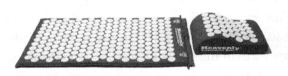 minutes, your body releases tension and drops into relaxation mode, likely through the release of pain modulating, feel-good endorphins, and oxytocin. I myself have benefitted with these mats and have consistently seen many people benefit from them too.

Floatation therapy, neurofeedback, and **sound therapy** are also well worth a try.

SUN: HELIOTHERAPY

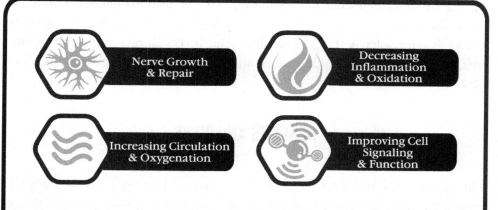

Heliotherapy

Benefits:

Sun exposure increases vitamin D levels (neuroprotective properties); stimulates beta-endorphin production (promotes healing and relaxation, reduces pain); regulates melatonin and serotonin levels; boosts mood; stimulates ATP cellular energy production.

Drawbacks:

Potential overexposure to UV rays (resulting in sunburn, premature aging and increased skin cancer risk).

Availability:

Sunshine is dependent on season and latitude.
Alternative light therapy boxes available for purchase.

Cost:

Great advantage – the sun is free!
Prices for high quality light therapy boxes are generally $300 – $500

Nearly every species on the planet benefits from exposure to sunlight, and we're no exception. But, between spending so much time indoors and slathering on the sunscreen when we do go out, many of us don't get *enough* sunlight.

Heliotherapy is the therapeutic use of sunlight. Although overexposure to the sun's ultraviolet A (UVA) and ultraviolet B (UVB) rays can cause premature aging, wrinkles, and skin cancer, smaller doses of UVB actually help our bodies function better.

BENEFITS AND RISKS

One of the benefits of heliotherapy is an increase in vitamin D. We naturally produce vitamin D in response to exposure to sunlight, and, in fact, most of the vitamin D in our bodies comes from this process, rather than from our diets. (You can find vitamin D in egg yolks, cod liver oil, and in oily fish like salmon, mackerel, and sardines. Also, milk, fruit juices, breads, and other food products are sometimes artificially enriched with vitamin D.[213]) *It is actually a hormone*, in that it is produced by a secretory gland (the skin) and has its effect elsewhere in the body (globally, and significantly in the brain and thyroid). Our cells need vitamin D to carry out key processes, and, without it, many cellular responses are impaired.[214] Shown to reduce inflammation in the brain and increase levels of the powerful antioxidant glutathione, vitamin D is super important neuroprotective agent.[215]

Vitamin D deficiency and decreased exposure to UVB rays can increase the risks of many forms of cancer, rheumatoid arthritis, type 1 diabetes, osteomalacia, hypertension, and multiple sclerosis.[216] Vitamin D deficiency also has been strongly correlated with depression.[217]

So, how do you know whether you have enough vitamin D? You can have your doctor check your blood levels with what's known as a **25-OH vitamin D test**. Results of this test are reported in nanograms per milliliter (ng/ml). Ideally, your vitamin D levels should be around 70 – 75 ng/ml—unless you have certain health conditions, that is. If you have had problems with bone spurs or if you have too much calcium in your blood, your vitamin D levels should be closer to 55 ng/ml. And, if your immune functioning is significantly depressed, your vitamin D levels may need to be as high as 80 – 90 ng/ml for the period of time necessary to support recovery and then closer to the 70 ng/ml level during the maintenance phase. Notably, this is significantly higher that the lower end of most laboratory's "normal" reference range set around

20 ng/ml, which is typically the level of vitamin D necessary to avoid the bone deformity condition known as Rickets. Throughout this entire Manual we are not only aiming to avoid disease, we are working toward repair and recovery of optimal function.

CASE REPORT:

While living in Portland, Oregon during one of the usual long, gray winters, the vast majority of clients I worked with were vitamin D deficient. One client in particular that comes to mind had a level of *only 9 ng/ml*. She had symptoms of chronic low-grade anxiety, severe depression, and experienced super low energy, motivation, and hope. Curiously, in a region known for its lack of winter sun, none of the previous practitioners she worked with had thought to check a vitamin D level. After seeing her very low results, we started her on a fairly aggressive supplemental vitamin D therapy for two months, and while she did feel better, after retesting her blood levels they had only increased to *19 ng/ml*.

This next time we started an omega-3 fatty acid support formula, and the next time I saw her was about two months later. She was glowing and positively radiant.

During that two-month period, not only had she continued the vitamin D and fish oil, she'd also decided to go to a tanning bed twice a week, only 10 minutes on each side each time she went. This small amount of UV exposure didn't change her skin tone, but it definitely improved her vitamin D levels. A new test revealed the increase from 19 to 54 ng/ml. Her symptoms of depression and anxiety were significantly better, her sleep and her libido improved, and she had more energy. It was as if a switch had been turned on for her. It taught me the value of full body sun/light exposure coupled with targeted fish oil supplementation and extra vitamin D supplementation when necessary or when sunlight or vitamin D beds are unavailable.

> **QUICK TIP** Want to use a vitamin D supplement to boost low levels? Your doctor can prescribe weekly vitamin D injections or you can opt for an over-the-counter supplement. If you go this route, take 10,000 units via liquid form or quick-dissolving tablets placed under your tongue every day for two to three weeks and then recheck your vitamin D levels.

But there's more to heliotherapy than increased levels of vitamin D. When exposed to UVB rays, our skin produces beta-endorphins, which boost the immune system, promote healing and relaxation and reduce pain. Light also helps regulate the production of melatonin and the neurotransmitter serotonin,[218] thus being significantly connected to mood.

Of course, if you've ever experienced a blistering sunburn, you know it's possible to get *too* much of a good thing. Overdoing it in the sun can increase your risk for melanoma, basal cell carcinoma and squamous cell carcinoma. (And, if you are fair-skinned, have many moles or a family history of skin cancer, your skin cancer risk is even greater.)[219] For those reasons, optimal sun exposure times vary from person to person, but some general guidelines follow.

Most glass blocks UVB rays, so sitting inside by a sunny window isn't going to work. Instead, plan to spend 10 – 20 minutes outdoors (depending on your skin tone and sensitivity), without any sunscreen, two to three times per week. For best results, expose as much skin as possible. The best times of day for heliotherapy are between 10 am and 3 pm—when the highest numbers of UVB photons can reach you—during the spring, summer, or fall.[220] Remember, you're aiming for *moderate* sun exposure, so head back inside after 10 – 20 minutes, or apply some type of effective sunscreen oil well before you have a chance to get a significant burn.[221]

HEADS UP! If you are taking any medications, ask your doctor or pharmacist before trying heliotheraphy. Some over-the-counter medications, as well as prescription antibiotics, antidepressants, chemotherapy regimens, and other drugs, can cause you to become more sensi-tive to the sun.

AVAILABILITY AND COST

Depending on your schedule and where you live, the sun's UVB rays can be a little difficult to come by. Working nights and sleeping during the day, for instance, will obviously cut down on your access to natural UVB. So will living above certain latitudes. (See image at left.)

From November through February, the number of UVB photons that reach the earth's surface are greatly reduced above the 37-degree latitude mark. (If you live in the northern latitudes, and it's wintertime, odds are high that your vitamin D levels are low. But, if you live below 37 degrees and closer to the equator, more of the sun's UVB rays can reach you year-round.[222])

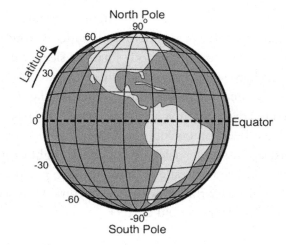

There are a few alternatives to natural sunlight you can explore, including short-term visits to a local tanning salon or low-level laser (light) therapy. (See Resources for LLLT details.)

And, for at-home use, light therapy boxes are convenient options. These are more for mood boosting than fully body exposure, and come in a variety of light types and intensities, typically positioned close to your face but just outside of your central vision. (For instance, you might place a full-spectrum light box on a table near your computer or work station.) When you begin using a light therapy box for the first time, you might experience eyestrain, headache or nausea. If so, you can vary the distance between you and the light or reduce your light exposure time.

- **White light** – Among the most common, full-spectrum light boxes you'll find are those that emit white light. These are frequently used to treat Seasonal Affective Disorder (SAD), and regular exposure to this kind of light has been shown to be as beneficial as medication for depression. In one randomized, placebo-controlled trial, researchers compared the effects of treatment with Prozac versus white fluorescent light at 10,000 lux. The treatments were equally effective, and patients responded to light therapy sooner and experienced fewer side effects than their medicated counterparts.[233] If you go with a white, full-spectrum light box, opt for a unit that emits 10,000 lux of white light.

- **Blue light** – In addition to white light units, there are full-spectrum lights that emit shorter wavelength, blue light. Blue light is observed to be good for restoring the body's natural sleep cycles, however exposure to this light spectrum is best when relegated to the daylight hours. Late evening and night exposure to the blue light spectrum can dysregulate circadian rhythms and appropriate melatonin-brain signaling. If you have been practicing good sleep habits and still have trouble falling asleep or staying asleep through the night or if you feel groggy, lethargic, confused or restless during the day, you might have a circadian rhythm disorder that exposure to daytime blue light exposure (and night time avoidance) could correct.

- **Combined full-spectrum/negative ion therapy systems** – You can also find full-spectrum light boxes which emit negative ions.

(Personally, I've had positive experiences with these, and I highly recommend them!) Exposure to high levels of negative ions has been shown to increase relaxation and improve mood and mental alertness,[224] and negative ion therapy has been effective in treating nonseasonal, chronic depression, too.[225] When thinking about negative ion generation, think of the energetic experience of rolling waves, waterfalls and the ambient air right after a heavy thunderstorm, all arenas charged with negative ions.

- **UVB lights** – Do a simple Internet search for "light therapy" and you'll also come across some systems which emit UVB. Unlike the white, blue and negative ion light boxes previously described, UVB lights *do* promote vitamin D production. UVB lights are frequently used to treat skin disorders like psoriasis, but, as with direct sunlight, overexposure can cause skin damage. Also, you should never look directly into a UVB light unit. (See here for more heliotherapy resources)

SEX

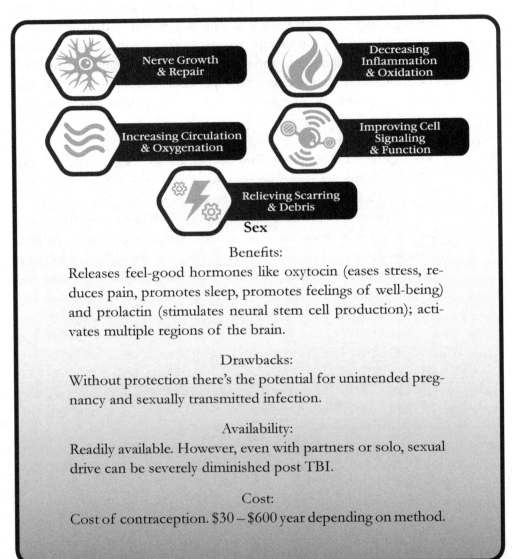

Nerve Growth & Repair

Decreasing Inflammation & Oxidation

Increasing Circulation & Oxygenation

Improving Cell Signaling & Function

Relieving Scarring & Debris

Sex

Benefits:
Releases feel-good hormones like oxytocin (eases stress, reduces pain, promotes sleep, promotes feelings of well-being) and prolactin (stimulates neural stem cell production); activates multiple regions of the brain.

Drawbacks:
Without protection there's the potential for unintended pregnancy and sexually transmitted infection.

Availability:
Readily available. However, even with partners or solo, sexual drive can be severely diminished post TBI.

Cost:
Cost of contraception. $30 – $600 year depending on method.

Sex not only makes life possible, ideally it also makes life loveable and livable. And any time there's a major challenge in a person's arena of sex and sexuality, it can deeply affect the sense of self-confidence, internal buoyancy and overall enjoyment in life. In the case of TBI this often becomes magnified because of the abrupt onset of symptoms and the deep neurological reparative work that can be required to correct the issues. From the experience of vulnerability after newly acquired cognitive difficulties, to the limitations in satisfaction and sexual performance after significant hormonal down regulation, the road to recovery can often seem a long-term struggle. This is exactly one of the main reasons to encourage hormonal evaluation and early intervention after TBI—to get *the juice* flowing again. Consistently those with healthy, active and fulfilled sex lives do better in the long term in terms of both reparative healing and general living outcomes.

Difficult sexual changes after TBI are actually more of the "norm" than most people would think, which can go far in validating one's own frustration while also highlighting the magnitude of the problem. For instance, after comparing 208 patients with moderate to severe TBIs with 150 control subjects who had no history of head trauma, researchers found that *more than half* of the TBI group experienced significant sexual changes. These included low libido, decreased enjoyment and frequency of sexual activity, and reduced ability to sexually please their partners. For 47% of the TBI patients, fatigue was the number one factor contributing to the changes in their sexual behavior and enjoyment.[226]

If you've noticed sexual changes since your own injury, there's no reason to feel embarrassed or ashamed—but there are plenty of reasons to work on reclaiming your active sex life. As is the case with sleep, sex happens to be very good medicine.

Besides putting the spring back in your step, having an orgasm can help rebalance hormone levels and causes the release of many beneficial chemicals in your brain, including prolactin and oxytocin.[227] Prolactin has been shown to stimulate the production of neural stem cells,[228] and oxytocin, also known as the "love molecule," eases stress, reduces pain, promotes sleep, and produces a general sense of well-being.[229] (By the way, it's worth noting that sex with a partner produces a much bigger oxytocin release than having an orgasm all by your lonesome. Connecting with a partner through bonding, cuddling, hugging, eye gazing, etc. all play their part!)

On the subject of **Vitamin O**, it's also my clinical experience (and yes, personal experience too) that—for men particularly—too many orgasms in a short period of time or climaxing when the hormones are severely depleted can leave one feeling pleased in the short term, but often drained for the longer term. In these cases, I usually encourage honest self-reflection to see if reaching ejaculation is feeding the longer term healing process or hindering it. If it is feeding it, then by all means go for it. If it's draining it, then a better sexual exercise is to learn the practice and art of cycling the breath to move the energy of the urge to climax throughout the body and prolong sex (akin to Taoist practices called Sexual Qi Gong), eventually getting to the point of being able to choose whether or not to ejaculate during sex, versus not having control of when ejaculation occurs. This can further lead one toward mastering the sexual response cycle and actually being able to reach greater fulfillment, satisfaction and confidence as a lover and partner.

Orgasm also activates many different areas in the brain. Researchers studying the effects of orgasm in women determined that up to 30 different parts of women's brains were stimulated. Some of these included the reward center, sensory cortex, and the areas responsible for emotion, pleasure, and memory.[230]

TOOLS AND TECHNIQUES

There are countless clinics, books, supplements, and other aids for sleep disorders, and there are easily twice as many of these kinds of resources to help with *sexual* function—far too many to detail here. Instead, I'll offer you a few tools and techniques to get you started. (And, for further reading and recommendations, you can check out the Resources section.

- **Personal reflection** – The first step towards improving (or restoring) your capacity for physical intimacy with a partner is taking stock of your feelings. Are you frustrated? Pissed off? Feeling less confident? Guilty or ashamed? Afraid? (Or all of the above and then some...?) These are all normal reactions to TBI and its resulting sexual changes.

- **Honest discussion** – The next step is being willing to have some difficult or uncomfortable conversations. Let your significant other know exactly how you've been feeling about the effect your TBI has had on your sex life and your relationship as a whole. Sharing your private thoughts to such a degree might make you feel even more vulnerable at first, but it can be a great way to reestablish some of the intimacy you and your partner have lost.

- **Examine medications** – A surprising number of physicians willingly ignore their TBI patients' sexual health, so you should also be prepared to broach the subject with your doctor on your own. Don't be afraid to ask about the sexual side effects of any medication you've been taking. (Many antidepressants negatively affect libido and sexual function, for example.) Weigh the pros and cons of your current medications with your doctor. Working together, you might explore ways to mitigate their side effects or you could decide to discontinue your meds in favor of alternative treatments.

HEADS UP! Quitting some antidepressants and other pharmaceuticals "cold turkey" can be dangerous. Consult your physician before discontinuing any prescribed medications. You should also task to your doctor before incorporating new supplements into your treatment plan

- **HRT** – Sexual side effects also can be caused by hormone deficiencies, so, if you haven't already done so, you should ask your doctor to check your hormone levels or refer you to an endocrinologist for a complete workup. If you're found to be deficient, supplemental hormone therapy can help get your system back in balance. (See the Hormone Replacement Therapy section to learn more.)

- **Maca** – Both a root vegetable and a medicinal herb, maca has been around for at least 3,000 years. It is native to South America and research has shown it can enhance sex drive and combat erectile dysfunction.[231] Maca also has helped alleviate antidepressant-induced sexual dysfunction in postmenopausal women.[232] Maca root is inexpensive and commonly sold in powder form and in capsules.

- **Sex therapy** – There's more to sex than physical performance. And there are many different ways to connect with your partner. Talking with a certified sex therapist can help you and your significant other to work through tough emotional issues, rebuild intimacy, and get your sex life back on track.

SOUND: MUSIC THERAPY — AUTHORED BY DR. ANDY SWANSON

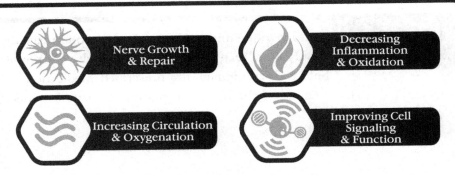

Nerve Growth & Repair

Decreasing Inflammation & Oxidation

Increasing Circulation & Oxygenation

Improving Cell Signaling & Function

Music and Sound Therapy

Benefits:

Significant improvement in relaxation and parasympathetic tone, lessening the stress response often associated with TBI, stimulating new neural networking patterns and improved mind-body connection.

Drawbacks:

None overtly.

Availability:

Trained practitioners readily available in most cities in U.S., home therapy support can be found in CD or audio file format.

Cost:

Variable depending on methodology type and/or therapist usage.

"Through studies of people with brain damage, we've seen patients who have lost the ability to read a newspaper but can still read music, or individuals who can play the piano but lack the motor coordination to button their own sweater. Music listening, performance, and composition engage nearly every area of the brain that we have so far identified, and involve nearly every neural subsystem."[233]

- Daniel J. Levitin

The use of sound to enliven the body, mind, and spirit has been a primary way in which human beings come together in community for as long as we've walked upright. The drum has been replicated across cultures and geography in various forms, from the simplest hoop drum of the Lakota people, to the Indian tabla and the drum kit of American rock. And where there's a drum, there's often a voice weaving its way into a rich tapestry of sound. When we look at EEG scans of people listening to music, we find that their brains begin to entrain with the musical rhythm. And when bands come together to jam, studies show that they not only entrain with the music, but each other as well.[234] "In such a situation, there seems to be an actual binding of nervous systems," observes the neurologist Oliver Sacks.[235]

Following brain injury, neurons may become stuck in a pattern of dysfunction. Damaged neurons have difficulty firing in synch with each other. Much like a band that has lost their rhythm, they create noise and chaos. In our chapter on Movement in this Manual, we discuss how the Thalamus assists in orchestrating neurons to restore rhythmic patterns. Another powerful tool for orchestration comes from the ear's unique ability to gather information from sound.

Our sense of hearing begins during fetal development. It is one of the first senses to develop, together with the sense of gravity. Sound and gravity are the first two sensory experiences we have, and they both transmit signals along the same cranial nerve.[236] Imagine what a fetus hears from the womb: mom's heartbeat, her blood circulating, her body digesting, her voice singing and speaking, and the voices of others close by, perhaps father and other family. Now imagine what the fetus feels when mom sits, stands, drives a car, or goes to yoga. As mother moves through the world, sounds emerge that establish our first relationships to loved ones, parents, family, and gravity.

Through sound and gravity, we establish our orientation in the world. Only then can we begin constructing our first images of the world beyond the salty waters of the womb. Other senses will soon build upon this structure, but sound and gravity are foundational. Without them, we struggle to maintain equilibrium.

Our sensory relationship with the world grows more intricate with each passing day, as finely tuned neuronal fabrics weave their way through every square inch of our body. When a traumatic brain injury occurs, it sweeps through like a violent storm with gale-force winds, tearing at the complex neural fabric and damaging axons, synapses, and dendritic connections. In the wake of such trauma, many struggle with orientation, which results in symptoms of vertigo and visual disturbance. Sounds and lights become louder than normal. Some of the most basic functions of daily living are lost, such as speech, language comprehension, emotional stability, and muscle coordination. These parts of life that normally occur with minimal effort, suddenly become exhausting and extremely difficult. After traumatic brain injury, equilibrium and orientation must be reestablished. We can do this by returning to the primary senses that establish these qualities: the ear and the vestibular system.

The combination of sound and movement offer a way to exercise the brain and the body. Many therapies for brain recovery bring these together. One example is the work of Albert Tomatis, who created the Integrated Listening Systems (ILS). His work is profiled in the book, *The Brain's Way of Healing* by Norman Doidge.[237] Tomatis was an otolaryngologist with a profound understanding of the ear and its relationship to the brain and body. He dedicated his career to exploring how sound and movement can be used to generate neuroplastic changes in the brain. Tomatis believed the ear was a battery to the brain, and that active listening aroused higher cortical areas of the brain. At the time, his ideas were revolutionary, and he achieved unprecedented results with patients. Only in the last 10 to 15 years have we developed technologies that affirm what Tomatis observed clinically.

The process of listening, Tomatis would surmise, requires one to distinguish the conversation at hand from background noise. The ear accomplishes this task through what he called "the auditory zoom," which allows us to tune into conversations occurring at specific frequencies. We do this by adjusting two muscles in the middle ear, the stapedius and the tensor tempani. The stapedius tenses to enhance our perception of medium-high frequencies, while muting bass tones. The tensor tempani adjusts the tension of the tympanic membrane, decreasing background noise and lower tones. Together, these two muscles allow us to actively select what we listen to, and protect us from sounds that could be damaging to the ear. Tomatis used this knowledge to develop the ILS program, which engages the listener in an "active" experience of learning.

Active listening, it turns out, triggers a cascade of activity throughout the body. Neuroplastic changes occur in the auditory cortex within minutes of applying focused attention.[238] Listening also involves a host of involuntary movements; to listen closer, we lean into conversation, and we tilt our head to bring our ear forward. We may even place our hand to our ear for better hearing, or to gesture that we didn't hear what was said. A deer in the wild uses active listening as a means of survival. Their large ears are designed to rotate in different directions, while the body assumes a vertical posture frozen in time. With active listening, sound and movement join in a dance as we gather information from the world around us.

Of course, it's appealing to just sit back and enjoy listening to music. And studies show that even the most passive experience with music reduces stress levels and lifts the spirits.[239] Passive listening activates the reward center of the brain, known as the nucleus accumbens, increasing dopamine levels.[240] The dynamic features of music, such as pitch and rhythm, enhance cognitive and emotional flexibility, in addition to sensorimotor development.[241]

Active listening, however, proves to be much more effective than passive.[242] It calls us to attention, promoting neuroplastic changes.[243] We see more neurogenesis and neuron repair mechanisms activated.[244] It enhances sensorimotor function, increases mobility, strength, endurance, and coordination of gross and fine motor movements.[245]

Visionaries, such as Tomatis, recognized early on that sound offered a vast array of clinical applications that could be applied to neurological healing and recovery. Advances in technology now allow us to gather more information, to see the effect of sound and music on the brain, which allows for more creative therapeutic applications.[246] Functional magnetic resonance imaging (fMRI), positron-emission tomography (PET), and electroencephalography (EEG) allow us to look deeper at systems of the brain previously inaccessible. Let's explore some of the information surfacing from the latest research on sound, music, and neurological response mechanisms.

LANGUAGE AND SPEECH

Our relation with "other" largely relies on our ability to communicate in words what we are thinking and feeling. I've heard many complain of partners that don't communicate their needs and feelings, and this can be a cause of strife in a relationship. Following injury to the brain, language and speech are often affected, and the loss of this ability leaves them feeling alone and isolated. It is a source of great frustration.

People who struggle with inability to speak have a condition called aphasia. Damage to a region in the left frontal cortex, called Broca's area, causes difficulty converting thoughts into spoken word. This region also processes the sequencing of musical rhythms and movement.[247] Studies show strong support for using movement and sound in speech recovery.[248]

Interestingly, many people unable to speak still have the ability to sing. Singing is largely a right-brained activity, and those with left-brained injuries often can carry a tune. In some cases, where speech therapy has failed, music and singing have offered an avenue to recovery.[249]

COORDINATION AND MOVEMENT

When listening to music, many people unconsciously begin tapping their feet, nodding their head to the rhythm, or drumming with their hands. The famous philosopher Nietzsche once said, "We listen to music with our muscles."[250] The best athletes and dancers infuse rhythmic movements together with agility and strength.

Muscle weakness and loss of coordination are common complications of TBI, and recovery can be very challenging. Studies show we can use sound to instill rhythm and timing into movement, and generate a neuromuscular response that is more reliable and fluid.[251] In one study, patients recovering from stroke utilized a therapy called rhythmic auditory stimulation (RAS). Results showed sustained long-term improvement of motor coordination, and outperformed standard methods of physical therapy.[252]

Elderly people that enjoy dancing decrease their risk of Alzheimer's by 76%, and those that play an instrument reduce it by 69%. Movement that is both musical and fun enhances neurogenesis and builds memory.[253]

EMOTIONAL REGULATION

Sound therapy has also been shown to establish better mood regulation.[254] The Prefrontal Cortex (PFC) lights up whenever we intently focus on something. It is an essential component to learning and brain arousal. By triggering activity in the PFC, we see greater executive function, in addition to better control of emotions and impulsivity. Therefore, musical interventions can affect non-musical cognitive functions.

Auditory and vestibular pathways also connect directly with the amygdala and paralimbic structures. These areas oversee the fight or flight response, and generate a state of fear in response to perceived danger. Overactivity in paralimbic structures causes a condition known as post-traumatic stress disorder (PTSD). By restoring balance in the vestibular system, we instill a sense of groundedness and safety.[255] We can do this by simply listening to sounds that generate a calm, pleasurable experience.

ENTRAINMENT

Sounds also have a global effect, synchronizing nerve patterns throughout the entire brain in a process known as entrainment. Entrainment occurs when one rhythmic frequency influences another until a synchronization occurs, just as waves of water influence one another when they meet. EEG scans confirm that when we listen to music, our neurons begin to fire in rhythm with the music.[256] In one study, the brain established a dominant brain wave frequency of 2.4 beats per second, exactly matching the waltz rhythm to which the participants listened.[257] These studies have been repeated with music by Mozart, and underscore the importance of choosing music to match the state of mind you desire to emulate.

THE RETICULAR ACTIVATING SYSTEM (RAS)

Alfred Tomatis was well-known for saying, "The Ear is a battery to the brain."[258] He was expressing his observation that the ear and other subcortical structures had the unique ability to awaken higher brain centers. We now know that sound entering through the vestibular system activates the Reticular Activating System (RAS) in the brain stem, arousing the higher cortex to attention. Arousal is essential for learning, and chronically low arousal limits recovery in those with TBI. Low arousal is also highly prevalent in people with ADHD. Sound therapies increase responsiveness and cognitive arousal in even the earliest stages of acute traumatic brain injury.[259]

CONCLUSION

Sound therapy offers a wide range of clinical applications for treatment of concussion and TBI. New technologies have expanded our awareness of how to use this powerful tool. We know that some approaches enhance motor recovery, while others focus on the development of speech[260], while still other methods stabilize mood and relieve anxiety. In the not-too-distant future, we may see that sound therapy becomes a standard protocol in neurological rehabilitation programs.

A couple of programs mentioned earlier successfully implement movement and sound to activate brain healing, such as the Integrated Listening Systems (ILS) and rhythmic auditory stimulation (RAS). Other schools of sound therapy exist, such as those of the Neurologic Music Therapy (NMT). Like any medicine, the selection and delivery of sound is an art, and the practitioners that provide this tool have cultivated their practice over years of schooling and clinical work. For best results, seek out a practitioner trained in the proper assessment and implementation of sound as a healing tool for the brain.

SKIN: EARTHING

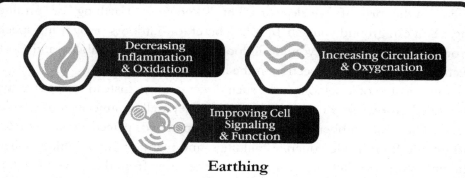

Earthing

Benefits:

Has been shown to improve sleep and blood pressure, reduce pain and inflammation, decrease cortisol levels and also thin the blood, which may help improve circulation and oxygenate tissue.

Drawbacks:

Indoor Earthing initially may cause flu-like symptoms in some people (generally as a transient healing response) and connecting to improperly grounded electrical outlets can cause injury.

Availability:

Outdoor Earthing can be practiced for free anytime Indoor Earthing products, including Earthing bands, patches, mats and bed sheets available for purchase.

Cost:

Prices for indoor Earthing products vary from $30+ (bands and patches); $75+ (mats) and $140 to $200 (bed sheets).

Walking barefoot in the grass or on a sandy beach feels good, helps reconnect us to the natural world, and can offer major health benefits, too. When we make direct, physical contact with the earth, our bodies pick up some of its energy in the form of free electrons. This is known as "Earthing" or "grounding." You can ground yourself by going barefoot outdoors or by using special grounding devices while you are indoors. (See above "Availability and Cost" section and "Resources" section in the back for more details.)

But most people seldom make such direct contact, instead remaining "ungrounded" for weeks or months at a time. They walk around in rubber-soled shoes. They drive rubber-tired cars. They sleep in beds placed a couple of feet off of the floor inside concrete buildings, and many of these buildings have multiple stories, stretching up and even further away from the nearest patch of soil, sand, or grass.

So, although our early, barefoot ancestors unwittingly practiced Earthing throughout their lives, this concept is relatively new in our modern age. There is much anecdotal evidence in support of Earthing, and small pockets of researchers have conducted some Earthing pilot studies with compelling preliminary findings. Ultimately, more study is needed to better understand Earthing's full potential, but, in the meantime, here's some of what we know.

BENEFITS

Earthing seems to have many therapeutic applications for the body and the brain. Research suggests regular Earthing may improve blood pressure, irregular heartbeat, and autoimmune conditions like rheumatoid arthritis and multiple sclerosis.[261] I first heard about Earthing (also called Grounding Technology) from Jeff Spencer, the chiropractic physician for the US Tour de France team when they had their long victory run, in a conference about healing technologies. He was using it for the team to significantly increase their recovery rates when the technology was still in its early testing phases.

When absorbed into the human body, the earth's electrons can cause a shift from the sympathetic state to a more relaxed, parasympathetic state.[262, 263] These free electrons also are thought to improve sleep, reduce pain,[264] and, by helping to neutralize reactive oxygen species, an influx of electrons may decrease acute and chronic inflammation as well."[265, 266] A study of 10 healthy subjects revealed that Earthing also can have a blood-thinning effect. This has positive implications for improved blood circulation and oxygenation of tissues.[267, 268]

And Earthing appears to affect levels of the stress hormone cortisol. In one study of 12 subjects who self-identified as having sleep disorders, pain, and stress, cortisol levels were tested before and after a six-week period of grounded sleep. *Before* grounded sleeping, the majority of subjects had exhibited high nighttime cortisol levels. *After* grounded sleeping, cortisol secretion normalized in all but two of the subjects. They also reported to researchers that, during the six-week period, they took less time to fall asleep, woke up less frequently at night, and had improvements in levels of pain and fatigue.[269]

AVAILABILITY AND COST

Taking off your shoes to stand on grass in the park or in your own yard costs nothing, and you can do it whenever you have decent weather and a little time to spare. If you go this route, try to maintain direct contact with the earth's surface for about 25 - 30 minutes each day.

If you aren't able to spend so much time outside, you can purchase an Earthing device designed to provide the benefits of grounding to you while you are indoors. Some of these include Earthing patches, mats and even bedding sheets which can be plugged into the bottom hole of a properly grounded electrical socket or connected to a grounding rod driven into the ground outside. When your skin makes contact with the conductive fibers woven into your Earthing product, you absorb free electrons from the earth's surface.

Earthing technology ranges widely in price. Wearable Earthing bands and patches cost about $30, mats retail for $75 and up, and individual Earthing bed sheets sell for between $140 and $200. (See the Resources section for more product information.)

RISKS

There are some potential risks associated with indoor Earthing products. For your safety and to ensure you fully benefit from your indoor Earthing device, you need to confirm that your electrical service and the individual outlets you plan to use are appropriately grounded. This is especially important if you live in an older home, because electrical safety grounds haven't always been required. Also, even if you do have updated wiring, some outlets in your home still may be ungrounded or improperly connected to the ground. Most of the new Earthing products on the market come with a plug-in unit to use for checking to make sure the outlet is appropriately grounded.

Ideally for simple home safety even outside of using any grounding equipment, you would have an electrician double check there is a functional ground system and check your individual outlets. You can also buy an electrical ground connection tester to check the outlets yourself. Just be aware that it is sometimes possible to get a "correctly grounded" reading from these even though the outlet being tested has a "false" or "bootleg" ground.[270] If you discover that your electrical wiring isn't connected to a functional ground, you can instead connect your Earthing device directly to a grounding rod driven into the earth outside. Most indoor Earthing products include grounding rods and installation instructions.

Whether you plan to connect your Earthing device directly to an outside grounding rod or to a grounded electrical outlet, you should avoid indoor Earthing during lightning storms.

Also, some people may feel flu-like symptoms when they begin grounding indoors. Often, this is a temporary reaction that can be managed. If you feel ill after, say, sleeping all night on an Earthing sheet, move the sheet to a chair or couch and try napping there for 45 minutes to an hour each day for about a week. If your symptoms subside, move the Earthing sheet back to your bed and try all-night Earthing again. Still having a negative response? Move the grounding sheet back to the chair or couch, continuing the daily naps there for a month. If, after that time, you continue to feel ill after longer-term exposure, indoor Earthing might not be for you. About one percent of the population doesn't respond well to the technology, and their sleep can become compromised.

Fortunately, many Earthing companies offer money-back guarantees on their products, so you can try them out, see how your body responds and return them as needed.

CHAPTER 5

PERSONAL PRACTICES

In This Section

You'll learn about:

- Balance and bodyweight training
- Qi Gong, Tai Chi, and Yoga
- Meditation
- Inversion therapy
- Faith and perseverance

Feeling a little low? Or simply not sure where to begin? In that case, start with Faith and Perseverance.

Perseverance is stubbornness with a purpose.
— *Josh Shipp*

CASE REPORT

The story to share here about Personal Practices is a particularly close one to my heart as it involves a dear friend I've known since childhood. Amanda has always been an avid dancer and artist, on the shy side, with extreme kindness towards life and to all whom she meets. She married in her early twenties after moving away from home to be closer to her extended family. She met her husband at the local church and were engaged, then married fairly soon afterwards. The honeymoon phase was easy and joyful, though unfortunately, after a year he was laid off from his job as a labor man and the stress took its toll. His previous alcohol addiction, which had been unknown to her, rekindled and it was not long before he was drunk most nights and becoming verbally abusive.

They had a daughter within a couple of years in the midst of the mounting stress, only adding more tension to an already volatile situation. Then one night in a drunken rage while in the street outside their house, he repeatedly hit her in the head until she passed out, further kicked her in the head and stomach while she was lying on the ground, then got in his truck and drove away. She lost consciousness almost immediately after the first blow and had no recall of the event. What is reported came from the next-door neighbor who heard the yelling and saw it occur. A police report was filed. He was later found, charged with multiple offenses and jailed. She was taken to the hospital, monitored for a week to treat brain swelling and internal bleeding, and required facial reconstructive surgery to repair the damage to her cheekbone and eye. Eventually, she was put into protective custody, and over the course of a year, he was sentenced to prison and she was able to divorce and safely leave the area. Her physical and cognitive recovery, however, would take much longer.

Her cognitive deficits were severe. She had to relearn to read, write, and talk and required assistance for most of her activities of daily living, including walking, eating, bathing, and taking care of her infant daughter. We spoke on the phone for the first time after the incident soon after she started her rehab course in physical, occupational, and speech therapies. When we talked on the phone, it was evident by her speech that something catastrophic had happened. Her speech was significantly delayed and slurred, and she was having major word finding difficulties.

As a religious woman, she was dedicated to her church and her faith. She didn't drink alcohol nor do any drugs, and she was mostly against taking any form of medication or supplementation. (She didn't even have anesthesia in the delivery of her daughter). Her path of healing was to be largely stoked from within, filled with relentless dedication to her rehabilitation program, her personal faith and forgiveness for what had happened. Over about a year, with multiple rehabilitation sessions per week her physical function fully returned. First standing unassisted, then walking at home, then walking in the woods near where she lived. Gradually, she relearned to cook, clean and do things around the house, much of which seemed re-stimulated by a motherly instinct to take care of her daughter.

However, it took over 5 years of consistent and intensive speech therapy for all her cognitive abilities, including speech pronunciation and full language, to come back to pre-injury levels. (The only remnant is a return of slightly slowed and slurred speech when she gets tired). Given her extended time in speech therapy, she took a deeper interest in the mechanics of language and used visualization strategies to reformulate words, sentences, and grammar. Then, to the surprise of her friends and family, she chose to engage language as a formal vocation by becoming a stenographer at the local courthouse. Shortly after starting her new job she visited her ex-husband in jail to forgive him for what he had done, to show him his daughter, whom he had not seen since court sentencing, and to pray for his life to head in a good direction.

Today she remains one of the brightest, most optimistic, humble, and sweet people I've had the pleasure to know. When I need a booster shot of faith and gratitude, I often think of her and smile. From her situation, I'm reminded of many lessons I've heard, personally lived, or witnessed over the years.

- We never know what life has in store.
- It is up to us to do the best we can.
- Faith is a choice
- The bigger healings in our lives take time, perseverance, and strength.
- Nobody can do it for us.
- It's for us to do ourselves.
- In the midst of it all, we can still try to make the world around us a better place.

Unlike some of the therapies introduced elsewhere in *The Concussion Repair Manual*, the concepts presented in this chapter don't require much at all in the way of professional assistance. But they *do* require a little motivation and self-discipline, as you work to create—and stick with—some new personal habits and practices.

Any new campaign in personal practice starts with some degree of motivation. Sometimes we're driven by fear, other times by inspiration and excitement. Whatever the motivation for addressing your target TBI related issues, rest assured many have come along the path before you, met their challenges, and mustered the will and determination to reclaim their lives and achieve their own degree of optimal function. The common theme in those finding success in their recovery largely rests in setting a plan and committing to see it through. Although you may not always feel motivated, it's important to "stay on target," which may include an occasional dosage of "fake it 'til you make it." It's also supremely helpful to enlist others to support your cause, which can include joining a gym or fitness center, finding a personal trainer or coach, signing up for an exercise class, finding a few training videos to help inspire you, and asking friends and family members to lovingly hold you accountable.

If your TBI has been classified as more severe, you might already have a physical or occupational therapist. For best results, you should be working with a professional who has been trained in TBI recovery. When in doubt, therapists with a designation and certification through the Academy of Certified Brain Injury Specialists is a good place to start.

HEADS UP! To ensure safety and "treatment team cohesion," consult your physician or primary practitioner before incorporating balance and bodyweight training, yoga, Qi Gong, martial arts or inversion therapy into your on-going treatment plan.

GYROSCOPIC REPAIR: BALANCE AND BODYWEIGHT TRAINING

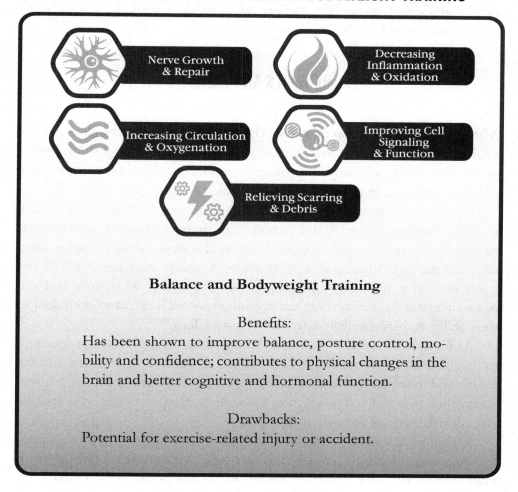

Nerve Growth & Repair

Decreasing Inflammation & Oxidation

Increasing Circulation & Oxygenation

Improving Cell Signaling & Function

Relieving Scarring & Debris

Balance and Bodyweight Training

Benefits:
Has been shown to improve balance, posture control, mobility and confidence; contributes to physical changes in the brain and better cognitive and hormonal function.

Drawbacks:
Potential for exercise-related injury or accident.

"You don't miss your water until your well runs dry."
— American singer William Bell

Your sense of balance and proprioception (your brain's ability to detect the position of your body in space) are two things you may not have considered much before a brain injury, but you will certainly notice when they've become impaired. TBI frequently affects both of these senses, which can cause unsteadiness on your feet and being more accident-prone.

The good news? There are many simple balance and bodyweight training exercises you can do to help improve your balance and restore your brain's ability to process your body's spatial orientation. And, because it positively affects the brain's physical structure, adding aerobic exercise to the mix can also provide functional benefits. Before we get to some of the specific exercises and activities you can try, let's explore some of the ways balance and body-weight training and aerobic exercise have been shown to help.

BENEFITS AND RISKS

After putting a small group of young TBI patients through just eight weeks of intensive balance training, researchers noticed structural changes in portions of the subjects' cerebellums—involved in coordination and motor control—and improvements in the subjects' balance and postural control.[271]

In another study, chronic TBI patients completed 50 hours of intensive mobility training over a 20-day period. The mobility training included gait training with a bodyweight-supported treadmill system, various balance activities and strength, coordination, and range-of-motion exercises. All TBI patients showed improvement in walking speed, mobility, and balance and, the researchers noted, "subjectively, participants reported being more confident in their ability to perform daily activities without falling."[272]

As for aerobic exercise? In animal studies, it has been shown to contribute to the growth of new capillaries in the brain[273, 274] as well as an increase in the length and number of dendritic interconnections between neurons.[275] It was also shown to boost cell production in the hippocampus,[276] the brain area involved with memory formation and storage.

In human research, aerobic exercise has been shown to improve cognitive function. This was certainly the case in a small study of patients with mild-to-moderate TBI. After performing 30 minutes of vigorous aerobic exercise three times a week for a total of 12 weeks, the subjects made strong gains in cardiorespiratory fitness levels as well as in cognitive processing speeds and many aspects of executive functioning.[277]

Aerobic exercise can even turn back the clock. As we age, some parts of our brains naturally shrink. For instance, in older otherwise healthy adults without dementia, the volume of the hippocampus tends to decrease by 1 – 2% each year.[278] This reduction in brain volume is directly related to the increased risk of developing cognitive impairments, and research has shown aerobic exercise can actually work to mitigate this tendency by increasing hippocampal volume and offsetting the losses typically associated with aging.

In one study, researchers randomly assigned 120 older adults to either an aerobic exercise group or a stretching (control) group. The study's subjects were between the ages of 55 and 80, and none had dementia. One year of

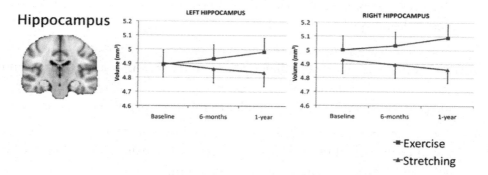

regular aerobic exercise training resulted in a 2% increase in hippocampal volume and improvements in spatial memory. Similar benefits were not seen in subjects in the stretching group.[279]

Whether it's pulling a muscle or falling off of the treadmill, there is always some risk associated with both aerobic exercise and balance and bodyweight training. Exercise-related injuries and accidents can happen to anyone—with or without a TBI—but TBI survivors do need to be extra careful. If you only recently sustained your TBI—say, within the last couple of weeks—it's too soon to start a balance and bodyweight training program. Instead, begin by taking regular walks, practice regular stretching of all the major muscle groups, try floatation therapy, and slowly experiment with balance training to assess where your starting point is currently. It's even more important here to work with a skilled trainer to get a baseline snapshot of present function: what's working well, what are the major areas of concern, and what is the degree of severity of any notable impairment. Develop a plan working towards measurable, obtainable goals, engage with optimism and dedication to make gradual improvement, and continue the support with your practitioner, trainer or physician to problem solve any challenges that may arise.

GETTING STARTED – BALANCE CHALLENGE EXERCISES

Once you're ready to try balance and bodyweight training, begin with the following exercises as a general guideline to progressively demanding exercises and practices. They are listed below in order from least to most difficult. Plan to work on just one exercise at a time, moving on to a new exercise only after you've mastered the previous one. Use a timer and aim for at least 30 seconds in each Balance Challenge Exercise.

1. Using a nearby wall to help stabilize yourself as needed, stand up and close your eyes. Keeping your eyes shut, see how long you can retain your balance without touching the wall.

2. With your eyes open, stand on one leg. See how long you can remain balanced on one leg without falling over. Then try the other leg. You may find one is easier to balance on one than the other. This is typically due to a side preference in footedness, similar to most people being right handed.

3. Now stand on one leg with your eyes closed. If you need to, use a nearby wall or chair for stability. See how long you can remain standing on one leg with your eyes shut—and without touching the wall or chair.

4. Stand with your feet together and look up at the sky. See how long you can retain your balance in this position.

5. Next, stand with your feet together, look up at the sky, this time closing your eyes. Again, if you need to, use a nearby wall or chair for stability. See how long you can retain your balance without touching the wall or chair.

6. For the finale, stand with your feet together, looking up at the sky with your eyes closed. Now try standing on one foot and touching your nose. Alternating with each index finger. Do this until you are able to easily keep your balance. (Yes indeed, this one is quite a bit tricky, even for healthy people not experiencing a TBI).

Finally, be patient and try not to get discouraged if you don't progress as quickly as you'd like. The degree of difficulty associated with each of these exercises will depend on the location and severity of your injury—as well as how physically fit and balance coordinated you were before you were hurt. Do these exercises a few times a day and monitor your progress. Results vary, and many people will experience noticeable steady improvement over time.

ADVANCED AND ELITE PRACTICES

In time, you may reestablish your pre-TBI levels of physical and mental functioning, but why stop there? I challenge you not only to *reach* those levels but to *surpass* them. The following tools can help you do just that. (See the Resources section for more information on these and other balance and bodyweight training optimizers.)

- **Jumping rope** – Jump ropes are inexpensive, portable, easy to use, and extremely beneficial. Jumping rope will improve your stamina, cardio, balance and hand-eye coordination. It also helps build your slow-, intermediate- and fast-twitch muscle groups and activates the parts of your brain that sense the position of your body in space. It's easily one of the cheapest, easiest, most effective exercises around.

- **Resistance bands** – If you've been in physical therapy before, you may already be familiar with resistance training with long, elastic tubes or bands. By providing varying degrees of resistance as they are stretched, Thera-Bands and similar resistance training products enable you to heal muscle as you exercise with them—but they aren't just for rehab anymore. There are high-level athletes who now train exclusively with resistance bands, rather than with traditional weights, to build muscle for a lower stress price point on the associated joints mobilized.

  Typically, resistance bands are color-coded to indicate the maximum degree of resistance they provide. (In the case of Thera-Bands, for example, yellow bands provide 3 pounds' worth of resistance when fully stretched, green bands offer 4.6 pounds', black bands represent 7.3 pounds', etc.)

- **Balance boards** – The average balance board is about the size and shape of a skateboard. Lacking skateboard trucks and wheels, the board is instead positioned atop a wooden or plastic cylindrical roller. To use, you practice balancing on top of the board with one foot on either side of the roller. Balance boards are great for improving agility, strengthening your core and stabilizer muscles and rebuilding your brain's ability to sense your body's position in space.

- **Slacklining** – Practicing on a slackline is another great way to work on your balance, core strength and your brain's body awareness. Made of strong, nylon webbing, slacklines are anchored between two sturdy points—most often trees or telephone poles. Most slacklines are between 5/8" and 2" wide.

Adjusting your slackline's tension and height will affect the degree of difficulty, so experiment to see what works best for you. In the beginning, you may find it difficult just to stand and balance on the line, but, eventually, with time and perseverance you should be able to walk across it. Props, such as tall poles or bamboo sticks can assist people who require support in order to get from one end to the other. This is a fairly advanced practice, so props should not be discouraged as this is still better than not doing it at all. With enough practice, many people are able to hold yoga poses while on the slackline perform other slacklining tricks.

MOVEMENT, QI GONG AND ENGAGING VESTIBULAR "FLOW"

COAUTHORED BY DR. ANDY SWANSON

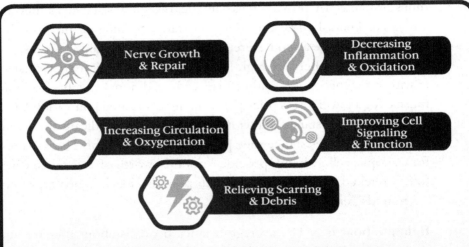

Movement & Flow: Qi Gong, Tai Chi and Yoga

Benefits:
Increased sense of freedom in the body and relaxation in the mind. Improved strength, breath awareness, flexibility and focus.

Drawbacks:
Although typically quite safe, these movement based practices still require individualized adjustment to a given person's physical ability.

Availability:
Classes widely available; personal practice can be anywhere.

Costs:
Classes are priced individually; personal practice has none.

Experience coupled with attention leads to physical changes in the structure and functioning of the nervous system.

— Michael Merzenich[280]

Imagine the structure of the brain as a tree, the brain stem as the trunk, with branches of neurons known as dendrites extending outwards like a tall oak, twisting and turning, reaching outwards for higher brain centers we know as the cerebrum. Like any tree, this brain has deep roots that extend down into the body along the spinal column, and out through nerve roots, creating a neuronal fabric known as the peripheral nervous system.

The body and brain share an intricate relationship. Essentially, the nervous system activates the body, and the body anchors the nervous system. They are symbiotic. Similar to the earth, the body feeds nutrients and oxygen to the brain and shapes neurological branching through sensory input. As we move through the world, smelling, tasting, seeing, hearing and touching, we generate a sensory experience that helps the brain draw conclusions about our environment. This in turn generates a corresponding action. Movement is the brain's response to incoming sensory data.

The research of Michael Merzenich of UCSF has helped unlock our understanding of how movement affects change in the brain, in a process known as neuroplasticity. His studies suggest that *attention* focused on movement promotes learning in the brain.[281] In our chapter on meditation, we discuss how attention activates the pre-frontal cortex (PFC), improving mood regulation, memory, comprehension, reasoning, and decision-making. When we apply attention to movement, PET scans show that the PFC actually grows in size.[282] We also see more differentiation and development of the sensorimotor cortex, which enhances coordination and balance, and reduces pain and muscle tension.[283, 284]

Regardless of skill level, when we approach a subject as though it is our first encounter, we pay closer attention. We leave the world of routine, and everything becomes novel. When we apply this to movement, we feel deeper into the body; we notice each muscle, ligament, and joint and how they interact. This enhances brain function globally and stimulates nerve regeneration. As brain activity builds, a new responsibility arises. Somehow we must organize these firing neurons. For this, we look a little deeper into the brain, to a region called the thalamus.

Studies suggest that the thalamus is the generator of rhythmic electrical activity in the brain—the orchestra conductor.[285] It relays all sensory information before it reaches the cortex. Then the cortex signals back to the thalamus in a feedback loop. The thalamus gathers this data, and together with the basal ganglia, sets the rhythm for neuron activity. Collectively, this calms the brain by reducing sensory stimulation and coordinating motor output. This theory was first proposed by Dr Rodolfo Llinas, a neuroscientist at NYU.

Imagine a conductor at the podium, waving a baton, directing the music of the brain. Just like an orchestra with many musicians, neurons must fire together rhythmically in order to create synchronized movements. After TBI, neurons have difficulty organizing, and instead generate noise in the brain.[286] According to Llinas, the thalamus solves this problem by creating fixed action patterns (FAPs). FAPs liberate us from spending unnecessary time and attention on every aspect of movement.[287] With the direction of the thalamus, the brain can once again create harmonious music.

What's the key to generating a FAP? Attention. Repetition. Through careful attention and repetition, we learn a new pattern of electrical activity that the brain recognizes, which eventually becomes a FAP. We can replace old patterns of movement and behavior, and restore function to damaged neurons, with attention and repetition. And we already know that this also activates the PFC, improving many other aspects of brain function.

The thalamus cannot work alone, however. There is another helper in the movement equation: the vestibular system. This system lies deep in the brain stem, and works with the thalamus to ensure smooth integration of sensory input. Imagine yourself in a conversation at a party. Unconsciously, the brain is processing large amounts of data at high speeds: such as observing gestures, filtering background noise, sensing the environment, and making postural adjustments. This requires an amazing amount of coordination between the vestibular system and other regions, which include the cerebellum, the eyes, the thalamus, the basal ganglia and cerebrum. Following head trauma, these connections are greatly hindered, negatively impacting balance, sensory processing, movement, and cognition. Without assistance, the vestibular system becomes easily overwhelmed, and sensory integration problems ensue.

Now imagine you are recovering from traumatic brain injury. You're holding a conversation at a party. Someone is speaking to you, but you are unable to process the words. It seems as though someone just turned the background noise up, and the lights in the room are brighter. A severe headache begins with a sense of pressure inside the head. And if that isn't enough, dizziness kicks in and your stomach begins to turn with nausea. You try to leave the room, but your legs are wobbly and you can't see straight. People assume you're drunk. What they don't know is that your vestibular system is completely overwhelmed and unable to process incoming data, resulting in cognitive decline, loss of gravitational sense and poor coordination.

If the thalamus is the conductor of the orchestra, establishing the rhythm of electrical activity through FAPs, the vestibula would be the sheet music, the stage and the auditorium. It ensures that, above everything, the body knows where the ground is. As we move, the vestibular system makes certain that we know where we are at all times, coordinating muscles to react to changes in the environment. We call this proprioception. It is like the Earth sensing its own orbit. With proprioception, we know whether we are standing or lying down, and we can differentiate the axial spin of the Earth from our own movement and position on its surface. It could be argued that proprioception is the body's most important priority second to breathing. It would follow then that movement exercises for TBI must also balance vestibular function.

To review, we know that movement depends on activation of higher brain centers, such as the PFC and the sensorimotor cortex. It also needs rhythmic organization in the form of FAPs from the thalamus. Finally, the vestibular system must be in balance for proper integration of sensory information and fluid movement response. Exercises must take all systems into account to restore balance and coordination post-TBI.

Weakness in sensory integration and muscle coordination requires a movement program with shorter periods of non-strenuous exercises that initially begin on the floor, and gradually increase in difficulty and duration. The practitioner should be trained to observe the body for signs of an overwhelmed vestibular system. These include: increased respiration, muscle tone, heart rate, dizziness, and flushed cheeks. If these signs present, exercise should be discontinued until balance returns.

Here we present Qi Gong as an intentional movement therapy ideal for the TBI community. Other movement traditions to consider include Feldenkrais, martial arts, yoga, Tai Qi, Pilates and Brain Gym. Find the tradition that best suits your belief systems, personal goals and health care needs. Then, find a practitioner in your area that can guide and teach you the precise movements necessary for creating a conscious experience.

QI GONG

The ancient people of China understood the importance of intentional movement. They lived close to the land, and made keen observations of nature and the inner workings of the body. From these insights, Chinese medicine was born. Acupuncture and herbal medicine are some of their most well-known contributions, but a lesser known medicine emerged from these observations called Qi Gong (pronounced "Chee Gong"). The practice of Qi Gong incorporates the understandings of Chinese medical theory with exercises that build a conscious experience with activities such as walking, moving, breathing, sleeping, and even drinking tea. Most forms involve repetitive, precise movements that engage specific systems of the body and draw energy from the surrounding environment. One who practices Qi Gong quickly realizes that most actions in life benefit from focused attention.

There are hundreds of schools of Qi Gong, each that offer differences in their instruction and approach. A Qi Gong provider may prescribe an exercise that specifically addresses the needs of the individual. As needs change, new exercises are implemented. In this case study, we discuss how Qi Gong assisted Steve in his recovery from TBI.

CASE STUDY

When Steve was 26 years old, he dreamed of pursuing the life of a financial analyst. He had one year left in a MBA program at a well-respected university. While at home visiting family, he went for a walk in a local city park. Crossing the street, he was broadsided by a SUV. He suffered major trauma to the brain, and would spend the next couple of years suffering from symptoms of post-TBI syndrome. When he first presented to the clinic, he expressed a fear of going outside; he felt danger all around, as though he was in a war zone. He suffered from agoraphobia, the fear of leaving the home. Most days, he chose to stay indoors, which facilitated the onset of depression and hopelessness.

The SUV had struck him on the right side of his body. He had chronic right-sided pain that was worse in the neck and head. He incurred right-sided hearing loss as well. He displayed poor balance, and intermittent dizziness. His memory was poor. He couldn't recall names of close friends or remember recent conversations. He experienced severe agitation and at times explosive anger, which was previously uncharacteristic of his personality. He dropped out of the MBA program due to his inability to read or process information, and was unable to carry a job. He required a caretaker for help with daily needs such as cooking, cleaning, and paying bills.

Steve suffered a major TBI. His prognosis was poor, and neurologists offered him little to no hope for healing. He was lucky to be alive, and after his eight-week recovery program, he was discharged with advise to accept his disability and learn to live with it. Steve hoped for more, and pursued second and third opinions.

When he finally arrived at the clinic two years later, he was skeptical of my optimism. I was recommending herbal remedies, nutrients, and an anti-inflammatory diet. This was a world of medicine Steve had never encountered. Nevertheless, he had exhausted other options, and reluctantly embraced the treatment plan. He initiated a course of regular acupuncture and Qi Gong. When I recognized his commitment, I decided to meet with him weekly at a local park to teach him Qi Gong. Our program started with simple movements, in order to avoid over-stimulating the vestibular system. As weeks passed, we increased the duration and complexity of exercises. He was losing excess weight and developing muscle tone. His balance improved from one week to the next. His vision improved, and pain levels dropped. Soon, he was going outdoors for walks around city blocks without anxiety.

A momentous day arrived when Steve decided to try riding his bike for the first time since the accident. With some practice, his body remembered what it once knew. It was like watching a bird learn to spread its wings again. Every time we met, he pushed the boundary a little further, and his confidence grew. At around 14 months into the program, he no longer needed a care provider at home. At 18 months, he announced that our work together would be coming to a close; that he would be boarding a flight for Costa Rica. It was a one-way ticket. He had decided to move there for four months to enjoy his newfound freedom, and to envision new dreams. At the writing of this book, 5 years later, he maintains an independent life, with a regular job and a long-term relationship.

CENTERING THE MIND, STRENGTHENING THE BRAIN — MEDITATION. COAUTHORED WITH DR. ANDY SWANSON

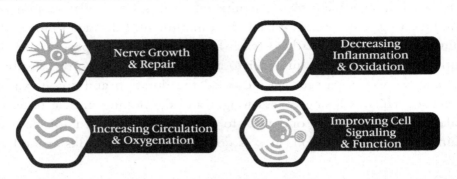

Meditation

Benefits:

Innumerable and immeasurable with additive effects over time.

Increased mind-body connection, calmness, centeredness, experience of Oneness; improved optimism, compassion and overall relaxation.

Drawbacks:

None, except from stiffness from sitting or kneeling too long.

If that happens, try walking meditation or Qi Gong; can also try floatation therapy as an alternative or adjunct to "standard" meditation.

It can take a while to find the "right" practice and therefore, diligence and perseverance along the path of quieting the mind.

MEDITATION FOR TBI

Behind each quiet moment lies a host of fears, anxieties, and to-do lists that pose a challenge to the desired peace of mind. Meditation and Qi Gong both offer daily exercises to practice the art of focus and learn to preserve stillness. Each thought is like a horse that wants to run; and the mind like a band of wild horses galloping in every direction. Meditation is the exercise of placing each horse back in its stable. Only then can stillness prevail. With this skill the mind becomes a tool, and at our choosing, we can select the horse we want to ride. When the mind is trained in such a way, it becomes a powerful tool for healing and manifestation of life goals.

So what happens in the brain during meditation that helps it establish a state of stillness? And how can we apply this knowledge to establish optimal function in recovery from TBI? Studies over the last four decades have sought to answer this very question. Herbert Benson, MD, author of the book, **The Relaxation Response**, pioneered some of the first scientific studies on meditation. Over the last 40 years, he and other scientists have amassed a large body of data in efforts to explain empirically what ancient peoples have observed for thousands of years—that meditation greatly enhances the brain's ability to regulate emotion, sustain attention, and build self-awareness.

Imagine looking out over a valley floor from atop a mountain. From here, we can see for miles and observe the various changes of landscape. In the distance, we see weather patterns developing, as dark clouds roll over neighboring mountains. A thunderous clap resounds as drops of rain begin to fall. A chill in the air sweeps in as the temperature suddenly drops. We decide it's a good time to seek shelter. The information we have gathered allows us to make conclusions that guide us away from the storm, towards a place of safety.

Similarly, we can look out over the internal landscape of our bodies by cultivating self-awareness. Looking deep within, we can feel and reflect upon the state of our internal health and well-being. With cultivation, we learn to scan our internal systems, and make adjustments to our thoughts and actions. We are no longer a ship flailing in the turbulent seas of emotion. We are a captain at the helm, maneuvering through the challenges of life with grace and ease. Self-reflection and awareness may be meditation's greatest gifts, as we are no longer subject to the spontaneous swings of emotion.

Self-regulation of emotion becomes particularly important following a traumatic incident, such as TBI. Following such severe trauma, a high percentage of people exhibit symptoms of post-traumatic stress disorder (PTSD).

In one assessment of soldiers returning from Iraq, 44% of those who had suffered a TBI also struggled with symptoms of PTSD.[288] The body and brain become locked in a pattern of fight or flight, as they seek to defend and protect against any further insult. Symptoms of PTSD include intense fear, hopelessness, and a range of other crippling emotions. In most cases of PTSD, the condition is chronic and difficult to treat. Anti-anxiety and sleep medications are offered to provide some relief. Fortunately, alternatives to medication exist. A number of studies suggest that meditation can assist in restoring emotional stability in those with PTSD.[289, 290] Strong scientific support exists showing a daily practice of meditation reverses sympathetic dominance, meaning the body and brain are no longer locked in a state of fight or flight.[291] With this stillness, we are better able to make adjustments in the moment, and thus be steered toward a place of safety.

The ability to steer emotion requires optimal function of the pre-frontal cortex (PFC). Unfortunately, the PFC is highly susceptible to TBI. Damage here results in deficits of memory, comprehension, reasoning, and decision-making.[292] Often with TBI, patients have difficulty with emotional turbulence and impulsive behavior. The PFC is also essential for learning, applying attention and focus to accomplish an objective. Research shows that meditation not only activates the PFC, but also physically grows the neurons in this region, allowing for a stronger transmission of nerve signals.[293] Therefore, following TBI meditation becomes an essential tool to restore emotional balance and optimize PFC function.

The usefulness of meditation in the medical setting is gaining momentum, largely due to the efforts of another pioneer, Jon Kabat-Zinn, who developed the *Mindfulness Based Stress Reduction (MBSR)* program at the University of Massachusetts Medical Center.[294] The program has been well-received by the medical community, and there is ample research supporting its use for a variety of conditions, including chronic pain, psoriasis, anxiety and depression.[295] Meditators who participated in an eight-week program exhibited a significantly greater antibody response to influenza vaccine.[296] Conversely, we know that stress, and more specifically the stress hormone cortisol, inhibits immune response.[297] As we meditate, stress levels drop as do cortisol levels. Subsequently, immune system function improves and we are better able to heal from injury.

The brain learns through repetition, and one benefits more from increasing the frequency of meditation rather than duration. In other words, 5 minutes of meditation three to four times daily would accomplish more stabilization than one 30-minute session. Forcing longer sessions prematurely will not offer the same benefit, and in fact may be counterproductive as the pressure to perform builds stress and tension. As we get stronger in our practice and focus, we strengthen the capacity of brains structures such as the prefrontal cortex (PFC), and we can increase the duration without overwhelming the brain. As relaxation and clarity build, it is natural that one will create more time for these positive sensations and teachings. This natural draw to sit for longer enhances the benefits of meditation. If time allows, it is recommended to sit in meditation following the completion of a Qi Gong session. Both practices offer time for quieting the mind, and strengthening focus.

There are many world traditions that have developed various ways of meditating. The word itself has a host of interpretations. Each practice varies in terms of their effects on the brain.[298] Herbert Benson distilled the practice down to its bare essentials, presenting a style that everyone can use. He called this style the "Relaxation Response." We offer this technique as a way of learning to cultivate relaxation, focus and attention, while reducing fear and anxiety.

MEDITATION EXERCISE:

Nature is our best teacher in the art of stillness, patience, trust, and surrender. If you can create an outdoor space for meditation, this would be ideal. Find a place where you will not be interrupted, away from the noises of city life, and one that offers a feeling of safety. A large stone or tree is recommended for grounding.

If an outdoor setting is not possible, then find yourself a quiet room with very little light. Natural morning light offers a gentle, inspiring sense of freshness and a reminder of new beginnings, as the sun slowly reaches for the sky. Those with sensitivity to sound and light may choose a darker room, or even a sleep mask to cover the eyes. Please read the chapter on sound healing for some recommendations on sounds that accommodate a healing meditative experience.

The following are instructions for meditation, as taught by Herbert Benson, MD, author of the book, *The Relaxation Response.*[299]

1. Repetition of a word, sound, praise, prayer, or muscular activity. Pick a focus word, short phrase, or prayer that is firmly rooted in your belief system.
2. Passively disregard everyday thoughts that inevitably come to mind, returning to your repetition.
3. Sit quietly in a comfortable position.

4. Close your eyes.
5. Relax your muscles, progressing from your feet to your calves, thighs, abdomen, shoulders, head and neck.
6. Breathe slowly and naturally, and as you do, say your focus word, sound, phrase, or prayer silently to yourself as you exhale.
7. Assume a passive attitude. Don't worry about how well you're doing. When other thoughts come to mind, simply say to yourself "Oh well," and gently return to your repetition.
8. Continue for 10 to 20 minutes. When finished, do not stand immediately. Continue sitting quietly for a minute or so, allowing other thoughts to return. Then open your eyes and sit for another minute before rising.
9. Practice the technique once or twice daily. Before breakfast and before dinner are good times.

Healing visualizations work well with meditation. This would be an example of focusing the mind by choosing the right horse to ride; the one that knows the healing path.

OPTIONAL VISUALIZATION:

Using your imagination, see a beautiful golden light building behind the center of your brow. Allow this light to wash over your brain, and down through your spine. Then guide this light through your body. Bring the light back to the head, and now go deeper. See your neurons and glial cells absorbing this light, and watch as they extend branches outward, growing, learning, expanding their network, transferring golden light throughout. See this network unify at the brain stem, into a golden river of light that flows down the spinal cord and washes out through the body. Guide this river wherever it needs to go, for cleansing and healing. With each breath, watch as the light expands further, deeper into the body, into each muscle, joint, organ, bone and to the deepest regions of the bone marrow. When you are finished with this visual exercise, return to the breath.

THE PUMP: INVERSION THERAPY

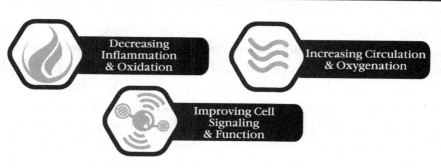

Inversion Therapy

Benefits:
Stimulates cerebrospinal blood flow; pumps cerebrospinal fluid to the brain and master glands; can help flush harmful debris out of the brain; improves anxiety and insomnia; has been shown to lower blood pressure and pulse rate; contributes to feelings of calm and relaxation.

Drawbacks:
May cause headaches, dizziness and sensations of head pressure; may not be suitable for people with a history of migraines, glaucoma, high blood pressure, heart disease or recently acquired, acute or actively bleeding TBI.

Availability:
"DIY" inversion techniques can be practiced easily.
Inversion or "gravity" boots and inversion tables available for purchase.

Cost:
$50 to $100 for inversion or "gravity" boots.
$150 to $500 or more for an inversion table.

For me, inversion therapy highlights *the core themes* of this entire Manual. It's an available modality, with a low risk profile, and can easily be incorporated into any program using other modalities with little interference and *most importantly* I consistently feel a beneficial effect. The key to any of the therapies listed in the entire Manual—does it work for you? The only way to know is to try it on for size, stay reasonably dedicated to assess its efficacy over time, manage any tendency to quit from lack of motivation, and then, after a good trial, if it doesn't work, leave it off the menu and keep trying other modalities.

Personally, inversion therapy has consistently worked for me, and it's been a staple in many of my client's Concussion Repair programs too. It can be used just about anywhere, at any time, whatever one's energy level is, and no matter how long you choose to "hang out" for, it's usually beneficial. Although scientific research has yet to be conducted on the effects of inversion on TBI patients specifically, there are many anecdotal reports supporting inversion therapy as an extraordinarily therapeutic for repairing the brain.

The leading theory about its efficacy involves working the brain's internal cerebrospinal fluid (CSF) like a pump. When you invert your body—by hanging upside-down from a chin-up bar or strapping yourself into a tilting inversion table, for example—you enhance the hydrostatic pumping action that stimulates increased cerebrospinal movement and blood flow. While your body is in an inverted position, and slowly opening and closing the jaw like a repeated yawn, the volumetric pressure of cerebrospinal fluid is increased and fluid is more actively pumped throughout the brain, including the master glands. This increased flow may give TBI associated, down-regulated master glands a boost, as well as helping open up previously held stagnant areas of circulation that have accumulated in the brain.

BENEFITS AND RISKS

In Chapter 4, I mentioned that inversion can improve anxiety and help with insomnia by putting the body in a more laid-back, parasympathetic state. (See the section in Chapter 4 on sleep for a before-bed inversion exercise to try.)

According to researchers examining the effects of "oscillating" inversion, inversion therapy can also reduce blood pressure and pulse rates and cause feelings of calm and relaxation as well. Using individual inversion tables, the study subjects were required to maneuver from an upright position to a fully inverted position and then back to the original, upright position between 80 and 150 times during a 15-minute period. The subjects' pulse rates and blood pressure readings dropped during periods of inversion and oscillation, and blood pressure readings taken during inversions became lower and lower with each successive recording.[300]

Inversion therapy offers musculoskeletal benefits, too. In a small study of patients with lumbar disc disease, inversion therapy, when paired with physiotherapy, greatly reduced the need for back surgery. Surgery was avoided in 77% of patients in the inversion group and in just 22% of the control group (patients who had had physiotherapy only.)[301]

HEADS UP! Inversion therapy may pose some risk if you are pregnant or if you have a history of migraine headaches, glaucoma, high blood pressure, or heart disease. Also, if you recently experienced a concussion and there is any possibility of having an active, bleeding TBI, you should definitely wait until your condition has stabilized before incorporating any inversion therapy into your treatment program. When in doubt, consult with your concussion care specialist.

AVAILABILITY AND COST

One of the most appealing aspects of inversion therapy is that you don't need to travel to a special facility or own a lot of expensive equipment in order to try it. As long as you are able to angle your body such that most of your weight is above your heart, you will get some benefit, and there are a few ways to achieve this.

If you're a do-it-yourselfer or you're on a tight budget, all you need to get started is a sturdy, wooden board and a chair, bedside, or even a heavy bucket. Position one end of the board on the seat of the chair, rest the other end of the board on the ground and recline on the board so that your legs and feet angle up, toward the chair. Although it's a start, this DIY setup doesn't afford you the full range of motion that a hinged inversion table does. Over time you can experiment with greater degrees of inclination, provided it's a sturdy set up and see how that feels. Typical lengths of sessions are anywhere from 30 seconds to 30 minutes.

Inversion Tables range in price from $150 to $500 or more. Their main benefit? The ability to move from an upright position to a fully inverted position—and all points in between—easily and at will. Your legs remain static, but you can change the angle of declination your body rests in by moving your arms as you would if you were doing jumping-jacks. (To invert your whole body, simply place your arms above your head. Want to be upright again? Just position your arms back down at your sides.)

Being able to change positions so easily is especially handy for those who are new to inversion. In the beginning, you may experience headaches, dizziness and a sensation of head pressure while you are inverted, so it's best to take things slowly.

Inversion or "gravity" boots which can be secured to a pull-up bar are another, less expensive option. You can pick up a pair for between $50 and $100. Just keep in mind that these don't enable you to fluidly change position like an inversion table can. And to give a sense of overall safety for this style of inversion, I've even fallen asleep for about a half hour completely inverted, Batman style, while wearing Gravity Boots on a pull-up bar without any problems or side-effects.

GETTING STARTED

Once you have the all-clear from your doctor, plan to start with just three to four minutes of inversion each day. Gradually add a couple of minutes, as you are able to, working your way up to a total of 20 minutes of inversion therapy daily.

Before each inversion session, make sure you are well hydrated, and, after each session, try to avoid standing up too quickly. If you've been upside-down for a long time—and particularly if you are dehydrated—you're much more likely to become light-headed due to inadequate blood volume in your brain (a phenomenon called orthostatic hypotension) and may faint. This happened to me after flying in an airplane all day and being super dehydrated. I was completely inverted for about 10 minutes before getting off the bar and walking away. Very shortly after that, I passed out and hit the deck. It was the one and only time that it's happened, and it does happen, so be cautious in the position transition. To avoid injury after long-term inversion, grab onto a solid piece of furniture, sit down or get your bearings with the help of a friend.

THE GATEKEEPERS: FAITH AND PERSEVERANCE

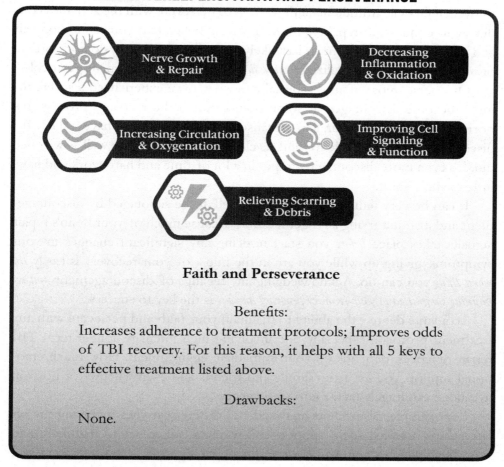

Nerve Growth & Repair

Decreasing Inflammation & Oxidation

Increasing Circulation & Oxygenation

Improving Cell Signaling & Function

Relieving Scarring & Debris

Faith and Perseverance

Benefits:
Increases adherence to treatment protocols; Improves odds of TBI recovery. For this reason, it helps with all 5 keys to effective treatment listed above.

Drawbacks:
None.

You can't rush your healing.
— American singer, Trevor Hall

Once your life has been upended by traumatic brain injury, having faith—and hanging onto it from day to day—can be one of the hardest things to do. Even so, I believe strongly that all TBI survivors need faith in order to fully heal and recover. Now, I'm not talking about *religious* faith here. Instead, I mean having faith in your own capacity to heal. That means maintaining the belief that, in time, your symptoms and your overall condition will improve. And, because this is *faith*, rather than *hope*, it also means maintaining that belief even if you lack hard evidence to support it. (After all, if you always have proof that you are, indeed, getting better, you wouldn't need faith, right?)

Just as it takes discipline to practice good sleep hygiene, exercise regularly and eat well, it takes at attitude of faith to *decide* to persevere with the activities conducive to concussion repair. Without a strong belief that your condition can and will improve, you're much less likely to comply with your doctor's orders or to stick to your personalized *Concussion Repair Manual* treatment protocols.

Of course, most of us—especially those who've experienced a severe injury—become discouraged at some points during the recovery process. It's normal to become discouraged, because it's discouraging to have a TBI! It's discouraging not to be able to think as clearly or to function as well as we once did. It's even more discouraging to put in a lot of time and hard work and have little to show for it.

It can be very tempting to allow yourself to be sabotaged by discouragement and just quit trying all together. But, because much of your brain's repair actually takes place *before* you start noticing any significant changes in your symptoms, giving up while you are in the midst of your recovery is easily *the worst thing* you can do. Acknowledging any feelings of discouragement *and remaining committed to your recovery program anyway* is the key to success.

To a large degree, the ability to maintain your faith and persevere with any treatment protocol, especially one involving high intensity, longer-term TBI repair practices, depends on your immediate environment. How much emotional support you get from family and friends and even whether or not you live alone can hugely factor into your success.

For example, researchers analyzed 122 different studies involving the relationships between social support and patients' adherence to treatment and found that patients who had close and cohesive family relationships were *more than three times* as likely to follow treatment guidelines than patients without strong family ties. And patients from high-conflict families were 2.35 times more likely to *fail* to comply with treatment protocols.[302]

The researchers also determined that patients who didn't receive adequate emotional support were 1.35 times more likely to ignore or neglect treatment requirements. Friends and family were recognized to contribute to patient adherence in treatment in many ways, including "encouraging optimism and self-esteem, buffering the stresses of being ill, [and] reducing patient depression."[303]

Along these lines, there is also something to be said for having a roommate. The odds of adherence to treatment among adults living with other people were 1.38 times higher than for people who lived alone.[304] We are social beings by nature and any sense of isolation typically leads to depressive tendencies, thus dampening the highly necessary motivation and optimism for active engagement in the repair process.

GETTING STARTED

Begin each day by taking stock of your faith. Is it as strong as it was yesterday? Or is it wavering a bit today? If doubt about your progress has crept in, your first priority should be restoring your faith. Here are a few ways to get started.

- **Friends and family** – Whether it's a quick call, text, email, video chat or in-person visit, reach out to a friend or relative you trust and let them know how you're feeling. This can be difficult, as the majority of people in our culture have trouble expressing vulnerability and asking for help. If and when this happens, try to recognize it, *move into the resistance*, and open up to those you feel safe with and are reliable. Feel as if there's no one you can turn to? Try social media. There are a growing number of TBI-related Facebook pages and private groups where you'll find other survivors you can relate to. (Search Facebook for "TBI Hope & Inspiration," "Traumatic Brain Injury Healing & Recovery Support Group" or "Life After Brain Injury—Friendship, Support, and Laughter" to see a few, and see the Resources section for more.)

- **Inspiring quotes** – Seek out famous quotes, poems or book excerpts that really move you. Print some out to hang up, carry in your wallet or just keep nearby.

> **"The best way out is always through."**
> **—Robert Frost**

- **Give back** – Volunteering your time and talents is a great way to gain confidence and a fresh perspective. Your local library, natural food store, rec center, and community newspaper should be able to provide you with a fairly comprehensive list of volunteer opportunities in your area. Or try an online search via sites like Volunteer Match (http://www.volunteermatch.org/) or All for Good (http://www. allforgood.org/).

- **Seek support** – For extra support, find a good counselor or support group. If you're a veteran or college student, you may have access to free or low-fee therapy options. Some employers also offer access to short-term counseling services. Teaching hospitals and large universities are another potential source for affordable counseling sessions. And there may be a traumatic brain injury support group nearby as well. (To get pointed in the right direction, check the Resources section for a list of national and regional TBI associations.)

CHAPTER 6

FOODS FOR RECOVERY

In This Section

You'll learn about:

- Ketogenic diet
- Oily fish
- Coconut oil
- Turmeric
- Egg yolks and lecithin

These foods can be introduced simultaneously for an additive effect in support of a more robust brain recovery program. See the Bringing it All Together chapter for a Foods Log tracking form.

There is also a note on vegetarianism, detoxification, and the growing field of Nutrigenomics.

"Let food be thy medicine and medicine be thy food."
— Hippocrates

It's a sad-but-true fact that most people routinely do the very *opposite* of what's good for their brains—especially when it comes to the foods they eat. High in carbohydrates and sugars and relatively low in fat, the standard American diet doesn't do much to accelerate neuronal healing, the production of new neural tissue, or overall cognitive recovery. Instead, it contributes to inflammation and the down-regulation of essential neurotransmitters. Fortunately, just as the wrong foods can have detrimental effects, the *right* foods can act as medicine, helping to speed your TBI recovery.

It's as much a personal journey to find the right dietary *approach* for any given person, as it is to live an authentically chosen *lifestyle*. Furthermore, it's not so important to necessarily "be" ketogenic, paleo, vegan, macrobiotic, pescatarian, lacto-ovo-vegetarian, omnivorous, or whatever, as much as it is to be nourished well through trying out a variety of styles of eating in order to know what works best. Just as with all the other mentioned approaches and technologies in this Manual, these dietary guidelines work best for the majority of people healing from concussion, and it's still necessary to put yourself "in the laboratory" and find the most appropriate, workable fit for you.

That being said, there are some general principles to keep in mind regarding food choices for improving and maintaining overall health and longevity, while considering sustainability and resource conservation. Ideally, one's diet comprises as many of these factors whenever possible:

- Locally sourced foods
- Seasonal
- Organic
- Rich in plant phytonutrients, healthy fats and usable protein
- Mindfully raised and sustainably harvested

Many people who know my background in "live food medicine" and raw food detoxification often ask me about the benefit of a plant based approach for healing a variety of conditions. Personally, I was raw vegan for about five years and medically directed one of the more preeminent live food vegan detox centers in the U.S., the Tree of Life Rejuvenation Center in Patagonia, AZ. It is true that the raw vegan diet is the best cleansing diet out there, hands down. When done well, it's the cleanest dietary approach to rid the body of built up toxins, and there's a good case to be made for the superior ecological footprint of a plant-based dietary focus over an animal-based one.

Some people ask the question, doesn't the body already have built in detox methods that helped us evolutionarily get this far? Yes, indeed, the body's blueprint is certainly built for detoxification on its own. However, with the advent of processed foods lower in nutritional value, increasing levels of environmental toxicity and a fast-paced life, over time the body gets saturated and requires concentrated, supported efforts to reduce the burden of inflammation and stress. Furthermore, it appears that generationally over time we are becoming collectively taxed in our ability to detoxify the body and brain, largely due to genetic influences.

One example of this growing trend can be seen with the epidemic of autistic spectrum disorders, and the improvement of such symptoms when targeted supplementation is utilized in accordance to one's genomic variation in the methylation cycles and detoxification pathways. This is the quickly emerging field of **Detoxigenomics** and **Nutrigenomics**, and it represents a potentially monumental piece of the individualized health puzzle, as optimizing genetic profiles is essential across the board for all people at any stage of healing and recovery.

Though unpacking this full discussion in much greater detail is outside the scope of this Manual, a brief overview will help. **Methylation cycles** are involved in every cell's function and their implications are wide reaching. A few notables include: immune regulation, neuronal myelination, making and repairing DNA and RNA, digestion, neurotransmitter balance, detoxification (for ex. heavy metals) and energy production. Suffice it to say it's a considerably important topic for the future science of medicine in general and a growing number of physicians and genetic specialists are working towards bringing this data into the mainstream of the field. (Please see the Resource Section for more information about detoxification science, methylation cycles, and approaches/strategies for testing and treatment).

There is little doubt that plant-based nutrients are a vital part of one's diet for ongoing health by providing many of the vitamins, minerals, micronutrients and cofactors necessary for key pathways and reactions in the body and brain. I've seen some people completely thrive on a fully raw, uncooked, live, plant-based diet, and although it's ideal for detoxification, it is not the best maintenance diet for most folks, particularly not for those healing from TBI. The healing brain requires essential amino acids and fats for repair and reconstitution, and in my experience this is most readily achieved through proper inclusion of animal based foods. While consulting many long-term vegetarians, it became evident that the gains made in the mind, heart and spirit by a plants-only approach, over time were typically not mirrored by the body.

My own case was a good example of the hormonal depletion and cognitive sluggishness that accompanies one through many years of veganism. At the time of being raw vegan, I was committed to seeing the 5-year experiment through, and although I was noticeably more centered in my mind and opened in my spiritual practice, I was consistently low in physical drive, mental stamina, and global energy, no matter how much I supplemented with herbs, amino acids, and other plant-based nutrients. Then when I chose to reintroduce eggs, fish, and organic raw goat's milk there was a massive increase across the board in vitality, mental acuity, strength, and overall body-mind performance. In seeing hundreds of clients, friends and family members over the years exhibit the same trend, I (and most of my colleagues) believe that a strictly vegetarian diet is not the best healing diet for the brain.

Of course this must all be *balanced with one's own personal values*. Many people have chosen a primarily plant-based approach as a maintenance diet as a statement in consideration to the Earth for more sustainable food practices, as well as the more spiritual and compassionate orientation to relationships with our animal friends. There is *no doubt* we humans as a single species on the planet have contributed to massive global shifts in climactic weather patterns, resource scarcity, wildlife species die-off and environmental pollution. Anyone that says otherwise is simply not paying attention. That being said, it is still possible, and some would argue imperative, that reengineering a sustainable relationship with animal husbandry is not only healthful, but a vital part of how we're genetically programmed to thrive and potentially even survive.

If one is **vegetarian**, supplementing the diet with lots of fats (coconut oil and fish oil) and protein (hemp, pea, and rice proteins are typically good plant sources of BCAA) is very likely to be of benefit; if one's vegetarian dietary preference allows, many people experience significantly improved health with raw goat's milk, butter and yogurt as it is more tolerable than cow's milk given the improved protein compatibility profile for the majority of people (then there's the whole discussion of potential bacterial load of unpasteurized milk that should be investigated so that your choice is an educated and informed one); if **vegan**, then also adding supplemental vitamins A, D, E and K, lecithin, bee pollen (some strict vegans will choose to avoid bee pollen all together), B12, and folate is likely to be warranted.

Probiotic rich foods are another important addition to any diet, particularly for the healing brain given the benefit of a healthy biome to the gut-brain connection. (See the Resources section for further reading on the subject).

HEADS UP! The list of foods included in this section represents some of the more impactful ones for brain repair and function, and it is not an exhaustive list. There are many foods that support the brain and can contribute to function and repair that were not listed here, for example: avocados, brightly colored berries, chocolate, lentils, beets, nuts and seeds and cruciferous vegetables. Feel free to explore and include all those that resonate with your own palate.

THE KETOGENIC DIET

In our culture, we've long been told that dietary fat and cholesterol are the enemy and that having a low fat diet will keep our cholesterol low and our waistlines slim. However, that approach definitely has not proved to be true. In the last 30 years since this movement has taken hold, the rates of obesity have continued to rise, heart disease is still the number one killer worldwide (according to the World Health Organization), and all of this is in the setting of cholesterol "Statin" medications still being the number one prescribed and used pharmaceutical group of meds on the market.

To better understand the relationship between food, fat, and health we need to look at an evolutionary picture. In reality, we evolved as a modern day species of man with the consistent utilization of fats (particularly omega-3 oils from sea and shell fish) to assist our brain in neurological development. In fact, the human brain is more than 60 percent fat. So it would stand to reason that our brains actually need healthy levels of both fats and cholesterol to function properly. Cholesterol is the building block for all other hormones in our bodies, governing sleep cycles, metabolism, cellular function, sexual arousal, neuronal synaptic formation and SO much more, and thus directly contributes to life and longevity.

Despite all we hear about the dangers of high cholesterol, the truth is that when inflammation is kept in check, it's actually *more problematic for blood cholesterol levels to be too low*. Multiple studies have associated low blood cholesterol levels with depression and increased risk of suicide. For instance, in one study of more than 11,000 people, those with a total blood cholesterol score of less than 165 were *six times* more likely to commit suicide than people with total blood cholesterol levels greater than 223.[305]

When taking your own cholesterol numbers into account, keep in mind that the ratio between your LDL and HDL levels is what matters most. You can calculate this ratio by dividing your total blood cholesterol score by your HDL number. (HDL, or high-density lipoprotein, is your "good" or healthy cholesterol, while LDL, or low-density lipoprotein, is the "bad" cholesterol often associated with increased risk of cardiovascular disease.) Ideally, your cholesterol ratio should be between 3.5 and 5. Many of the fat-based foods that make up a ketogenic diet will contribute positively to your HDL levels and, as a result, to this overall cholesterol ratio.

Taking a more **ketogenic dietary approach** that's weighted much more heavily towards healthy fats, moderate protein intake and relatively low in carbohydrates can go a long way to provide your brain with what it needs to repair itself. It's actually been studied and successfully used since 1921 as a beneficial aid in treating childhood epilepsy. In animal models it's been shown to be neuroprotective against TBI, as well as several other diseases of the central nervous system including Parkinson's and Alzheimer's Disease, glutamate toxicity, hypoxia, and ischemia.[306] As with many beneficial treatments in medicine, research science is still not exactly sure what makes a ketogenic diet supportive in healing the brain. It could have to do with upregulated genetic profiles via using alternative energy pathways, increased mitochondrial production and function and improved resistance to metabolic stress.

> **Ketogenic diet**—a selection of foods high in healthy fats, moderate in proteins and low in carbohydrates causes the body to burn fats, rather than glucose, for energy.

In the *strict* ketogenic diet, about 70 to 75 percent of overall calories will come from fats, another 20 to 25 percent will come from proteins, and less than 10 percent will come from carbohydrates. Going "strictly ketogenic" can be a process, and it doesn't have to happen overnight. Even going *more* ketogenic, which many would correlate with "**Paleo**" is a step in the right direction, as *slow change is lasting change* and moving more consistently towards a positive outcome is usually more sustainable than an "immediate makeover." This is why most crash diets don't work and why most people who win the lottery lose the majority of what they won. This is a journey of brain recovery from TBI, and as such the goal is long-term improvement, not up and down yo-yo win-losses that can be more trouble than they're worth.

Looking at it on the physiological level, over time eating a more ketogenic diet causes the body to convert glycogen—the energy stored in your liver—into glucose that it can use for energy. During prolonged states of ketosis, your body will also break down fat stores, resulting in the production of organic compounds called "ketones" which replace blood glucose as the brain's energy source. This highly efficient metabolic state is known as "ketosis."

Of course, it's important to note that *not all dietary fats are created equal.* (For examples of healthy sources of fats and proteins, see the "Tools and Techniques" section below.) Commonly found in heavily processed fried foods, unsaturated "trans fats" made from PHOs (poly-hydrogenated oils) have been linked to greater risk of heart disease, obesity, liver dysfunction, and other health problems. Unlike healthier fats, which have a more slippery consistency and move through easier, trans fats are sticky. Think of trying to push mud through a screen (not very easy) versus through chicken wire (a lot easier). In the brain, these trans fats are almost glue-like, and plugging up the neuronal membrane causes interference with the natural flow of nutrients *into* brain cells, while also blocking the removal of toxins *out of* the cells, further causing oxidative stress, inflammation, and even cell death. So, it goes without saying that a diet laden with trans fats isn't the best option for your neuronal repair menu. Replacing the sticky trans fats that have built up in your brain with these more pliable, healthy fats will take time—not to mention diligence and discipline on your part as you change your eating habits—but it is a necessary key to brain repair and well worth it.

A deeper exploration of further fat differences: *saturated* fats have no double bond between molecules, leaving the fat saturated with hydrogen molecules and are typically solid at room temperature (these include most animal fats and coconut oil); *unsaturated* fats have a double bond between the molecules creating gaps between the hydrogen molecules, leaving them liquid at room temperature (these include your fish based oils and plant based ones like olive, hemp, sunflower and others). Generally, the fish-based unsaturated oils are preferentially focused on in brain recovery protocols because of the higher concentration of neuronal reparative omega-3 fatty acids. That isn't to say the plant-based oils are bad and should be avoided. Many people are simply too overly concentrated on the omega-6s and 9s from plant sources (with an omega 6:3 ratio greater than 10:1) and would do better with more balance between the two in order to optimize nervous system function and healthy mood (omega 6:3 ratio closer to 3:1). For those curious to know, this is assessed by looking at a specialized blood EFA—essential fatty acid—panel. (See the following sections on Fish Oil and Coconut Oil for more information on these fats).

BENEFITS AND RISKS

The ketogenic diet has many applications. Because it up-regulates metabolism, it is frequently used for weight loss. It also has been successfully used to control difficult cases of epilepsy,[307] to stabilize mood,[308] and even to improve symptoms of autism in children.[309]

In the context of traumatic brain injury and the cascade of harmful effects that can ensue weeks, months, or years later, eating a diet that's high in healthy fats and low in carbohydrates can make a substantial, positive impact. (For a refresher on the mechanics of brain injury and how and why TBI sufferers are more predisposed to cognitive impairment, dementia and Alzheimer's disease, see "The Injured Brain" and "Genetics and the Alzheimer's" sections).

Just how positive can the impact of a high-fat, low-carb diet be? Well, consider a 2012 study published in *The Journal of Alzheimer's Disease* in which researchers examined and reported on the diets of 937 elderly people.[310] In the beginning, each of the study subjects was cognitively normal, but, over time, 200 people developed mild cognitive impairment or dementia. Researchers followed all of the subjects during an average period of nearly four years, carefully analyzing the percentages of fats, proteins, and carbohydrates eaten. They discovered that subjects who ate high-carb diets had *double* the risk of mild cognitive impairment or dementia, compared to people who ate fewer carbohydrates. And people who consumed higher percentages of healthy fats and proteins greatly reduced their risk of mild cognitive impairment or dementia.

Despite its potential benefits, the ketogenic diet isn't recommended for people who have weakened kidney function or only one working kidney. It is also not ideal for people who have had their gallbladders removed or those with poor gallbladder function, given that bile acids stored in the gallbladder are necessary for fat digestion and utilization. Notably, oral supplementation with bile salts when eating fatty meals has been beneficial for many with their gallbladders removed.

Although rare, it is possible to develop kidney stones while on a ketogenic diet. Other side effects may include constipation and increased cholesterol levels, and, as a result of shifting dietary fat ratios and the associated hormonal changes, some women may also experience temporary menstrual irregularities.

HEADS UP! If you're not sure whether a ketogenic diet is right for you, check with your doctor before you make any sweeping dietary changes. Going "strict ketogenic" here is not the goal. It is a goal to work towards, and one that has to work for you. Make gradual, sustainable changes over time and track your progress. This will give you a better idea if it's the right dietary approach to support your recovery program.

TOOLS AND TECHNIQUES

Good fats and proteins can come from a variety of animal and plant sources. Here are just a few of them, along with some tips to help you achieve and maintain the beneficial metabolic state of ketosis. We'll go into more detail about ketogenic staples like coconut oil in the next sections of this chapter, and, for further reading and recommendations, see the Resources section.

- **Dairy products** – Butter, whole milk, and cheeses are rich sources of fat and protein for the ketogenic diet. Opt for certified organic dairy goods made from the milk of grass-fed cows or goats that have been humanely stewarded. (Note: Having trouble digesting dairy products? If you haven't tried goats' milk, you should. Not only does goat milk have less of the alpha-s1-casein protein molecule implicated in cow's milk allergies, it also contains less lactose and smaller fat particles than cows' milk does, making it much easier for the human body to assimilate.)

- **Nuts and seeds** – Another good source of healthy fats are organic nuts and seeds, but to get the most nutritional benefit, you should soak or sprout them before eating. The outside layer of most nuts and seeds contain enzyme inhibitors, which contributes to their shelf life but limits their digestibility. Soaking these in warm water for several hours helps dissolve and remove this outside layer and essentially start the "sprouting" process. (For certain nuts—like almonds—soaking may make it possible to remove these outside skins entirely.) After a long soak, skinned almonds and other nuts and seeds can be blended into smoothies, chopped up for use in salads or added to stir-fried dishes.

- **Quality oils** – When purchasing healthy fats like coconut or olive oils, don't settle for that discount store's cheapest, one-gallon jug. Instead, choose only organic, high quality oils from reputable distributors, and, whenever possible, ask to sample the product for freshness and taste before you buy. Most oils are sensitive to light and heat. As a result, they can become rancid in high heat, long-term, poor storage conditions, and when consumed contribute to greater inflammation down the road.

- **Raw meats** – When meat is cooked, protein, vitamins, and minerals are lost. The biochemical profile of fats in the meat also changes with cooking. Raw meat, by contrast, is rich in protein, minerals, and free-form amino acids which are much more accessible to the body. The same can be said for raw, unpasteurized milk and eggs. This nutritional profile makes raw meat a brain-regenerative food that can boost neurotransmitter levels, improve cognition and normalize hormones.

Wondering whether or not it's safe to eat raw meat? Preparing raw meat dishes is a time-tested tradition in many cultures. A few examples include South American *ceviche*, a dish of raw, citrus-cured fish, Italian *carpaccio*, thinly sliced, raw meats prepared with lemon, vinegar and assorted seasonings, French Alsatian/German *parisa* (my personal favorite as it is popular where I was born and raised in south Texas), made of raw ground red meat cured in lime juice, jalapeno and onion, and Ethiopian *kitfo*, chili-marinated, raw beef. To kill off any pathogens and parasites they may contain, raw meats are typically cured or marinated in natural acids like lemon juice, lime juice or apple cider vinegar, as seen in all the above mentioned traditional foods. They may also be heavily seasoned with hot peppers, garlic, and onions or cumin, cardamom, cloves, and other spices. (See the Reference Section for examples of food information and preparation books).

HEADS UP!   Be aware that eating raw meats is not without risk. There is a reason the U.S. FDA's Food Code says "consuming raw or undercooked meats, poultry, seafood and eggs can increase your risk of foodborne illness." It does, especially if you're not the one preparing it. That's why it's best to know what you're doing, prepare it yourself, avoid the dangers and then reap the benefits. If you are in doubt, get support. And officiall , if you are pregnant, elderly or have a significantly impaired immune function, consult with your medical provider before eating raw meat.

If you plan to make a raw meat dish on your own, choose only the freshest, fatty meats from hormone-free, grass-fed animals. When preparing the meat, be sure to keep your hands—and all kitchen surfaces and utensils with which the meat comes into contact—very clean and sterilize utensils in a high heat dishwasher after use. And lastly, according to the US Dept of Agriculture using meat that has been previously frozen for more than 3 weeks will have killed off most if not all the potential parasites.

- **Early morning protein** – Getting protein first thing in the morning—especially protein containing free-form amino acids—will help to balance your blood sugar, support adrenal functioning and build neurotransmitters. Need some high-protein examples? Begin your day with a couple of raw egg yolks, a quarter pound of hormone-free, pasture-raised meat, or a low-sugar smoothie made with pea, chia, whey or rice protein powder blended into almond milk or whey isolate.

- **Fasting** – Regular fasting is an important component of the ketogenic diet, because it helps the body prolong its state of ketosis. Ideally, fasting periods should last between 12 and 16 hours, but fasting doesn't have to be complicated. One of the simplest ways to fast is to refrain from eating anything after dinner and then to sleep through your fasting hours. (So, if you last ate at 7 p.m., you wouldn't eat again until at least 7 a.m. the next day when you have breakfast.) Fasting before (and during) sleep means that, instead of spending energy digesting a heavy meal, your body will be able to direct all of its energy to recuperation and repair. Incidentally, that's how breakfast derived its name—*Breaking the Fast*.

QUICK TIP When it's time to break your fast, start with the juice of half of a lemon and a pinch of Himalayan crystal salt mixed into one liter of spring or filtered water. (And, to really get your lymphatic system moving, add 10 minutes of vigorous exercise like a brisk walk, yoga, a few minutes of inversion or jumping—using a jump rope or on a mini trampoline!).

If you make the switch to a ketogenic diet, don't expect to see benefits overnight. Although you may start to see *some* improvement in your target symptoms within one or two weeks, it will take a few months to realize the ketogenic diet's full potential effects on your recovery.

OILY FISH

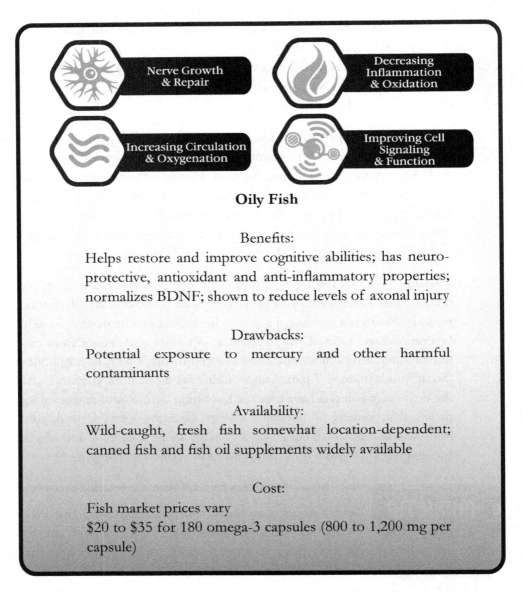

Nerve Growth & Repair

Decreasing Inflammation & Oxidation

Increasing Circulation & Oxygenation

Improving Cell Signaling & Function

Oily Fish

Benefits:
Helps restore and improve cognitive abilities; has neuro-protective, antioxidant and anti-inflammatory properties; normalizes BDNF; shown to reduce levels of axonal injury

Drawbacks:
Potential exposure to mercury and other harmful contaminants

Availability:
Wild-caught, fresh fish somewhat location-dependent; canned fish and fish oil supplements widely available

Cost:
Fish market prices vary
$20 to $35 for 180 omega-3 capsules (800 to 1,200 mg per capsule)

Adding oily fish like sardines, herring, anchovies, and salmon to your diet will provide your body—and brain—with more than just a little protein. You'll also get vitamin D, some B vitamins, essential minerals and lots of omega-3 fatty acids. Comprised of alpha linolenic acid (ALA), eicosapentaenoic acid (EPA) and docosahexaenoic acid (DHA), the omega-3s are vital for healthy brain function and, as you will see, they can pay particularly large dividends for TBI survivors.

BENEFITS AND RISKS

Inflammation in the brain, whether from the natural aging process or the result of a TBI, impairs our cognitive abilities, but there is strong evidence to suggest that omega-3 fatty acids can help restore and improve cognition. Omega-3s have antioxidant potential, making them effective anti-inflammatory agents.[311] They're also believed to normalize the levels of brain-derived neurotrophic factor (BDNF), which is critical for the survival of neuronal cells and necessary for normal synaptic transmission.[312]

In a study of rats with TBI, supplementation of dietary omega-3 fatty acids counteracted the effects associated with their brain injuries. The fatty acids reduced oxidative damage and improved the rats' spatial learning ability.[313] During a similar study of rats with TBI, post-injury administration of fish oil rich in EPA and DHA greatly reduced the number of injured axons in their brains.[314] Omega-3s have also been shown to provide robust neuroprotective effects when used prophylactically. Researchers first gave a DHA supplement to healthy rats for 30 days and then induced TBIs in the animals. DHA decreased the levels of cell death and axonal and cellular injury, and the DHA-treated rats performed better during maze memory testing than did rats from the unsupplemented control group.[315]

Omega-3s—and DHA, in particular—have also been shown to protect the structure and function of *human* brains.[316] During one study of 280 people between the ages of 35 and 54, researchers took blood samples and assessed the subjects' performance on a battery of cognitive tests, including nonverbal reasoning and mental flexibility, attention and concentration, general or episodic memory, working memory and verbal knowledge and processing. People with higher blood levels of DHA consistently performed better in the areas of nonverbal reasoning and mental flexibility, working memory, and vocabulary. (Interestingly, high blood concentrations of EPA were only marginally associated with working memory, and high ALA levels seemed to have no bearing on the participants' cognitive performance.)[317]

And researchers studying the effects of DHA supplementation on 485 older adults with "mild memory complaints" (like forgetting names or appointments) demonstrated that the participants taking 900 mg of DHA per day improved in the cognitive areas of episodic memory and learning. Over a 24-week period, when compared to the placebo-controlled group, the DHA-supplemented group showed a twofold reduction in the number of visuospatial learning and episodic memory errors during testing.[318]

There are also more long-term human studies, including one spanning five years. For that study, researchers examined 210 men between the ages of 70 and 89, noting that the men who regularly consumed more fatty fish and other foods containing EPA and DHA, experienced less cognitive decline during that five-year period.[319]

Despite all of those benefits, you do have to exercise caution when choosing which kinds of oily fish to eat. Aside from the good omega-3 fatty acids, many fish sources also contain harmful toxins like the heavy metal mercury. After sampling freshwater fish from 367 sites, the U.S. Geological Survey reported, "[Mercury] concentrations in freshwater fish across the United States are often greater than levels specified in various criteria for protection of fish-eating wildlife and humans." At 27% of the sites sampled, the mercury concentrations found were either equal to or greater than the human health standard set by the Environmental Protection Agency.[320]

To mitigate your exposure to mercury and other toxins, choose fish that live near the bottom of the food chain. Because they don't live as long, little guys like anchovies and sardines don't have as much time to accumulate toxins into their bodies. By contrast, the bigger fish like king mackerel, sharks and swordfish live longer and travel long distances to feed on many other fish, thereby building up higher concentrations of contaminants. As such, these and other very large fish should be avoided.

AVAILABILITY AND COST

The nutritional profiles of fish caught from the wild are often better than those of farmed fish, but your access to really fresh fish depends, in part, on your geographic location. If you're in a land-locked region, you may have to pay a premium for wild-caught. Fortunately, canned sardines, herring and anchovies are widely available and comparatively inexpensive.

Eating one serving of oily fish every other day is ideal to meet brain reparative requirements. In addition, it's a good idea to take an omega-3 supplement daily. Before you buy, make sure the manufacturer routinely assays its fish oil-based products for heavy metals and other contaminants. Choose a supplement that's high in both DHA and EPA. Omega-3 supplements often come in 800 – 1,200 mg capsules with a target dose range of 1,200 to 3,000 mg per day. A bottle of 180 capsules may cost between $20 and $35.

COCONUT OIL

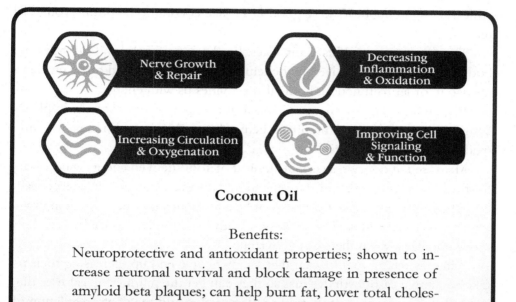

Coconut Oil

Benefits:
Neuroprotective and antioxidant properties; shown to increase neuronal survival and block damage in presence of amyloid beta plaques; can help burn fat, lower total cholesterol and improve cholesterol ratios.

Drawbacks:
Some people have a food sensitivity to coconut products, and using too much coconut oil can cause diarrhea.

Availability:
Widely available in grocery and health food stores.
Also sold in capsule form as a dietary supplement.

Cost:
.40 to .70 per ounce for virgin coconut oil.
$20 to $35 for one-month supply of capsules (1,000 to 1,300 mg).

COCONUT OIL

You've likely heard countless diet "experts" promoting low-fat diets as the key to good health, but as mentioned in the Ketogenic diet section, this is a little misguided. While there are certain *types* of fats that should be kept to a minimum in your diet (as we've talked about extensively before), *good fats* are essential for a healthy body and a high-performance brain. That's why it's critical to get enough of these good fats—like coconut oil—during your TBI recovery.

The food we eat fulfills many roles. For basic survival, food provides our bodies with neuroprotective phytochemicals, amino acids, and other nutrients needed in order to function. Food also provides us with energy.

Phytochemical – a chemical compound which occurs naturally in plants. When we ingest them, some phytochemicals provide us with medicinal, anti-oxidant and other benefits.

Measured in calories, a certain amount of food-derived energy is necessary for the human body's day-to-day operation. However, engaging in energetically "expensive" activities like exercise—or healing from a traumatic brain injury—requires us to take in *additional* calories. With this in mind, it's easy to see how those popular low-fat diets can go wrong.

After switching to a low-fat diet, many people end up increasing their intake of simple carbohydrates just so they can get the number of calories they need. But, because it contributes to inflammation and the down-regulation of essential neurotransmitters, a high-carb diet is a poor choice for TBI survivors. By eating a diet rich in healthy fats, you can keep your carbohydrate intake to a minimum.

One of the very best of these healthy fats is coconut oil. A great source of neuroprotective phytochemicals, coconut oil is a nearly magical ingredient with myriad benefits.

BENEFITS AND RISKS

In some animal studies, ingesting coconut oil has been shown to help burn fat, lower total cholesterol, and increase the ratio of good-to-bad cholesterol.[321]

Some of the benefits of coconut oil are the result of its special chemical structure. Coconut oil is comprised primarily of medium-chain triglycerides (MCTs), which are shorter than the chemical chains found in other dietary fats. Their shorter length makes MCTs easier to metabolize, and they are more rapidly absorbed by the liver. The fatty acids from these MCTs are converted to acetoacetate and hydroxybutyrate—two great sources of fuel for the brain.[322]

By contrast, consumption of *long*-chain fatty acids is associated with larger concentrations of "bad" cholesterol particles.[323] Even worse are industrially synthesized, unsaturated trans fats (see the section above on Ketogenic Diet for review). Not found in nature, these trans fats are poorly metabolized by the body. Plugging up the neuronal membrane, they block the exchange of nutrients into the brain and hinder the removal of toxins from it.[324]

The benefits of coconut oil extend beyond its role as a great energy source. In addition to the MCTs, coconut oil has lots of dietary fiber, vitamins, minerals, and phytochemicals with medicinal properties, many of which have been studied over the course of many years. Researchers have documented the health benefits of coconut oil on human cells grown in petri dishes, as well as in animal subjects and human patients. In human cell studies, coconut oil has been shown to increase neuronal survival in the presence of harmful amyloid plaques,[325] and can actually block the damage from these amyloid beta plaques once they've formed.[326] (As you read in the Introduction, amyloid beta plaques are protein deposits that clog the space between brain cells. These plaques underlie Alzheimer's disease, and they are a dangerous component of the cascade of additional damage that accompanies TBI).

And, in animal studies, a diet rich in coconut oil was shown to provide significant neuroprotection. For example, after being fed coconut oil, brain-injured rats retained much more of their mobility than did rats in the control group.[327] New data suggests that this neuroprotective effect results from the antioxidant properties of coconut oil.[328]

There is less data on the use of coconut oil in human TBI patients, but we have every reason to suspect that the same neuroprotective properties seen in animal studies may apply to people, and there *is* abundant research showing that coconut oil is great for human health in general.[329]

The only caveat? For millennia, coconut oil has been a major food source for some of the healthiest populations on the planet, and it is known to be very safe. However, it is also very calorically dense. As with all high calorie foods, if you eat more than your body needs without exercising and utilizing it, you may gain weight.

AVAILABILITY AND COST

Considering coconut oil's many potential benefits and its relatively low risk, it's well worth incorporating into your TBI treatment protocol. For best results, you should ingest a few tablespoons of coconut oil per day. You can do this by replacing your current cooking oil with coconut oil, slathering it on toast in place of butter or simply eating it raw.

Expect to pay between 40 and 70 cents per ounce for bulk, whole virgin coconut oil. It also comes as a dietary supplement. Most commonly available in 1,000- to 1,300 mg capsules, the cost for a one-month supply ranges from $20 to $35.

Lastly, in taking a deeper look at coconut oil, we can see similar implications for food utilization in general. The recent demand on coconut oil has started to impact supply chains. As a result, some manufacturers have lessened the reigns on proper handling and storage practices, and thus much of the coconut oil on the market is either rancid or severely limited in its shelf life. A good test is *smelling* it. If it smells off it usually is off. If it's from one of the more reputable, organic and "fair trade" companies *and* it smells good then it probably is.

A brief and necessary soap-box moment in terms of sustainable food sourcing: To unpack this entire discussion would take us down a long and passionate road and is generally not the focus of this book (although it has been the focus of other writings and blog entries I've written elsewhere). Suffice it to say, *our food choices and dollars matter!* Often times one of the very best ways we can support total planetary health as well as our own is to buy organic and "fair trade" whenever possible. These designations verify that a higher degree of mindful assessment in food growth, processing, manufacturing and sustainable community wage practices have been honored. 9 times out of 10 the food just plain tastes better too.

TURMERIC

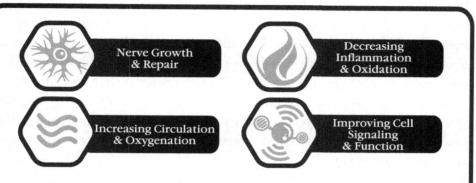

Turmeric

Benefits:
Natural antioxidant, anti-inflammatory, and antidepressant properties; has been linked to retention of cognitive function; increases dopamine and serotonin levels.

Drawbacks:
High doses may cause diarrhea; may not be appropriate for people taking blood thinners or those undergoing surgery or chemotherapy.

Availability:
The spice is widely available in grocery and health food stores. Turmeric's active ingredient, curcumin, is also available in capsule form.

Cost:
$4 for one ounce to $10 to $15 for bulk purchases.
(16+ ounces) of the spice.
$25 to $40 for 120 capsules (500 to 1,000 mg).

A key ingredient for Indian and south Asian curries, turmeric happens to be a great addition to the neuroprotective diet. The bright yellow spice can help heal your brain *while minimizing* the risk of further damage caused by your initial TBI.

Before we see how turmeric can help, here's a quick review about what I mean by "further damage." In the Introduction section of this Manual, you learned that a single incident of moderate or severe traumatic brain injury often marks the beginning of a chronic injury. This is the result of the blood-brain barrier becoming permeable, allowing toxic substances to reach the brain. Swelling and scarring can disrupt your synaptic connections, interfering with memory, learning and cognition. TBI also results in an overproduction of highly unstable, chemically reactive free radicals called reactive oxygen species (ROS). While reactive oxygen species are important for signaling in a healthy brain, having too many can cause oxidative stress—a major cause of secondary damage following TBI.[330]

> **QUICK TIP** Adopting a neuroprotective diet as early as possible after your initial TBI can help slow or stop the progression of additional, secondary damage to your brain. But, if you are trying to address the chronic symptoms of a past TBI, eating turmeric and other neuroprotective foods will still provide benefit, because many of the same principles that help to stabilize an acute injury will also promote long-term healing.

BENEFITS AND RISKS

The active ingredient in turmeric, curcumin, gives it the distinct orange-yellow color and acts as a major antioxidant, thus a neural protective agent. Frequent turmeric consumption has been linked to retention of cognitive function in the elderly,[331] and as a key component of Indian *Ayurvedic* medicine, turmeric has been used for millenia to treat a variety of ailments.[332] Acting as an anti-bacterial,[333] anti-cancer[334] agent, as well as a natural antioxidant,[335] curcumin's medicinal property arsenal provides a treasure trove of benefit from a single food source.

As mentioned earlier in this section, excessive quantities of ROS and other signaling molecules combine to form oxidizing agents and result in oxidative stress.[336] Healthy brains have mechanisms in place to keep the amounts of ROS in check, however after a TBI, the brain's natural protections become overwhelmed. Introducing curcumin into your diet can replenish the antioxidant stores and help neutralize more of these dangerous ROS before further damage occurs.[337]

Curcumin also has anti-inflammatory properties[338] and has been shown to reduce acute inflammatory injury associated with TBI.[339] With a significant brain injury, shearing forces cause swelling and scarring that can obstruct the growth of new axons and interfere with your synaptic connections. Interestingly however, researchers studying the effects of curcumin on animals with a TBI found that the anti-inflammatory agent significantly reduced scarring and aided in recovery.[340]

Turmeric's active ingredient has antidepressant properties as well.[341] Ingesting curcumin triggers increased production of an important protein called brain-derived neurotrophic factor (BDNF), which is thought to be responsible for curcumin's antidepressant effects.[342] Curcumin has also been shown to increase dopamine and serotonin levels.[343]

Some people should avoid curcumin, however. Because it is a blood thinner, it may not be appropriate for people undergoing surgery in the near future or those taking blood-thinning medications.[344] High doses of curcumin may also interfere with other medications, such as chemotherapy agents,[345] and can cause diarrhea in people unaccustomed to taking it. When in doubt, ask your doctor before adding it to your TBI treatment protocol.

AVAILABILITY AND COST

Turmeric is available in most grocery stores and can easily be incorporated into soups, curries, and meat dishes, but its bioavailability may be an issue. (**Bioavailability** is the degree to which your body can process and use an ingested compound). Very little curcumin will dissolve in water or watery solutions like blood or gastric juices. Instead, it breaks down much more readily in vegetable oil or other fats. Traditional Indian and South Asian cooking uses turmeric in curries prepared with coconut milk. Because coconut milk has a higher fat concentration than other foods, it may improve curcumin's bioavailability.[346] Combining black pepper with it (as "piperine") will also boost bioavailability.[347] There is a potential caveat to using black pepper for upregulating bioavailability, however. Theoretically the piperine could also increase the absorption of undesirable elements and environmental toxins too. More studies are necessary to evaluate this further.

Alternatively, nanoparticle preparations of curcumin will dissolve more easily in the gastric juices or blood,[348] so you could cover your bases by ingesting this active ingredient as a dietary supplement, too. The FDA has approved curcumin's use, labeling it "generally regarded as safe."[349] It has been shown to be nontoxic in cancer treatment at doses as high as 2,500 mg per day,[350] and single doses as high as 12,000 mg are well-tolerated by healthy individuals.[351]

Curcumin is commonly available in 500 to 1,000 mg capsules, and a bottle of 120 capsules averages between $25 and $40.

EGGS

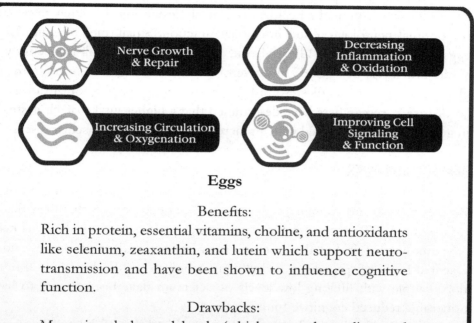

Eggs

Benefits:

Rich in protein, essential vitamins, choline, and antioxidants like selenium, zeaxanthin, and lutein which support neurotransmission and have been shown to influence cognitive function.

Drawbacks:

May raise cholesterol levels (which as we have discussed above, may not be a bad thing). Some people have a food allergy or sensitivity to eggs and should therefore, avoid them or consume sparingly.

Availability:

Widely available from grocery stores and farmers' markets; lecithin supplements can be substituted for eggs.

Cost:

Market prices for eggs may range from $2 to $4 per dozen. Liquid, powdered, or granulated lecithin costs about $1 per ounce.

$20 for 400 capsules (1,200 mg).

Eggs have been given a rotten reputation over the years. It's a real shame, because eggs have a lot going for them. They're an amazing source of protein, B vitamins, and the fat-soluble vitamins A, D, E and K, and they represent a very sustainable food source when stewarded with humanitarian care and vigilance. This however, is far from the standard in current care of most chickens utilized for egg production.

That being said, these nutritional powerhouses can be an anchor for a rehabilitative and peak performance diet. Yes, eggs do contain cholesterol, and as previously mentioned a healthy dose of cholesterol is absolutely necessary for optimal neurological and hormonal function. Small, medium, and large eggs each contain about 141, 164, and 186 mg of cholesterol, respectively.[352] While low levels of "good" cholesterol (HDL) and high levels of both triglycerides and "bad" cholesterol (LDL) *are* known risk factors for cardiovascular disease,[353] researchers have determined that a higher intake of cholesterol, in general, is not associated with an increased risk of cardiovascular disease.[354]

BENEFITS AND RISKS

Besides protein and vitamins, eggs contain other compounds that provide extra benefits to TBI survivors. One such compound is selenium. We don't need *large* amounts of it, but this micronutrient has antioxidant properties and is essential for some processes, including metabolism and healthy thyroid function. People with lifelong low levels of selenium have been shown to have noticeably reduced cognitive function.[355, 356]

Eggs are also rich in the antioxidants, zeaxanthin, and lutein. Protecting against macular degeneration and cataract formation, both are important for eye health,[357, 358] and they are thought to be neuroprotective too. Zeaxanthin and lutein naturally accumulate in neural tissue, and research indicates that high concentrations of these compounds in neural tissue may influence cognitive function in the elderly.[359] In one study of 108 adults in their late 70s, researchers tested the subjects' memory and processing speed via eight cognitive tests. Subjects with high levels of zeaxanthin and lutein in their neural tissue exhibited better global cognition, verbal learning and fluency, recall, processing speed, and perceptual speed.[360]

Important for neurotransmitter support, choline is another compound found in eggs. In human and animal studies, dietary intake of choline has been linked to improved cognition.[361, 362] Researchers evaluated the cognitive effects of dietary choline intake in 1,391 people between the ages of 36 and 83 and determined that subjects with choline-rich diets performed better on tests of verbal memory, visual memory, verbal learning, and executive function.[363]

AVAILABILITY AND COST

When adding eggs to your TBI recovery diet, it's best to include the yolks, since these have more protein and other nutrients per gram than egg whites. One dozen eggs may cost between two and four dollars, depending on where you live—and whether you pick up whatever's on hand at the grocery store or you spring for free-range, organic eggs from your local farmers' market.

But, because eggs can cause inflammation in some people, they aren't for everyone. If that's the case for you, consider substituting a lecithin supplement. Extracted from eggs, milk, soybeans and many kinds of seeds, lecithin provides some of the same benefits that eggs do and is a good source of choline.

Lecithin is frequently used to make commercially prepared salad dressings and other foods creamier. You can purchase a one-pound container of liquid, powdered or granulated lecithin for about $15. To use lecithin in these forms, just add a little to your yogurt or blend into a smoothie.

You can also purchase lecithin capsules. A 400-count bottle of 1,200 mg capsules usually costs about $20.

CHAPTER 7

WHAT TO AVOID

In This Section

You'll learn about:

- Repeat TBI
- Sugar consumption
- Obesity and gluttony
- Alcohol

Looking for maximum impact with minimum effort? Both eliminating sugar from your diet and avoiding repeat TBIs will contribute massive benefits.

An ounce of prevention is worth a pound of cure.
—*Benjamin Franklin*

Benjamin Franklin was originally referring to fire safety when he wrote, "An ounce of prevention is worth a pound of cure,"[364] but the old adage certainly applies to recovery from traumatic brain injury as well. If you are able to steer clear of the harmful elements and practices outlined in this chapter, you are nearly guaranteed to heal your brain more quickly—and experience more significant symptom relief and improved functionality in the process.

And, as with the "Personal Practices" we covered in Chapter 6, you're going to need to draw upon your self-discipline again to make the concepts presented here work for you. To help you strengthen your resolve as you work to establish new habits, consider enlisting the support of a trusted friend or fellow TBI survivor.

REPEAT TBI

REPEAT TBI   Drawbacks: Increased susceptibility to programmed cell death or cell "self-destruction;" higher likelihood of cognitive impairment and memory problems; possibility for earlier onset of Alzheimer's disease and development of chronic traumatic encephalopathy.

There is nothing more damaging to recovery from a TBI than *sustaining another TBI*. That's why, no matter how much you (understandably) may want to get right back to playing your favorite sport or engaging in all of your pre-injury activities, you're definitely going to need to take time off and do everything you can to avoid inflicting additional damage. In the worst-case scenario **Second Impact Syndrome** occurs when there's another TBI stacked on the still recovering brain. The brain swelling that can follow as a result may lead to out of control intracranial pressure and has led to death in athletes from the high school level up to the pros.

Recall that sustaining a single TBI sets off a chain reaction in your brain, including the release of large amounts of damaging free radicals, neuroinflammation, damage to the protective blood-brain barrier, build-up of harmful debris and more. (We detailed the cascade of negative effects that take place in an injured brain beginning in the Introduction, so if you skipped that part or just need a reminder, I encourage you to read or re-read that part. Really this cannot be stated enough as it's the major issue in the entire arena of concussion related medicine). In short, your brain doesn't just respond to its *initial* injury. Your brain also reacts to the byproducts caused by *its own response* to the initial injury. This sets up a vicious cycle that can last for weeks, months, and, sometimes, years.

Your injury also makes your brain cells more susceptible to a natural process of programmed cell death known as **apoptosis**.

> **Apoptosis**—a naturally occurring process of programmed self-destruction in a cell. This may simply be the end of its natural life cycle or can be hastened by the trigger of a virus, genetic mutation, or other stressor.

Under most normal circumstances it is actually beneficial for many of the cells in our bodies to choose to naturally die off. This is a part of the natural life cycles of cells, just as it is for all other aspects of life in nature. For other reasons, this cell death signaling is called for in order to remove a potential offender. An example of this is when cells contain a problematic genetic mutation or virus. Premature initiation of this self-destruct sequence may be in order for protection of healthy, neighboring cells that have not yet been affected.

Exposure to large amounts of reactive oxygen species and other environmental stressors can also cause cells to self-destruct. So, as you heal from your TBI—especially during the first few weeks after the initial injury—you may continue to lose brain cells as they undergo apoptosis. What's more, even the cells that *haven't* self-destructed may be poised to do so. In their pre-apoptotic state, such cells teeter on the brink of programmed cell death, and it doesn't take much to push them over the edge. In this post-injury environment, *any* repeat damage to your brain can be devastating.

> **HEADS UP!** Since every case is different, it's best to ask your doctor when you can safely return to sports and other strenuous activities. Ideally this evaluation contains some form of quantitative, functional neurological assessment to help gauge "return to play" readiness. At minimum, be prepared to take at least three weeks off from participating in sports or other strenuous activities after a significant TBI.

The National Football League (NFL), National Hockey League (NHL), and other professional sports organizations have only recently begun to take TBI more seriously by implementing new head trauma protocols for their players' protection.[365] On average, there was one player concussion for every 149.5 games played in the National Basketball Association between 2013 and 2014, but the risk rises precipitously for high contact sports like in the NHL and NFL.[366] Between 2009 and 2014, NHL players averaged one concussion for every 20 games played, and, in 2013 alone, there was an average of one concussion for every 1.4 NFL games played.[367]

In the past, it was common practice for players in many different sports—and at levels from peewee to professional—to take a "dinger" (common parlance for a heavy blow to the head), "shake it off," and get right back into the game. But they may have done so at a steep price. For example, researchers studying more than 2,500 retired, professional football players determined that players who had sustained three or more concussions were *five times* more likely to have been diagnosed with mild cognitive impairment than were retired players without histories of concussion. The multiple-concussion group was also *three times* more likely to have significant memory problems than their non-concussed counterparts. The researchers also noticed an earlier onset of Alzheimer's disease in the retirees than in the general population of American males.[368]

A recently found massive correlation between long-term football play and major brain damage has rocked the sport. After examining the brains of 128 deceased football players, researchers with the Department of Veterans Affairs' brain repository in Bedford, Massachusetts discovered that nearly 80 percent of them had a serious neurodegenerative condition called chronic traumatic encephalopathy (CTE). Although these past football experiences ranged from playing in high school and college to playing semi-professionally and professionally, 79 of the subjects had formerly played for the NFL. *Of those 79 players, 76 tested positive for CTE.*[369] While this is an extraordinarily high correlation, it is in the context of self-selection. This means those football players that sensed there was neurological damage willingly donated their brains to science for examination. Consequently, these findings do not mean that 90-plus percent of those playing competitive football for year will get CTE.

Much more study is currently underway, and the recently released movie *Concussion* with Will Smith further encourages deeper examination into the nuances that correlate brain trauma to long-term degenerative conditions, as well as the implementation of neuroprotective rules and methodologies that can be put into place for the sport to maximize safety while keeping the essential nature of its play and popularity intact. As a result of the increased awareness of potentially life-altering long term consequences of repeat TBI, some players are even opting out of the game all together even after early success in their careers. Notable examples were the full retirements from the 49ers squad alone in 2015, Chris Borland (leaving after an excellent rookie year), and Anthony Davis after 5 strong years in the league.

It is known that CTE can cause depression and other mood disorders, confusion, poor or lost memory, and dementia. Unfortunately, however, the presence of CTE can only be positively confirmed postmortem (after death) on autopsy. As a result, increasing numbers of professional athletes, suspecting they might have the condition, have chosen to donate their brains to researchers for posthumous analysis. Just one of many examples is former Chicago Bears Player Dave Duerson, suffering from headaches, blurred vision and a deteriorating memory, committed suicide in 2011 by shooting himself in the chest, ostensibly to preserve his brain for study. *The New York Times* reported, "His final note to his family finished with a handwritten request: 'Please, see that my brain is given to the N.F.L.'s brain bank.'"[370]

REAL WORLD EXAMPLE: REPEAT TBI IN MMA

The rate of traumatic brain injury amongst mixed martial arts (MMA) athletes is also being scrutinized. TBI rates for MMA fighters appear to be higher than those of practitioners of individual martial arts and even boxers. This is not super surprising given the growing popularity of a sport whose frequent end outcome is to cause submission in one's opponent, often done by inflicting a TBI. Notably, the incidence of TBI in MMA often occurs during training periods (when less people may be watching) and not even so much in the ring on

Fight Night. Consequently, to minimize the risk, many of the top fighters are opting for less intense head combat sparring sessions during these pre-fight training periods.

After studying 844 Ultimate Fighting Championship MMA events taking place between 2006 and 2012, researchers found a combined incidence of match-ending head trauma in *31.9 percent* of matches. They also noted an average time of 3.5 seconds between the delivery of a knock-out strike and stoppage of a match, with bout losers sustaining nearly three *additional* blows to the head *after* the knock-out strike. And, regarding technical knock-outs, bout losers received an average of 18.5 strikes—with 92.3 percent of these being direct head strikes—in the 30-second period just before the fight was stopped.[371] As with the NFL, the UFC and Bellator (the two biggest MMA card holders) are feeling the pressure to up the protective rules and regulations of fighters returning to the ring after a noticeable concussion, as well as the protection of fighters in the ring before taking such a major head beating.

Bottom line? After your initial injury, plan to take a minimum of three weeks off before returning to sports or any activity that could put you at risk for sustaining additional head injuries. Ideally, you should ask your doctor to weigh-in on your individual case and recommend a personalized timeline for your safe return to each of your pre-injury activities.

SUGAR

SUGAR Drawbacks: Suppresses immune function; promotes chronic inflammation; contributes to oxidative stress in the brain; interferes with neurotransmission, memory and cognitive function; deregulates mood, hormone levels, and more.

With sugar hidden in so many processed foods, it can be difficult to avoid, but, next to repeat brain injury, sugar is one of the *worst* things you can expose yourself to during your TBI recovery. (As you'll see, sugar is pretty lousy for people *without* brain injuries, too.)

Sugar weakens the body's immune system and promotes chronic inflammation and has also been directly linked to cancer.[372] Nevertheless, the average American eats more than 126 grams—or 31.5 teaspoons!—of sugar *every day*.[373] That's just over 100 pounds of sugar per year! It's not that people don't know that sugar is bad for them. The challenge in removing it from one's diet lies not only in its prevalence in all of the most common foods on the market, but also in its highly addictive nature. It's the most common (and likely detrimental) addiction on the planet, making it essentially public enemy number one for societal health, and as we will see shortly, it's also chemical enemy number one for neurological repair.

Much of what comes in the form of sugar is not even sugar in its most natural, pure form. The sweet fix is most often satisfied in foods through the modified sugars like high-fructose corn syrup, a cheap filler routinely included in pre-packaged and heavily processed foods. (Regular table sugar is, itself, made up of about half glucose and half fructose.) While glucose can be metabolized throughout the body, fructose is metabolized primarily in the liver. To state the case, the negative effects of fructose on the liver are said to be comparable to those of alcohol.[374] This is because, when your liver is taxed with breaking down large quantities of fructose, fats called triglycerides are produced.[375] Long-term exposure to these can cause liver dysfunction, hardening of the arteries, high blood pressure, and metabolic syndrome, leading to diabetes and cardiovascular disease.

And what were we saying about addiction? Sugar stimulates the same pleasure centers that heroin and cocaine do.[376] Sugar also scrambles the hormones that signal hunger and those that produce feelings of satiety, causing you to crave more and more of the sweet stuff.[377]

Eat too much of it, and sugar takes a toll on your mood and cognitive function. Sugar forms free radicals in the brain, contributing to oxidative stress and interfere with neurotransmission.[378] In a study of 141 people between the ages of 50 and 80, researchers found a significant association between high blood sugar levels and poor memory performance. Higher glucose levels were also correlated with decreases in hippocampus volume in the subjects' brains.[379] (The hippocampus is a region of the brain involved with memory formation and storage.)

Sugar consumption has even been linked to antisocial behavior. Over a two-year period, researchers studied a sample of 276 incarcerated juveniles ages 12 to 18 and found that simply replacing "junk food" and sodas with fruits and more nutritious snacks, and eliminating sugary cereals and desserts all together, caused a *48% drop* in formal disciplinary actions. To further assess this correlation, the researchers compared two groups, including 102 offenders who had had access to sugary snacks, sodas and desserts prior to the institution of a reduced-sugar menu throughout the juvenile detention center and 174 offenders who had only been exposed to the reduced-sugar menu. The outcome was a significant *56% decline* in the problematic behaviors in the percentage of offenders considered to be "chronic offenders."[380]

TOOLS AND TECHNIQUES

If you haven't already been paying attention to your daily sugar intake, start by reading the nutrition labels on all of the pre-packaged, processed foods you eat, and try to stay under 40 grams of sugar per day. Cooking more meals "from scratch," rather than relying on these pre-packaged foods will help cut down on the amount of sugar in your diet. (For further reading and recommendations about sugar and sugar substitutes, see the Resources section.) Here are a few other ideas to try:

- **Beverages** – Eliminating soft drinks, switching to unsweetened tea, and drinking your coffee black can also make a huge dent in your daily dose of sugar.

- **Whole grains** – You should watch your intake of refined carbohydrates like white bread, pasta and white rice, because these essentially turn into sugar in the body and cause blood sugar levels to spike. Opt for high-fiber, whole grains like whole wheat breads and pastas instead.

- **Natural fruit sugars** – When you *have* to have something sweet, reach for fresh fruit. The sugars naturally found in fruits are easier for your body to process and they create less inflammation. Also, fruits contain fiber, helping you to feel more satisfied and slowing the absorption of sugar into the bloodstream.

- **Sugar substitutes** – Although each has its limitations, there are many all-natural sugar substitutes on the market you can try. Some of these include:

- **Glycine** – A naturally sweet-tasting amino acid, glycine has been shown to reduce insulin sensitivity in mice and improve immune function in people with diabetes.[381]

- **Stevia** – Said to be 300 times sweeter than sugar, stevia is extracted from *Stevia rebaudiana,* a cultivar of the chrysanthemum plant.[382] Stevia has improved metabolic syndrome in animal studies, and it has been shown to enhance glucose tolerance in both animal and human studies.[383] Some people experience a slightly bitter aftertaste.

- **Monk fruit** – Originally harvested by monks some 800 years ago, this small, Asian gourd, also known as *luo han guo,* really packs a punch. An antioxidant compound called mogroside makes this sugar substitute between 200 and 500 times as sweet as sugar. Mogrosides have improved blood sugar levels and increased good cholesterol in animal studies.[384] As with stevia, some people detect a slightly bitter or "off" aftertaste when using monk fruit-derived sweeteners.

- **Xylitol** – Xylitol is an alcohol sugar extracted from the fibrous parts of sugar cane refuse, corn husks, birch trees and other hardwoods. It has about 33 percent fewer calories than sugar, has been shown to reduce the occurrence of tooth decay and is a common ingredient in sugar-free gum and candies.[385] Because it's absorbed by the body more slowly than sugar, xylitol doesn't cause blood sugar to spike and is well-suited for use by people with diabetes.[386] Some people report symptoms of bloating, gas, and diarrhea after ingesting xylitol, so use caution until you know how well your body will tolerate it.

- **Erythritol** – Found in certain fruits and fermented foods, erythritol is another sugar alcohol. Although it is 60 to 70 percent as sweet as sugar, erythritol has 95 percent fewer calories than sugar does. Like xylitol, erythritol also inhibits tooth decay and won't spike blood sugar;[387] however, some people have experienced nausea and gastro-intestinal upset after eating too much.[388]

OBESITY

OBESITY Drawbacks: Can contribute to longer hospital stays and greater complication rates; associated with abnormal neuronal activity; correlated with poor memory, deteriorating cognitive and motor functions; and may increase risk of Alzheimer's disease and dementia.

If sugar is public enemy number one, one of its main down streams detriments is obesity. We live in a culture of excess and privilege, and these "first world problems" have led to a tidal wave of obesity and an epidemiological metabolic catastrophe.

If you've been carrying around some extra pounds, you're not the only one. According to the Centers for Disease Control and Prevention, more than 35 percent of adults in the U.S. are obese and another 34 percent are overweight.[389] (For people ages 20 and older, "obesity" is defined as having a **body mass index** (BMI) greater than or equal to 30 and "overweight" is defined as having a BMI greater than or equal to 25 but less than 30.[390])

> **Body mass index** – a calculation involving a person's weight and height that is used to estimate amount of body fat.
>
> BMI = (Weight in Pounds / (Height in inches × Height in inches)) × 703

But being obese doesn't just increase your risk of coronary heart disease, diabetes or cancer.[391] It can also interfere with your recovery and can negatively affect long-term outcomes. In a study of 1,153 blunt force trauma patients, for instance, people who were obese suffered more complications and required longer hospital stays than non-obese patients.[392]

Obesity has been associated with abnormal neuronal activity in both animals and people,[393] and, in animal studies, overeating has been shown to make the nervous system less able to defend against stress and more susceptible to dysfunction and degeneration.[394] There is also a strong correlation between high body weight and poor memory, as well as deteriorating cognitive and motor functions.[395]

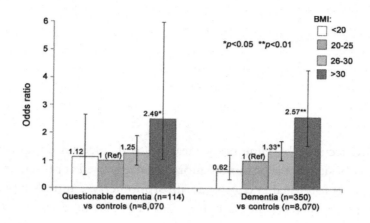

After studying 4,267 sets of twins aged 65 or older, researchers found a clear association between abnormal BMI and Alzheimer's Disease and vascular dementia. Among all participants, dementia was diagnosed in 350 people, and 114 others had "questionable dementia." People in these groups were much more likely to have had BMIs in the "overweight" or "obese" ranges during middle age.[396] And, in a later, follow-up study, researchers tracked 392 non-demented women from the original study over an 18-year period. Women with higher BMIs had a greater risk of developing Alzheimer's Disease. In fact, their Alzheimer's Disease risk jumped by 36% for every one-point increase in BMI score at age 70.[397]

Because obesity has become such a pervasive problem, Alzheimer's Disease is expected to become much more prevalent in the coming years. Also, because people are becoming overweight at younger ages, what was once considered a geriatric disease may strike people earlier in life.[398]

HEADS UP! Remember, if you've had a moderate TBI, your risk of devolping Alzheimer's is doubled—and even higher, if you had a more severe injury. Add a genetic predisposition to the mix, and you are even more likely to develop the disease. (See Genetics for more detail.) Being overweight or obese, under these circumstances, definitely adds insult to injury!

If you don't already know your BMI, take the time to calculate it using an online BMI calculator or the above included formula. Next, check your BMI score against the ranges below to see where you fall.

The standard weight status categories associated with BMI ranges for adults are shown in the following table.

BMI	Weight Status
Below 18.5	Underweight
18.5 – 24.9	Normal or Healthy Weight
25.0 – 29.9	Overweight
30.0 and Above	Obese

A more accurate baseline body measure to deduce fat composition, and thus assess obesity, that is becoming more popularly used at present is a **DEXA scan**. It stands for "dual energy x-ray absorptiometry", and it's typically used as a bone mineral density measure. It comes in to play here as it has the ability to better measure body composition while not being dependent on weight. Frequently when someone starts an up-leveled dietary and exercise regimen, the transition from fat stores to muscle mass is not reflective on the scale, thus using DEXA before and during a metabolically scripted therapeutic regimen can offer better assessment of progress.

If you're overweight or obese, you can examine your activity levels and eating habits. You might also consider intermittent fasting and moving towards a low carbohydrate, more Paleo/Ketogenic dietary approach. Now, we already discussed these briefly in the last chapter (See Ketogenic diet) but it's worth revisiting again here, because of the massive potential benefits and neuroprotective effects.

In animal studies, *alternate-day fasting* has been demonstrated to delay the onset of Alzheimer's, Parkinson's, and other neurodegenerative diseases.[399] And, in humans, fasting can reduce inflammation and decrease oxidative stress.[400] It also increases brain activity and ramps up production of a protein involved in neural cell growth, learning and memory.[401, 402]

ALCOHOL

ALCOHOL Drawbacks: Slows neuronal activity; impairs memory and cognition; disrupts sleep architecture; dysregulates mood, and has been shown to contribute to mood disorders in TBI patients.

Maybe it's not being able to return to school or work. Maybe it's missing out on your favorite activities. Or maybe it's not being able to play the sport you've devoted your life to. As you recover from your TBI, there may be plenty of reasons to *want* to drown your sorrows in the bottle, and it's *totally* understandable to be frustrated and wanting to take a mental break from it all. And in the end, the vast majority of people will conclude you'll be much better off resisting that temptation to dive into drinking for very long.

Sure, when consumed in moderation, alcohol has been shown to offer many general health benefits, but in the context of traumatic brain injury repair, alcohol will only set back your progress. It does this in several ways.

First, although alcohol may make you feel more animated and sociable, it is actually a central nervous system depressant. Alcohol slows neuronal activity, impairing memory, cognition, reaction time and much more. It can also cause you to make super poor choices that can tend to be flavored with frustration and acting out of anger, further negatively impacting your TBI recovery.

And remember how important sleep is for a healing brain? During the deep REM stage of sleep, your glymphatic system clears away harmful cellular debris, tau tangles, and amyloid beta plaques. However, alcohol disrupts your sleep architecture. It may encourage "passing out" or more quickly falling to sleep, but it severely interferes with the healing REM stage of sleep, consequently the sleep you get is not as restful, deep or rejuvenating.

What's more, alcohol further compounds the mood dysregulation that often accompanies traumatic brain injury, especially if the TBI is moderate to severe. This is because alcohol can damage the brain's dendrites—the parts of your neurons which receive signals.[403] This interferes with neurotransmission and can significantly alter your thinking patterns and moods.

To understand the effect excessive alcohol consumption can have, researchers compared 158 TBI patients—some with and some without a history of alcohol abuse or dependence. They discovered that patients who had had prior problems with alcohol were much more likely to develop mood disorders during the first year following their TBIs. And those patients with a history of alcohol abuse or dependence who *continued* to drink after sustaining their TBIs experienced an even higher frequency of mood disorders during the first year following their injuries.[404]

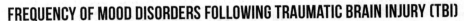

FREQUENCY OF MOOD DISORDERS FOLLOWING TRAUMATIC BRAIN INJURY (TBI)

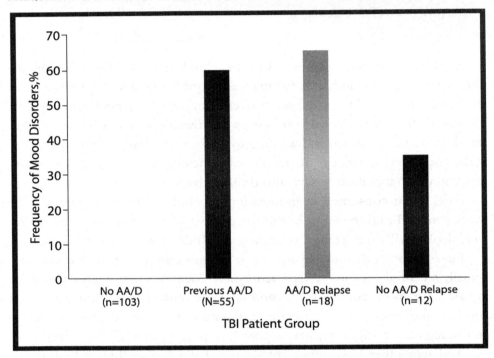

The first two columns show the frequency of mood disorders among patients with or without a history of alcohol abuse and/or dependence (AA/D) during the year before TBI.

The second pair of columns shows the frequency of mood disorders among patients with a history of alcohol abuse and/or dependence who either relapsed or did not relapse into alcohol abuse during the year following TBI.

RELATIONSHIP OF MOOD AND ALCOHOL USE DISORDERS WITH VOCATIONAL OUTCOME

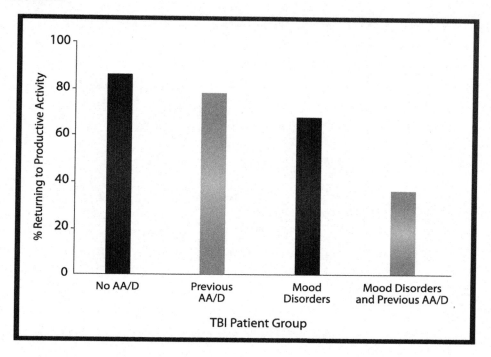

The researchers also concluded, "Previous alcohol abuse increases the risk of developing mood disorders after TBI, and emotional disturbance, in turn, increases the risk of alcohol abuse relapse." As noted in the above chart, patients with a history of alcohol abuse and/or dependence (AA/D) who developed mood disorders during the year following traumatic brain injury (TBI) were least likely to resume a productive life.

CHAPTER 8

TBI ASSESSMENT TOOLS

In This Section

You'll learn about:

- Brain Imaging: particularly SPECT—Single Photon Emission Computer Tomography
- EEG based computerized tools: Brain Network Activation (BNA) testing and Cognison
- Non-EEG based computerized tools: Immediate Post-Concussion Assessment and Cognitive Testing (ImPACT) and ANAM
- On-Field assessment tools– SCAT3, SCRT, VOMS, and more

To get the most out of this section:

At minimum, the On-Field assessment tools can be used in any situation to get a sense of the level of severity of symptoms after head injury. Please do get support from a concussion care specialist for assessment and any necessary treatment if there's ANY concern about the severity of an injury.

Progress is impossible without change; and those who cannot change their minds, cannot change anything.
— George Bernard Shaw

If you're reading this Manual because of your own experience with TBI, you may already have some inner sense of the extent of your injury and the way it has affected you. However, if you haven't had any formal neurological assessment of the health, integrity, and performance of your nervous system, that inner sense is largely subjective. A big reason for this is that we as humans are notoriously lousy at self-assessment. Your own personal assessment may be based on your *perception* of your pre-TBI level of physical and cognitive function, as well as being biased by the frustration of current symptoms and the desire for a speedy, full resolution of the TBI itself. The perceptions and collective memory of friends and family also may come into play. But in the end, how truly accurate are all these perceptions?

There are several layers and levels to the comprehensive neurological assessment for TBI.

1. Neurological examination looking at alertness and orientation, cognition, and overall mental function, balance, coordination, and focal neurological signs of any impairments in function or weakness
2. Neuro-Imaging – taking a look inside the head to evaluate structural and/or functional brain anatomy
3. EEG supported, and non-EEG supported computerized cognitive assessment tools
4. Paper forms – typically clinician directed standardized assessments
5. Mobile App devices for the layperson and clinician to use for acute evaluation and for tracking recovery over time

As with a good portion of medicine, multiple approaches and perspectives add more information from which to make an accurate diagnosis and appropriate treatment plan. So is the case here with the assessment of the injured brain. At present, there is no computerized neurological assessment device that replaces the skilled neurological examination of a trained concussion care clinician, and it is this clinical skill that guides the methodological evaluation of the client at hand. Advanced brain imaging and functional tests have evolved rapidly, and it's now possible to get a truly objective evaluation of your injury status in the present moment (particularly as they are associated with neurological impairments), while also using it to track progress in therapies over time. Offered by specialized head trauma centers and clinics, these assessment technologies can afford you with a more complete and accurate picture.

A brief note on a specific part of the neurological examination - the **Vestibulo-Ocular Motor System**: Persistent vestibulo-ocular motor symptom impairments occur when the areas of the brain connecting balance and coordination to eyesight and visual input are damaged. This can result in common symptoms such as vertigo, dizziness, imbalance, and vision changes. The impairments can be peripheral, affecting the inner ear itself, or central affecting the nervous system. Benign paroxysmal positional vertigo, characterized by acute nystagmus (small eye tracking twitches that occur when the eye follows an object in space), disorientation and nausea, is the most common cause of post-traumatic vestibular dysfunction. Pervasive vesibulo-ocluar symptoms require an appropriate history, visual acuity tests, extra-ocular muscle range of motion, light sensitivity, pupil response, motion sensitivity, and visual field testing. Functional changes in vision may require referral to an opthomologist.

Video nystanography (VNG) is a rapidly growing computerized tool for analyzing guided eye movements while tracking an object in motion. It has been used to support rehabilitation of oculomotility and improve cognitive and general performance in a variety of case reports, and it is expected to further evolve as a potent assessment and treatment modality. However, at present the broad scope research has yet to show proven clinical usefulness in identifying causative lesions, and it does not consistently differentiate between injured patients and healthy controls. Further along in this section we overview the VOMS screening protocol for use in the neurological physical exam assessment and evaluation of TBI.

BRAIN IMAGING

Functional neuroimaging and its recent advances in the last twenty years has been monumental in helping to identify significant abnormalities that contribute to diagnosis, symptoms, prognosis and treatment of TBI. One particular imaging technology—SPECT—stands above the rest. A comprehensive review of functional imaging modalities reported the superiority of Single Photon Emission Computed Tomography (SPECT) over either CT or MRI. While CTs (cat scans) can help identify bony structural impairments (like a skull fracture) and MRI (magnetic resonance imaging) assists in looking at the soft tissue anatomy of the brain, SPECT provides a true 3D image of the brain's metabolic activity as measured by radioactively traced blood flow.

OTHER CONSIDERATIONS:

The continued advances in brain imaging and functional neurological research are promoting further discoveries in the field of TBI recovery on an almost daily basis. Similar to the wide variety of treatments, the wide variety of assessment tools utilized to complement the integrative assessment and treatment of brain trauma is expanding and growing consistently. CT, MRI, computerized assessments, EEG, ERP, and SPECT imaging have become the current cornerstones of evaluation for the injured brain, and they will be added to by yet unforeseen iterations and types of advancements in technology for the ongoing contributions in the wealth of knowledge yet to be uncovered in the field.

SPECT IMAGING

Single Photon Emission Computer Tomography (SPECT)

Benefits:
Provides 3D view of blood flow to different brain regions to help identify areas of impairment, highly accurate and specific.

Drawbacks:
More invasive procedure which requires injection of radioactive substance and nuclear imaging equipment.

Availability:
Limited to specialty clinics.

Cost:
Typically around $3000 - $5000.

SPECT IMAGING

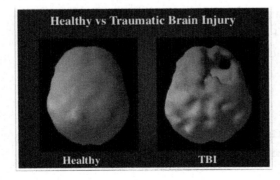

Healthy vs Traumatic Brain Injury

Healthy   TBI

Single Photon Emission Computer Tomography or SPECT is the holy grail of TBI assessment tools, because it provides a clear, three-dimensional view of blood flow to different regions of the brain. It requires the injection of a radioactive substance and the use of sophisticated nuclear imaging equipment to detect that substance within the body and brain. This technology creates supremely colorful anatomical pictures used to highlight regions of the brain that are significantly impaired in function.

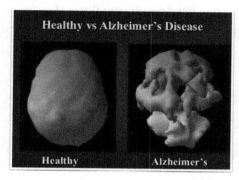

Healthy vs Alzheimer's Disease

Healthy   Alzheimer's

Dr. Daniel Amen is a pioneer in the use of SPECT imaging for brain injury, PTSD, depression, and other conditions. He operates several SPECT clinics in the U.S. and has been using this technology for more than 25 years. He also maintains the largest brain-mapping library in the world, with more than 100,000 scans, a few of which are shown here.

As you can see above, the healthy brain appears to have well-distributed blood flow, while the other brains have obvious detriments. These "holes" are more functional than structural (i.e. thankfully, there aren't literal holes in the brain). Looking at these two examples, the TBI brain shows poor flow to the right frontal lobe, and the brain of the advanced Alzheimer's patient shows an obvious and diffuse, significant number of holes, indicating more global system impairment in multiple lobes and areas.

While these images are impressive, SPECT scanning also provides promising clinical utility as a longitudinal measure for assessment over time. Its high specificity and positive predictive values correlate well with follow up assessments, and its negative predictive value approaches 100 percent, meaning it hardly ever shows something that is not there. As a result, it provides excellent accuracy as a reliable tool to discriminate brain trauma and PCS (post-concussive syndrome) from other clinical diagnosis where a client may have similar symptoms to concussion but in reality has something else going on.

As mentioned before, and as with any tool discussed here for assessment, its value becomes magnified when used as a part of a comprehensive plan evaluating progress over time. However, unique to SPECT in this case is its supremely colorful neuro-anatomical images. We humans receive about 80 percent of the information they take in through visual cues, and clients often appreciate the views of progress that SPECT offers, while treatment providers appreciate the high degree of sensitivity in marking functional changes to literally *see* how the brain is responding to treatment. The downsides are that it's relatively uncommonly used at present, being utilized in highly specialized clinics and it is more expensive than traditional scanning techniques.

The SPECT imaging process takes a couple of hours and can cost between $3000 - $5000.

HEADS UP! If you are pregnant or nursing, consult your doctor before under-going SPECT imaging.

EEG SUPPORTED TESTING

EEG guided cognitive evaluations - BNA (Brain Network Activation) and Cognison

Benefits:
Provides quantitative, highly accurate, objective data about functional status at time of assessment and for ongoing recovery progress.

Drawbacks:
No obvious risks are associated.

Availability:
Typically available in major metropolitan areas and brain clinics.

Cost:
$200 to $250 per 30-minute session.

Computerized neuropsychological testing is an increasingly popular primary method of assessing concussions in the global arena of sports, particularly at the college and professional levels. Its sophistication, plus relative ease of use and expanding availability is making it more widely appreciated throughout the sports world. There are a number of advantages to computerized testing including the large amount of information obtained electronically, reduction of administrative costs, the gathering of baseline cognitive data, and the ability to measure time sensitive tasks, such as reaction time.

A potential challenge with computerized testing is that baseline assessments may not be a full and totally accurate representation of the athletes' neurological skills and abilities. So, as mentioned before, each assessment has strengths and limitations, and determining the utility of information from computerized testing in determining "return-to-play" recommendations remains a major part of the art, science and practice of neurological recovery oriented physicians and practitioners.

Brain Network Activation (BNA) testing uses electroencephalography (EEG) and special software to assess the brain state and brain changes over time by tracking evoked related potentials (ERPs). You may recall that EEG is a non-invasive technology that measures the brain's electrical activity with a series of small sensors placed on the outside of the scalp. During BNA testing, the patient wears a snug head covering made up of hundreds of these sensors. As the patient completes specific cognitive exercises, the sensors record the brain's responses as ERPs and create a kind of heat map of brain function.

This emerging neurophysiologic objective tool gives considerable insight into actual synaptic function, as ERPs are measured electrical responses to specific sensory, cognitive, or motor events. More specifically, this type of testing uses a classic "two-oddball" paradigm to measure changes in electrical potential where the subject attends to an auditory *target tone* followed by affirmatively responding with a button click, while ignoring *non-target tones* without a button click response. Insights into synaptic activity can be correlated with this test in auditory attention by measuring the electrical potentials time locked to the auditory tone. Further useful measures are geared more specifically to performance, such as reaction time and button click accuracy. Current studies using ERP as a diagnostic and assessment tool for TBI show superiority over EEG alone, with good test-retest reliability. There have been proposals for specific markers for cognitive dysfunction resulting from TBI, and while more research is required for their validation, early results are promising.[405]

Developed by ElMindA, one of the companies behind the technology, "the BNA algorithms use innovative sets of signal processing and pattern recognition techniques to seek and map activated neural pathways in task-related data points with respect to time, location, amplitude and frequency. By projecting the individual data points into clusters, BNA reveals three-dimensional images of Brain Network Activation patterns (or BNAs in short) which represent high resolution functional neural pathways."[406]

The FDA has cleared BNA testing for use in adolescents and young adults, and some physicians now rely on BNA testing when deciding when a TBI patient may safely return to sports and other activities. It's also become increasingly common for professional athletes to undergo BNA testing before starting each new season. This enables them to establish baseline maps of their brains' normal functionality. Should an athlete sustain a head injury during the season, he then would undergo additional BNA testing, and his physician would compare the new results with the original baseline map to gauge which neural networks the injury has affected and to what degree. Periodic BNA testing is also used during an injured athlete's recovery as a quantitative monitor of overall progress.

Even if you don't have a baseline map of your brain's pre-injury level of function, you can still use BNA testing to track your recovery and offer insights about the effectiveness of a particular course of treatment. The average BNA test session takes about 30 minutes and costs between $200 and $250.

Another similar tool in the advancement of QEEG and ERP analysis is the Cognison made by Neuronetrix. It too has started to become popular in a similar utilization manner for baseline cognitive testing prior to injury, as well as testing post injury to assess present state limitations and obtain baseline information for monitoring progress over time. Companies, such as Neuronetrix who make the Cognison, are manufacturing these battery-powered EEG headsets with built in ERP protocols, all of which can be transported by a small briefcase. Collecting EEG activity was once limited to highly specialized technicians with costly and cumbersome equipment. Now EEGs can be recorded in the field, with data captured and uploaded wirelessly. The ease of portability of these technologies, along with the down trending cost of purchase and growing wide spread use will continue to support the accumulation of more concussion related data, and thus continue to advance the field of TBI associated rehabilitation medicine.

NON-EEG-BASED COMPUTERIZED ASSESSMENTS

Non-EEG based computerized assessments – ImPACT (Immediate Post-Concussion Assessment and Cognitive Testing) and ANAM (Automated Neuro-psychological Assessment Measures developed by the Army)

Benefits:
Provides quantitative, objective data about ongoing recovery progress, easier to use, less expensive than EEG-based.

Drawbacks:
Not as specific as EEG based testing.

Availability:
Widely available across the country.

Cost:
$10 – $20 per exam.

Immediate Post-Concussion Assessment and Cognitive Testing, also known as ImPACT, is perhaps the most affordable of the advanced TBI assessment tools mentioned in this section. It is a comprehensive, computerized test, which measures current symptoms, verbal and visual memory, cognitive processing speeds, reaction times, and impulse control. On average, testing costs around $20 and the test takes about an hour to complete.

Test-takers begin by entering basic descriptive information such as height, weight, and details about any prior head injuries and cognitive impairments. Next, they answer questions about their health status, including the date they sustained their injuries, amount of sleep they've recently had and what medications they may be taking. They also rate the severity of more than 20 concussion symptoms.

Up next are the neurocognitive test modules, including "Word Discrimination," "Design Memory," "X's and O's," "Symbol Matching," "Color Match," and "Three Letter Memory."[407] In addition to measuring attention processes, "Word Discrimination" and "Design Memory" evaluate verbal and visual recognition memory, respectively. The "X's and O's" module tracks visual working memory and visual processing speeds. Visual processing speed, learning and memory are further assessed via the "Symbol Matching" module. The "Color Match" portion gauges reaction time, impulse control and response inhibition, and the "Three Letter Memory" task measures working memory and visual-motor response speeds.

Test-takers then get standardized scores for verbal and visual memory, cognitive processing speed, reaction time and impulse control. Like the other TBI assessment tools, ImPACT results can be used for monitoring overall cognitive recovery and evaluating the effectiveness of individual treatment methods. To find a credentialed ImPACT consultant near you, visit www.impacttest.com/findcareprovider.

ON-FIELD AND AT-HOME PAPER FORM ASSESSMENTS:

> **On-Field & At-Home Testing – Paper forms (SCAT3, SCRT, PCSS), Mobile Apps (CRR and CAR), Eye specific exams (VOMS and King-Devick), Novel assessment devices (Infrascanner)**
>
> Benefits:
> Ability to use quickly on-site and in the field, leading to more immediate triage, more immediate treatment leads to improved outcomes.
>
> Drawbacks:
> Some are practitioner oriented and others require some basic training.
>
> Availability:
> Widely available for immediate use.
>
> Cost:
> Variable depending on test; many are free.

While there is no substitute for a proper neurological examination, the tools overviewed in this section have provided considerable support for on-field assessments. With greater accuracy in triage management for acute concussion comes improved immediate care treatment and ultimately better overall outcomes. The **SCAT3** (Sports Concussion Assessment Tool) is a clinician directed assessment battery developed from the Zurich 2008 3rd International Commission on Concussion in Sports. It clinical validity has been verified throughout the sports arena for use in teenagers and adults, and it's been formally adopted by many of the bigger international sports agencies including the Olympic Committee and the hockey, rugby and soccer federations. There is also a SCAT3 for children that is more age specific to kids 5 – 12 years old. The pocket **SCRT** (Sports Concussion Recognition Tool) is a similar assessment tool that is non-clinician based and to be used by the average person when a qualified and trained clinician using the SCAT3 is not available. Lastly, there is a **PCSS** (Post-Concussive Symptom Scale), which is a basic self-report measure that can be used as a baseline measure and over-time comparative to assess improvement in symptoms. See the Resources Section at the end of the Manual for more information on the On-Field and At-Home Assessment tools.

MOBILE DEVICE APPS:

In the digital age of the "quantified self," it makes sense that there would be a growing number of at home assessment tools available for mobile app devices. There are a growing number of these, and one of the more popular ones that is free, quite in depth and easy to use is the **CRR** – Concussion Recognition and Response. It gives guidelines for ACE (Acute Concussion Evaluation) in the home and school setting, gives basic information about concussions and answers questions from the parent and coach perspective. While some of these instructions are geared more for parents of children that may have had a concussion, it is good information for the adult assessment too. There is also a paid $5 version by the same makers of the CRR. This one is the **CAR** – Concussion Assessment and Response. It gives more in depth look at personal cognitive function through evaluation tools, as well as a Return to Play guide.

SPECIALIZED NEUROLOGICAL EXAMINATION FOR VISUAL PATHWAYS

In addition to the more comprehensive medical examination of acute brain injury, there is one more particular clinician-driven neurological exam focus that provides a high degree of sensitivity for brain trauma. Using the **VOMS** (Vestibular Ocular-Motor Screening) augments current methods for assessment as it specifically assesses the integrated functions of balance, vision and movement. The vestibular (balance) system is associated with the inner ear function and it has a direct relationship to the ocular-motor (eye movement) function of the brain connected to performance tracking of objects moving in space and the body's associated, coordinated movement. The five main areas of V-O system testing include: smooth pursuits, saccades (rapid eye movements), horizontal vestibular ocular reflex, visual motion sensitivity, and near point-of-convergence sensitivity. As mentioned previously in the Manual, the vast majority of concussions resolve in a few weeks (approximately 75 – 80 percent), and interestingly those that continue into chronic TBI related symptoms often have a VOM component.[408]

Another visual specific test that has been adopted by many teams at the level of high school to professional athletics as a remove-from-play tool is the **King-Devick**. It's a two-minute test that screens for saccades (eye movements), attention, and focus/concentration by having the athlete read single digit numbers displayed on an iPad or paper tablet. The on-field test time is used in comparison to the athlete's previous baseline time to completion, and if there's significant delay in response time then removal from play is recommended along with a further acute-care assessment by a concussion care specialist.[409]

NOVEL ASSESSMENT TOOLS

One particular novel tool of note is the handheld **Infrascanner**. It has been used with increasing frequency on the field, on the sidelines, and in the locker rooms to assess internal head bleeding and therefore, help to direct more appropriate critical care measures, especially when head imaging (CT, MRI, fMRI, SPECT) is not available. This device, developed by the Office of Naval Research, uses near infra-red light held on preselected cranial points for about 10 seconds each in order to differentiate between pooled and circulating blood. A separate unit in the development phase from the NIH (National Institute for Health) is a bit different in that it moves continuously over the skull and uses a noise signal in recognition of changes in blood volume in and around the dura (the protective membrane covering the brain), as well as distinguishing between three different types of hemoglobin to assess the time signature (acute vs. chronic) of any bleeds. These particular units highlight the burgeoning field of in-hand, on-field brain injury assessment tools that will continue to support advancement in the field of acute concussion management.

CHAPTER 9

PUTTING IT ALL TOGETHER

In This Section

You'll learn about:

- *Big 5* — to Do, Take, and Avoid — Immediately after a concussion
- Identifying your symptom baselines
  - Creating your own TBI treatment protocol
  - Monitoring and analyzing your progress
- Top 10 Rules of Engagement

In order to get the most out of this chapter, read through all the worksheets, print them out to have on hand and make it interactive. The more engaging the process of recovery becomes, the more you'll be able to get out of the information provided in the Manual.

There is a difference between knowing the path and walking the path.
— *Morpheus, the Matrix*

By now you've familiarized yourself with the TBI treatment tools and techniques I outlined in the first eight chapters of this *Concussion Repair Manual*. If so, I expect by knowing more about all the options that the growing field of integrative medical neurology has to offer, you will gain a modicum of both inspiration and empowerment to support your healing journey ahead. And now it's time to put it all into action.

For some of you, taking the next steps will include seeking an advanced TBI assessment (as outlined in Chapter 9) from a specialized practitioner or head trauma center. It cannot be stated enough, that I highly recommend this degree of formal assessment for anyone suspecting a clinically significant TBI has taken place, recently or in the distant past. After undergoing functional testing and brain mapping, you'll have greater detail about the extent of your injury and any associated impairments you will choose address. Both you and your primary care doctor will then use this information as you plan and manage your TBI treatment together.

In this chapter, we will go over the top five things to do immediately after a suspected concussion or TBI. You'll also learn how to establish a symptom severity baseline, identify the symptoms you wish to tackle first, and systematically track your recovery progress using the Comprehensive Symptoms Log. And by regularly using the diet, sleep, exercise, and other logging worksheets provided, you'll also be able to establish and continually refine your own personalized TBI treatment protocol.

Finally, I'll leave you with the Top 10 Rules of Engagement that I developed during my own recovery. They have also served as a support for countless clients along their own healing paths, and I believe they will benefit you too.

HEADS UP! You shouldn't put your own TBI treatment protocol together until you have been fully evaluated and stabilized in a medical environment. When you do begin evaluating new therapies, tools and techniques, do so only with the awareness, support and supervision of a local physician or primary care provider, ideally one skilled in properly assessing working with TBI.

TO DO, TAKE & AVOID CHECKLIST IMMEDIATELY AFTER A SUSPECTED TBI OR CONCUSSION

TO DO:

1. Get a thorough examination by a medically trained concussion care specialist ASAP
   a. Neurological exam to include physical exam, VOMS and CBCs
      1. VOMS – vestibular oculo-motor system
      2. CBCs – cognition, balance and coordination
   b. Brain Imaging - Severity of concussion related symptoms will dictate necessity
   c. BCT – *baseline cognitive testing* to measure baseline functional status, and, if a post-concussion care plan is implemented, this can serve as a comparative for progress assessment
2. REST and optimize healthy sleep patterns
3. FLOAT – Floatation tank therapy
4. Consider acupressure and/or acupuncture with someone experienced in TBI Rx
5. Ketogenic diet – primarily for the neurological benefit

TO TAKE:

1. Glutathione – major brain antioxidant and reparative factors
2. Vitamin D – neuro-protectant, anti-inflammatory
3. Melatonin – anti-oxidant hormone, helps to establish healthy circadian cycles
4. CBD – neuro-protectant and antioxidant
5. Curcumin – anti-inflammatory, neuro-protectant, promotes plasticity and growth factors

TO AVOID:

1. ANY kind of contact sports, especially involving the head. Return to play ONLY after full clearance by a concussion care specialist. Avoid any more TBIs in the future!
2. High sugar diet
3. Stress – physical or emotional
4. Bright light/loud noise/excessive EMF (ex. cell phones, computer work, video gaming)
5. Excessive pain meds (the potential sedative effects of these meds can mask the underlying symptoms of post concussive altered states of awareness and cognition)

ESTABLISHING SYMPTOM BASELINES

Your symptom severity baseline is the map you'll refer to again and again during your TBI recovery journey. In the beginning, you'll use it to identify each of your symptoms and measure their severity on a scale of 0 to 10. This, subsequently, will help you to prioritize which areas of healing you will choose to focus on first.

To get started, you'll need to complete the **Comprehensive Symptoms Log.** Take plenty of time to consider each of the symptoms listed in the "Cognitive," "Physical," "Mood," and "Social" sections. If you aren't experiencing a particular symptom, give it a "0" score. For each symptom that you *are* experiencing, you'll enter a score between 1 and 10, depending on its severity. You will score mild symptoms between 1 and 3, moderate symptoms from 4 to 6 and severe symptoms between 7 and 10. Here are some guidelines to help you:

The scores you enter for each symptom will serve as your initial point of reference. Together, they make up your baseline functioning, similar to a "You are Here" marker on a map.

MILD 1 – 3	MODERATE 4 – 6	SEVERE 7 – 10
1—very mild 2—somewhat mild 3—mild	4—moderate but tolerable 5—moderate 6—less moderate/interferes with day-to-day life	7—somewhat severe 8—severe 9—very severe 10—debilitating/nearly debilitating

CREATING YOUR TREATMENT PROTOCOL

Once you've established your baseline, you can begin creating your personalized TBI treatment protocol. First, isolate the symptoms on your Comprehensive Symptoms Log that have the highest severity scores and choose five of these to start with.

Armed with your list of initial target symptoms, go back through Chapters 1 through 8 to see which TBI treatment approaches are the most available, well suited, and matched for your needs. This can be tricky at first and takes some personal research on your part, getting a sense of which ones make "sense" to you or just seem to "fit" for any reason. This is also where it can be helpful to have a guide or someone with experience in one or more of these modalities give you their impression on whether or not a given approach is a good "match" for you. Generally, the first couple of therapies included in each chapter are the ones that I feel most strongly about and tend to recommend to someone as a starting point. Some of these are my top picks because my own clients and patients saw results with them more quickly and robustly, while others are at the top because I know through research that they're relatively safe and already helped a ton of people.

As we have mentioned many times up to this point… *everybody is different*, and what works well for one person might not work as well for you. So, when selecting treatments for yourself, be realistic about the amount of time, effort, and money you are willing (and able) to spend. Also, keep in mind that certain therapies might not be available where you live.

After deciding which TBI treatments you want to try, you will then choose which one (or multiple) of them to try first. And, while trying out that one therapy, plan to give it a solid month to work. You'll also be getting into the habit of logging your symptoms and scoring their severity every day. Once the 30-day trial period ends, you can then analyze your data to determine whether or not that therapeutic tool or technique has helped you. If it hasn't helped, discontinue it and test a different therapy for the next 30 days. Notably, the areas included in the section on "Things to Avoid" can generally all be done concurrently, as well as those under the heading Foods to Utilize.

In time, you may find that some of the symptoms you initially targeted have significantly improved or disappeared altogether. When that happens, you can work on lowering the severity scores for some of the *next* high-scoring symptoms on your list. Systematically continue to look at the top 5 high-scoring symptoms, trying different therapies and monitoring your responses to them. Stick with this process until the severity of each of your symptoms has been reduced to a score of 0, 1, or 2.

In addition to the Comprehensive Symptoms Log, at the end of the chapter you'll find some supplemental logging worksheets to help you monitor your sleep architecture, activity levels and diet.

QUICK TIP Make several blank copies of the Comprehensive Symptoms Log and other personal assessment worksheets included here, so that you'll have plenty to use as you apply and monitor your TBI treatment plan.

TOP 10 RULES OF ENGAGEMENT

As I mentioned earlier, following these 10 guidelines has helped me personally and many of my clients, patients, friends, and family. They are not only for guiding and supporting the recovery from TBI or concussion; these guidelines are also applicable for the healing process in rehabilitation of just about any acute or chronic condition. I'm confident that by following these Top 10 Rules of Engagement, you'll also make better progress in your recovery.

And if you *really* take them to heart on your path to healing? In time, you might not simply *regain* each of the abilities you had lost as a result of your injury. You just might discover you've *surpassed* your pre-TBI levels of cognitive or physical function in the process.

1. Be curious

Scientific and medical research evolves quickly, so you should do your best to stay up to date. Websites like sciencedaily.com and eurekalert.org are good examples of places to investigate and keep up with new developments.

2. Stack therapies

Once you determine which tools and techniques from each chapter are most beneficial for you, you may want to use two, three, or even more of them simultaneously. Layering multiple therapies in this way can help you target your symptoms more aggressively and efficiently, but also be mindful. Not all therapies work well with one another. When adding techniques, try to do so one at a time with a week or more in between so that you can have a better sense of what is creating any change (better or worse), and therefore be a better detective in maximizing benefits while minimizing the complexity of the entire treatment protocol.

3. Remember, the first 1 or 2 in each chapter are likely the best places to start

When evaluating new TBI therapies, I weigh several criteria, including potential efficacy, risk-benefit ratios, clinical track record, practicality, availability, cost, and ease of use. And, as a general rule, *the first 1 or 2 therapies* mentioned in each chapter are usually the ones I believe to be the most promising. These are therapies that I've personally observed to be the most effective for the largest numbers of people or which appear to have particular efficacy within a short period of time.

4. Start with symptoms and severity

Before you try any of the therapies in this Manual, you should first establish your symptom baselines. Having a clear understanding of your symptoms and their severity levels will help you decide which symptoms you actively wish to target first and which therapies to use along the way.

5. Give it 30 days

Determining whether a new therapy (or therapies) benefits you often takes time. As a result, I recommend about 30 days when trying a new tool or technique. Yes, sticking with it for a solid month and staying disciplined about tracking your response to the therapy during this 30-day evaluation period can take a lot of patience, and I can understand the desire to move through the trial period more quickly. This has to be a personal choice. I am specifically being a bit more judicious in the time recommendation here, so as to encourage more specific personal investigation into the benefit of the protocol. When you're working with a skilled treatment provider who knows how these technologies work together, the likelihood of choosing complimentary methods that "play well together" goes up, so the process can therefore be streamlined.

6. Keep moving

Once a 30-day evaluation period is up, analyze your data. If you failed to see significant benefit from a particular treatment, discontinue it and begin a new 30-day trial for another therapy.

7. Maximize methods that work

When you notice benefits from a therapeutic activity, step up your intensity. For instance, if you were receiving a certain treatment once or twice a *month*, you might bump that up to once or twice a *week*. And, in the case of dietary supplements and nootropics that are giving you good results? If you aren't already taking the maximum dosage, consider increasing to the maximum, if it is safe to do so.

8. Find the right fit

Conflict with your healthcare providers and practitioners can be an added source of stress. Your doctor's attitude towards you—and your feelings about your doctor and his or her methods—can even affect your treatment outcomes. Think of it a bit like dating. You don't necessarily marry the first person you go on a date with, nor would you do so after only one date. If the fit is not a good one after a few visits and you don't see eye-to-eye, move on and find someone new.

9. Everyone is unique

Every TBI survivor is unique, and each individual's recovery is a highly personal journey. As best you can, try to avoid comparing yourself to others, and, instead, focus on your own progress. Looking over your original symptom baselines, highlight your areas of improvement and celebrate! Be grateful for any of the "small victories" along the way. They will accumulate over time and add up to monumental ones.

10. Keep the Faith!!!

There is no methodology stronger than faith. Period. So do all that you can to keep yours strong. Maintaining a strong belief in your own capacity to heal is *critical* to the mission. Should doubt about your progress creep in, seek inspiration and encouragement from trusted sources, including support groups, family and friends. Also try to avoid those who may instill doubt or pessimism, lest one rotten apple spoiling the whole bunch.

Everything can be taken from a man but one thing: the last of the great human freedoms — to choose one's attitude in any given set of circumstances, to choose one's own way.
— Viktor Frankl

WORKBOOK SECTION

How to best use the provided tracking sheets below
in this Workbook Section:

Below are worksheets for tracking your symptom recovery over a 30 day period. These sheets cover the most common symptoms in the areas of — cognition, body, mood, relationships and sleep. You can make the process even more personal by writing in your own target symptoms at the bottom of the worksheets and following those. Print out or copy as many additional sheets as is necessary to cover the entirety of your healing process.

For each of the symptoms listed, enter a score between 1 and 10. See the severity scale below for guidance. If you aren't experiencing a particular symptom, give it a "0" score.

Remember, for the majority of people it's easiest to track the "Top 5" most severe or bothersome symptoms over the 30 day period. And if you prefer, you can always choose to follow more. Adapt the process to make it work best for you. If you don't track it, you won't know.

To assist in tracking symptoms you may also choose to use one of several popular brain training mobile apps (such as Lumosity, Peak or Elevate - subscription based from the internet). They help assess baseline cognitive measures that can be followed over the course of your personalized Recovery Regimen.

Also included is an Activities Log. There you can track all of your major and consistent daily activities so as to follow progress and gauge progressive change (ex. exercise / endurance or work / focused productivity).
You can also use this section to track your treatment days and which ones you used (ex. Day 1: floatation - 1 hour; body weight training - 30 min; music meditation - 20 min at night).

Lastly, there is a Nutrition & Supplementation Log to help you track and correlate these with the fluctuation and improvement of your target symptoms.

MILD 1 – 3	MODERATE 4 – 6	SEVERE 7 – 10
1—very mild 2—somewhat mild 3—mild	4—moderate but tolerable 5—moderate 6—less moderate/interferes with day-to-day life	7—somewhat severe 8—severe 9—very severe 10—debilitating/nearly debilitating

COGNITIVE SYMPTOMS

Enter severity scores for each symptom. Use extra rows to track any additional cognitive symptoms you're experiencing

	DAY 1	DAY 2	DAY 3	DAY 4	DAY 5	DAY 6	DAY 7
Enter date and/or day of week here							
Problems with memory							
Poor attention/ concentration							
Poor reasoning/ problem-solving							
Poor planning/ organizational skills							
Poor reading, writing and/or speaking							

COGNITIVE SYMPTOMS

Enter severity scores for each symptom. Use extra rows to track any
additional cognitive symptoms you're experiencing

	DAY 8	DAY 9	DAY 10	DAY 11	DAY 12	DAY 13	DAY 14
nter date and/or ay of week here							
roblems with memory							
or attention/ oncentration							
or reasoning/ oblem-solving							
or planning/ ganizational skills							
or reading, writing d/or speaking							

COGNITIVE SYMPTOMS

Enter severity scores for each symptom. Use extra rows to track any
additional cognitive symptoms you're experiencing

	DAY 15	DAY 16	DAY 17	DAY 18	DAY 19	DAY 20	DAY 2
Enter date and/or day of week here							
Problems with memory							
Poor attention/ concentration							
Poor reasoning/ problem-solving							
Poor planning/ organizational skills							
Poor reading, writing and/or speaking							

COGNITIVE SYMPTOMS

Enter severity scores for each symptom. Use extra rows to track any
additional cognitive symptoms you're experiencing

	DAY 22	DAY 23	DAY 24	DAY 25	DAY 26	DAY 27	DAY 28
Enter date and/or day of week here							
Problems with memory							
Poor attention/ concentration							
Poor reasoning/ problem-solving							
Poor planning/ organizational skills							
Poor reading, writing and/or speaking							

COGNITIVE SYMPTOMS

Enter severity scores for each symptom. Use extra rows to track any additional cognitive symptoms you're experiencing

	DAY 29	DAY 30	DAY 31
Enter date and/or day of week here			
Problems with memory			
Poor attention/ concentration			
Poor reasoning/ problem-solving			
Poor planning/ organizational skills			
Poor reading, writing and/or speaking			

PHYSICAL SYMPTOMS

Enter severity scores for each symptom. Use extra rows to track any physical symptoms you're experiencing

	DAY 1	DAY 2	DAY 3	DAY 4	DAY 5	DAY 6	DAY 7
Enter date and/or day of week here							
Headaches							
Dizziness							
Poor balance and/or coordination							
Sensitivity to light							
Insomnia and/or poor sleep quality							
Low energy levels/ feelings of fatigue							
Decreased libido							
Poor appetite and/ or digestive problems							
Reduced muscle strength							

PHYSICAL SYMPTOMS

Enter severity scores for each symptom. Use extra rows to track any physical symptoms you're experiencing

	DAY 8	DAY 9	DAY 10	DAY 11	DAY 12	DAY 13	DAY 1
Enter date and/or day of week here							
Headaches							
Dizziness							
Poor balance and/or coordination							
Sensitivity to light							
Insomnia and/or poor sleep quality							
Low energy levels/ feelings of fatigue							
Deereased libido							
Poor appetite and/ or digestive problems							
Reduced muscle strength							

PHYSICAL SYMPTOMS

Enter severity scores for each symptom. Use extra rows to track any physical symptoms you're experiencing

	DAY 15	DAY 16	DAY 17	DAY 18	DAY 19	DAY 20	DAY 21
Enter date and/or day of week here							
Headaches							
Dizziness							
Poor balance and/or coordination							
Sensitivity to light							
Insomnia and/or poor sleep quality							
Low energy levels/ feelings of fatigue							
Deereased libido							
Poor appetite and/ or digestive problems							
Reduced muscle strength							

PHYSICAL SYMPTOMS

Enter severity scores for each symptom. Use extra rows to track any physical symptoms you're experiencing

	DAY 22	DAY 23	DAY 24	DAY 25	DAY 26	DAY 27	DAY 28
Enter date and/or day of week here							
Headaches							
Dizziness							
Poor balance and/or coordination							
Sensitivity to light							
Insomnia and/or poor sleep quality							
Low energy levels/ feelings of fatigue							
Deereased libido							
Poor appetite and/ or digestive problems							
Reduced muscle strength							

PHYSICAL SYMPTOMS

Enter severity scores for each symptom. Use extra rows to track any physical symptoms you're experiencing

	DAY 29	DAY 30	DAY 31
nter date and/or ay of week here			
eadaches			
izziness			
oor balance and/ coordination			
ensitivity to ht			
somnia and/or or sleep quality			
ow energy levels/ elings of fatigue			
ecreased libido			
oor appetite and/ digestive oblems			
educed muscle rength			

MOOD SYMPTOMS

Enter severity scores for each symptom. Use extra rows to track any additional mood-related symptoms you're experiencing

	DAY 1	DAY 2	DAY 3	DAY 4	DAY 5	DAY 6	DAY 7
Depression and/or hopelessness							
Low motivation							
Mood swings							
Anxiety							
Irritability							
Hypervigilance/ PTSD							
Poor impulse control							
Agitation and/or combativeness							

MOOD SYMPTOMS

Enter severity scores for each symptom. Use extra rows to track any additional mood-related symptoms you're experiencing

	DAY 8	DAY 9	DAY 10	DAY 11	DAY 12	DAY 13	DAY 14
Depression and/or hopelessness							
Low motivation							
Mood swings							
Anxiety							
Irritability							
Hypervigilance/PTSD							
Poor impulse control							
Agitation and/or combativeness							

MOOD SYMPTOMS

Enter severity scores for each symptom. Use extra rows to track any additional mood-related symptoms you're experiencing

	DAY 15	DAY 16	DAY 17	DAY 18	DAY 19	DAY 20	DAY 21
Depression and/or hopelessness							
Low motivation							
Mood swings							
Anxiety							
Irritability							
Hypervigilance/ PTSD							
Poor impulse control							
Agitation and/or combativeness							

MOOD SYMPTOMS

Enter severity scores for each symptom. Use extra rows to track any additional mood-related symptoms you're experiencing

	DAY 22	DAY 23	DAY 24	DAY 25	DAY 26	DAY 27	DAY 28
epression and/or opelessness							
ow motivation							
ood swings							
nxiety							
itability							
pervigilance/ SD							
or impulse ntrol							
itation and/or mbativeness							

MOOD SYMPTOMS

Enter severity scores for each symptom. Use extra rows to track any additional mood-related symptoms you're experiencing

	DAY 29	DAY 30	DAY 31
Depression and/or hopelessness			
Low motivation			
Mood swings			
Anxiety			
Irritability			
Hypervigilance/ PTSD			
Poor impulse control			
Agitation and/or combativeness			

SOCIAL SYMPTOMS

Enter severity scores for each symptom. Use extra rows to track any additional social symptoms you're experiencing

	DAY 1	DAY 2	DAY 3	DAY 4	DAY 5	DAY 6	DAY 7
Enter date and/or day of week here							
Desire to isolate myself							
Problems experiencing/ expressing emotions							
Difficulty maintaining relationships							
Frequent arguments							

SOCIAL SYMPTOMS

Enter severity scores for each symptom. Use extra rows to track any additional social symptoms you're experiencing

	DAY 8	DAY 9	DAY 10	DAY 11	DAY 12	DAY 13	DAY 14
Enter date and/or day of week here							
Desire to isolate myself							
Problems experiencing/ expressing emotions							
Difficulty maintaining relationships							
Frequent arguments							

SOCIAL SYMPTOMS

Enter severity scores for each symptom. Use extra rows to track any additional social symptoms you're experiencing

	DAY 15	DAY 16	DAY 17	DAY 18	DAY 19	DAY 20	DAY 21
nter date and/or y of week here							
esire to late myself							
oblems periencing/ pressing notions							
fficulty aintaining ationships							
equent guments							

SOCIAL SYMPTOMS

Enter severity scores for each symptom. Use extra rows to track any additional social symptoms you're experiencing

	DAY 22	DAY 23	DAY 24	DAY 25	DAY 26	DAY 27	DAY 28
Enter date and/or day of week here							
Desire to isolate myself							
Problems experiencing/ expressing emotions							
Difficulty maintaining relationships							
Frequent arguments							

SOCIAL SYMPTOMS

Enter severity scores for each symptom. Use extra rows to track any additional social symptoms you're experiencing

	DAY 29	DAY 30	DAY 31
Enter date and/or day of week here			
Desire to isolate myself			
Problems experiencing/ expressing emotions			
Difficulty maintaining relationships			
Frequent arguments			

SLEEP SCHEDULE AND HABITS

	DAY 1	DAY 2	DAY 3	DAY 4	DAY 5	DAY 6	DAY 7
Enter date and/or day of week here							
I went to bed last night at:	_____a.m./ _____p.m		_____a.m./ _____p.m		_____a.m./ _____p.m		_____a.m. _____p.m
Number of times sleep was disturbed:							
I woke up this morning at:	_____a.m./ _____p.m		_____a.m./ _____p.m		_____a.m./ _____p.m		_____a.m. _____p.m
Number of hours slept:							
Number of naps taken today:							
Total duration of nap(s)	_____hr _____min		_____hr _____min		_____hr _____min		_____hr _____mir

SLEEP SCHEDULE AND HABITS

	DAY 8	DAY 9	DAY 10	DAY 11	DAY 12	DAY 13	DAY 14
nter date and/or ay of week here							
vent to bed st night at:	_____a.m./ _____p.m		_____a.m./ _____p.m		_____a.m./ _____p.m		_____a.m./ _____p.m
umber of times sleep as disturbed:							
voke up this orning at:	_____a.m./ _____p.m		_____a.m./ _____p.m		_____a.m./ _____p.m		_____a.m./ _____p.m
mber of hours pt:							
mber of naps en today:							
al duration nap(s)	_____hr _____min		_____hr _____min		_____hr _____min		_____hr _____min

SLEEP SCHEDULE AND HABITS

	DAY 15	DAY 16	DAY 17	DAY 18	DAY 19	DAY 20	DAY 21
Enter date and/or day of week here							
I went to bed last night at:	____a.m./ ____p.m		____a.m./ ____p.m		____a.m./ ____p.m		____a.m./ ____p.m
Number of times sleep was disturbed:							
I woke up this morning at:	____a.m./ ____p.m		____a.m./ ____p.m		____a.m./ ____p.m		____a.m./ ____p.m
Number of hours slept:							
Number of naps taken today:							
Total duration of nap(s)	____hr ____min		____hr ____min		____hr ____min		____hr ____min

SLEEP SCHEDULE AND HABITS

	DAY 22	DAY 23	DAY 24	DAY 25	DAY 26	DAY 27	DAY 28
Enter date and/or day of week here							
I went to bed last night at:	_____a.m./ _____p.m		_____a.m./ _____p.m		_____a.m./ _____p.m		_____a.m./ _____p.m
Number of times sleep was disturbed:							
I woke up this morning at:	_____a.m./ _____p.m		_____a.m./ _____p.m		_____a.m./ _____p.m		_____a.m./ _____p.m
Number of hours slept:							
Number of naps taken today:							
Total duration of nap(s)	_____hr _____min		_____hr _____min		_____hr _____min		_____hr _____min

SLEEP SCHEDULE AND HABITS

	DAY 29	DAY 30	DAY 31
Enter date and/or day of week here			
I went to bed last night at:	_____a.m./ _____p.m		_____a.m./ _____p.m
Number of times sleep was disturbed:			
I woke up this morning at:	_____a.m./ _____p.m		_____a.m./ _____p.m
Number of hours slept:			
Number of naps taken today:			
Total duration of nap(s)	_____hr _____min		_____hr _____min

SLEEP SYMPTOMS

Enter severity scores for each symptom. Use extra rows to track any additional sleep-related symptoms you're experiencing

	DAY 1	DAY 2	DAY 3	DAY 4	DAY 5	DAY 6	DAY 7
Enter date and/or day of week here							
Insomnia							
Problems staying asleep at night							
Difficulty waking up							
Problems staying awake during day							
Low energy levels/ feelings of fatigue							
Mood quality							

SLEEP SYMPTOMS

Enter severity scores for each symptom. Use extra rows to track any additional sleep-related symptoms you're experiencing

	DAY 8	DAY 9	DAY 10	DAY 11	DAY 12	DAY 13	DAY 1
Enter date and/or day of week here							
Insomnia							
Problems staying asleep at night							
Difficulty waking up							
Problems staying awake during day							
Low energy levels/ feelings of fatigue							
Mood quality							

SLEEP SYMPTOMS

Enter severity scores for each symptom. Use extra rows to track any additional sleep-related symptoms you're experiencing

	DAY 15	DAY 16	DAY 17	DAY 18	DAY 19	DAY 20	DAY 21
Enter date and/or day of week here							
Insomnia							
Problems staying asleep at night							
Difficulty waking up							
Problems staying awake during day							
Low energy levels/ feelings of fatigue							
Mood quality							

SLEEP SYMPTOMS

Enter severity scores for each symptom. Use extra rows to track any additional sleep-related symptoms you're experiencing

	DAY 22	DAY 23	DAY 24	DAY 25	DAY 26	DAY 27	DAY 28
Enter date and/or day of week here							
Insomnia							
Problems staying asleep at night							
Difficulty waking up							
Problems staying awake during day							
Low energy levels/ feelings of fatigue							
Mood quality							

SLEEP SYMPTOMS

Enter severity scores for each symptom. Use extra rows to track any additional sleep-related symptoms you're experiencing

	DAY 29	DAY 30	DAY 31
nter date and/or ay of week here			
somnia			
roblems staying sleep at night			
ifficulty aking up			
roblems staying wake during day			
w energy levels/ elings of fatigue			
od quality			

ACTIVITIES LOG

Track your major and consistent daily activities and the time spent in each one.
(ex. Day 1: body weight exercise - 30 min; focused reading - 1 hour).
You can also use this to track treatment days and which ones used.
(ex. Day 1: PEMF - 30 min; acupuncture - 45 min).

	_hr_min	_hr_min	_hr_min	_hr_min	_hr_min	_hr_min	_hr_m
DAY 1							
DAY 2							
DAY 3							
DAY 4							
DAY 5							
DAY 6							
DAY 7							

ACTIVITIES LOG

Track your major and consistent daily activities and the time spent in each one.
(ex. Day 1: body weight exercise - 30 min; focused reading - 1 hour).
You can also use this to track treatment days and which ones used.
(ex. Day 1: PEMF - 30 min; acupuncture - 45 min).

	_hr_min	_hr_min	_hr_min	_hr_min	_hr_min	_hr_min	_hr_min
DAY 8							
DAY 9							
DAY 10							
DAY 11							
DAY 12							
DAY 13							
DAY 14							

ACTIVITIES LOG

Track your major and consistent daily activities and the time spent in each one.
(ex. Day 1: body weight exercise - 30 min; focused reading - 1 hour).
You can also use this to track treatment days and which ones used.
(ex. Day 1: PEMF - 30 min; acupuncture - 45 min).

	_hr_min	_hr_min	_hr_min	_hr_min	_hr_min	_hr_min	_hr_min
DAY 15							
DAY 16							
DAY 17							
DAY 18							
DAY 19							
DAY 20							
DAY 21							

ACTIVITIES LOG

Track your major and consistent daily activities and the time spent in each one.
(ex. Day 1: body weight exercise - 30 min; focused reading - 1 hour).
You can also use this to track treatment days and which ones used.
(ex. Day 1: PEMF - 30 min; acupuncture - 45 min).

	_hr_min	_hr_min	_hr_min	_hr_min	_hr_min	_hr_min	_hr_min
DAY 22							
DAY 23							
DAY 24							
DAY 25							
DAY 26							
DAY 27							
DAY 28							

ACTIVITIES LOG

Track your major and consistent daily activities and the time spent in each one.
(ex. Day 1: body weight exercise - 30 min; focused reading - 1 hour).
You can also use this to track treatment days and which ones used.
(ex. Day 1: PEMF - 30 min; acupuncture - 45 min).

	_hr_min	_hr_min	_hr_min	_hr_min	_hr_min	_hr_min	_hr_min
DAY 29							
DAY 30							
DAY 31							

NUTRITION & SUPPLEMENTATION LOG

	FASTING? (a.m./p.m.)	MEALS AND SNACK(S) CONSUMES	WATER INTAKE	SUPPLEMENTS
Enter date and/or day of week below **DAY 1**				
		Breakfast:		
		Lunch:		
		Dinner:		
		Snack(s):		
Total duration	___hr___min		(cups/ounces)	
DAY 2				
		Breakfast:		
		Lunch:		
		Dinner:		
		Snack(s):		
Total duration	___hr___min		(cups/ounces)	

NUTRITION & SUPPLEMENTATION LOG

	FASTING? (a.m./p.m.)	MEALS AND SNACK(S) CONSUMES	WATER INTAKE	SUPPLEMENTS
Enter date and/or day of week below **DAY 3**				
		Breakfast:		
		Lunch:		
		Dinner:		
		Snack(s):		
Total duration ___hr___min			(cups/ounces)	
DAY 4				
		Breakfast:		
		Lunch:		
		Dinner:		
		Snack(s):		
Total duration ___hr___min			(cups/ounces)	

NUTRITION & SUPPLEMENTATION LOG

	FASTING? (a.m./p.m.)	MEALS AND SNACK(S) CONSUMES	WATER INTAKE	SUPPLEMENTS
Enter date and/or day of week below **AY 5**				
		Breakfast:		
		Lunch:		
		Dinner:		
		Snack(s):		
Total duration	___hr___min		(cups/ounces)	
AY 6		Breakfast:		
		Lunch:		
		Dinner:		
		Snack(s):		
Total duration	___hr___min		(cups/ounces)	

NUTRITION & SUPPLEMENTATION LOG

	FASTING? (a.m./p.m.)	MEALS AND SNACK(S) CONSUMES	WATER INTAKE	SUPPLEMENTS
Enter date and/or day of week below **DAY 7**				
		Breakfast:		
		Lunch:		
		Dinner:		
		Snack(s):		
Total duration ___hr___min			(cups/ounces)	
DAY 8				
		Breakfast:		
		Lunch:		
		Dinner:		
		Snack(s):		
Total duration ___hr___min			(cups/ounces)	

NUTRITION & SUPPLEMENTATION LOG

	FASTING? (a.m./p.m.)	MEALS AND SNACK(S) CONSUMES	WATER INTAKE	SUPPLEMENTS
Enter date and/or day of week below **DAY 9**				
		Breakfast:		
		Lunch:		
		Dinner:		
		Snack(s):		
Total duration ___hr___min			(cups/ounces)	
DAY 10				
		Breakfast:		
		Lunch:		
		Dinner:		
		Snack(s):		
Total duration ___hr___min			(cups/ounces)	

NUTRITION & SUPPLEMENTATION LOG

	FASTING? (a.m./p.m.)	MEALS AND SNACK(S) CONSUMES	WATER INTAKE	SUPPLEMENTS
Enter date and/or day of week below **DAY 11**				
		Breakfast:		
		Lunch:		
		Dinner:		
		Snack(s):		
Total duration	___hr___min		(cups/ounces)	
DAY 12				
		Breakfast:		
		Lunch:		
		Dinner:		
		Snack(s):		
Total duration	___hr___min		(cups/ounces)	

NUTRITION & SUPPLEMENTATION LOG

	FASTING? (a.m./p.m.)	MEALS AND SNACK(S) CONSUMES	WATER INTAKE	SUPPLEMENTS
ter date and/or of week below				
AY 13				
		Breakfast:		
		Lunch:		
		Dinner:		
		Snack(s):		
tal duration ___hr___min			(cups/ounces)	
AY 14				
		Breakfast:		
		Lunch:		
		Dinner:		
		Snack(s):		
al duration ___hr___min			(cups/ounces)	

NUTRITION & SUPPLEMENTATION LOG

	FASTING? (a.m./p.m.)	MEALS AND SNACK(S) CONSUMES	WATER INTAKE	SUPPLEMENTS
Enter date and/or day of week below **DAY 15**				
		Breakfast:		
		Lunch:		
		Dinner:		
		Snack(s):		
Total duration	___hr___min		(cups/ounces)	
DAY 16		Breakfast:		
		Lunch:		
		Dinner:		
		Snack(s):		
Total duration	___hr___min		(cups/ounces)	

NUTRITION & SUPPLEMENTATION LOG

Enter date and/or day of week below	FASTING? (a.m./p.m.)	MEALS AND SNACK(S) CONSUMES	WATER INTAKE	SUPPLEMENTS
DAY 17				
		Breakfast:		
		Lunch:		
		Dinner:		
		Snack(s):		
Total duration	___hr___min		(cups/ounces)	
DAY 18				
		Breakfast:		
		Lunch:		
		Dinner:		
		Snack(s):		
Total duration	___hr___min		(cups/ounces)	

NUTRITION & SUPPLEMENTATION LOG

	FASTING? (a.m./p.m.)	MEALS AND SNACK(S) CONSUMES	WATER INTAKE	SUPPLEMENTS
Enter date and/or day of week below **DAY 19**				
		Breakfast:		
		Lunch:		
		Dinner:		
		Snack(s):		
Total duration ___hr___min			(cups/ounces)	
DAY 20		Breakfast:		
		Lunch:		
		Dinner:		
		Snack(s):		
Total duration ___hr___min			(cups/ounces)	

NUTRITION & SUPPLEMENTATION LOG

	FASTING? (a.m./p.m.)	MEALS AND SNACK(S) CONSUMES	WATER INTAKE	SUPPLEMENTS
nter date and/or y of week below **DAY 21**				
		Breakfast:		
		Lunch:		
		Dinner:		
		Snack(s):		
tal duration	___hr___min		(cups/ounces)	
AY 22		Breakfast:		
		Lunch:		
		Dinner:		
		Snack(s):		
al duration	___hr___min		(cups/ounces)	

NUTRITION & SUPPLEMENTATION LOG

	FASTING? (a.m./p.m.)	MEALS AND SNACK(S) CONSUMES	WATER INTAKE	SUPPLEMENTS
Enter date and/or day of week below **DAY 23**				
		Breakfast:		
		Lunch:		
		Dinner:		
		Snack(s):		
Total duration ___hr___min			(cups/ounces)	
DAY 24				
		Breakfast:		
		Lunch:		
		Dinner:		
		Snack(s):		
Total duration ___hr___min			(cups/ounces)	

NUTRITION & SUPPLEMENTATION LOG

	FASTING? (a.m./p.m.)	MEALS AND SNACK(S) CONSUMES	WATER INTAKE	SUPPLEMENTS
Enter date and/or day of week below **DAY 25**				
		Breakfast:		
		Lunch:		
		Dinner:		
		Snack(s):		
Total duration ___hr___min			(cups/ounces)	
DAY 26				
		Breakfast:		
		Lunch:		
		Dinner:		
		Snack(s):		
Total duration ___hr___min			(cups/ounces)	

NUTRITION & SUPPLEMENTATION LOG

	FASTING? (a.m./p.m.)	MEALS AND SNACK(S) CONSUMES	WATER INTAKE	SUPPLEMENTS
Enter date and/or day of week below **DAY 27**				
		Breakfast:		
		Lunch:		
		Dinner:		
		Snack(s):		
Total duration ___hr___min			(cups/ounces)	
DAY 28				
		Breakfast:		
		Lunch:		
		Dinner:		
		Snack(s):		
Total duration ___hr___min			(cups/ounces)	

NUTRITION & SUPPLEMENTATION LOG

	FASTING? (a.m./p.m.)	MEALS AND SNACK(S) CONSUMES	WATER INTAKE	SUPPLEMENTS
ter date and/or y of week below				
AY 29				
		Breakfast:		
		Lunch:		
		Dinner:		
		Snack(s):		
tal duration	___hr___min		(cups/ounces)	
AY 30				
		Breakfast:		
		Lunch:		
		Dinner:		
		Snack(s):		
al duration	___hr___min		(cups/ounces)	

NUTRITION & SUPPLEMENTATION LOG

	FASTING? (a.m./p.m.)	MEALS AND SNACK(S) CONSUMES	WATER INTAKE	SUPPLEMENTS
Enter date and/or day of week below **DAY 31**				
		Breakfast:		
		Lunch:		
		Dinner:		
		Snack(s):		

Total duration ___hr___min   (cups/ounces)

ACKNOWLEDGMENTS

There are too many to fully include and so many to be yet remembered.

To all my teachers for helping support my place of standing on the shoulders of giants who have come before:
Roger Bell for being the great channel for deep wisdom and constant inspiration. Rob Cass for carrying forth the Legacy with honor and brilliance. Gabriel Cousins for unrelenting faith, dedication and perseverance.

To all my colleagues for helping keep it light and real in the midst of stellar work in the trenches:
Andy Swanson for showing me the art of healing as a way of life. Jason McNeil for bringing the warrior heart into the practice of medicine. Scott Sherr for an immediate fellowship and lighting the way for the next generations. Matt Cook for excellence in pioneering the realms of frontier healing.

To all my production team:
Jesse Krieger for constantly fielding my barrage of questions with patience and ease. Kristen Wise for managing an incalculable amount of details and my rookie mistakes. Susan Brackney for the many hours behind the scenes with research and fact checking.

To all my friends who have already witnessed and supported several of my lifetimes in this one body:
Aubrey Marcus for brotherhood and badassary in all its forms. Morgan Langan and Puma St Angel for providing open arms to wayward souls. Samantha Sweetwater for brilliance in the weaving of feminine magic. Sonya Stewart for beauty and grace in all Her forms.

To all the Indigenous Medicine carriers of the Amazon:
Thank you for staying true to the wisdom lineages of our beloved forests, for teaching me the rituals of soul centered medicine, for tending to the hearts of our collective grief and for staying light-hearted in the midst of constant threat from a reckless world.

RESOURCES

GENERAL RESOURCES

The Brain Injury Network (BIN)—The first brain-injury-survivor-operated, nonprofit advocacy organization
http://BrainInjuryNetwork.org/
https://www.facebook.com/BrainInjuryNetwork/
(707) 544-4323
707 Hahman Dr., #9276
Santa Rosa, California 95405-9276

The Brain Injury Association of America (BIAA)—The oldest, largest brain injury advocacy organization in the U.S.
http://www.biausa.org/
See also https://www.facebook.com/BrainInjuryAssociationofAmerica
(703) 761-0750
(800) 444-6443—National Brain Injury Information Center (Brain Injury Information Only)
1608 Spring Hill Road, Suite 110
Vienna, VA 22182
Visit http://www.biausa.org/state-affiliates.htm to find a BIAA affiliate in a specific U.S. state

National Intrepid Center of Excellence (NICoE)—U.S.-based military health system institute for treating active-duty service members who have experienced combat and mission-related TBI. "Service members must be capable of participating in an intensive outpatient level of care for up to four weeks and engaging in a structured post-NICoE recovery care plan at their home station."
http://www.nicoe.capmed.mil/
(301) 319-3600
dha.bethesda.ncr-medical.mbx.nicoe@mail.mil
4860 South Palmer Road
Bethesda, MD 20889-5649

International Brain Injury Association (IBIA)—"Dedicated to the development and support of multidisciplinary medical and clinical professionals, advocates, policy makers, consumers and others who work to improve outcomes and opportunities for persons with brain injury."
http://www.InternationalBrain.org/
See also https://www.facebook.com/IBIA123
(703) 960-0027 (U.S. Eastern Time Zone)
(713) 526-6900 (U.S. Central Time Zone)
congress@InternationalBrain.org
5909 Ashby Manor Place
Alexandria, VA 22310

European Brain Injury Society (EBIS)—"Dedicated to activities for traumatic brain injured persons and victims of acquired cerebral lesions: stroke, anoxia, encephalitis, brain tumour. EBIS brings together the many professionals involved in the field and the associations of people with a head injury and their families."
http://www.ebisSociety.org/
+32 (0)2 522 20 03
ebis.secretariat@skynet.be
Rue de La Vigne 56 B
1070 Bruxelles
Belgium

International Brain Research Foundation, Inc.
http://www.ibrfInc.org/
(732) 494-7600
pdefina@ibrfinc.org
227 Rout 206 N Building #2, Suite 101
Flanders, NJ 07836

Kevin Pearce—Former professional snowboarder who spent years in recovery after sustaining a TBI
http://KevinPearce.com/
See also http://KevinPearce.com/story.html
Love Your Brain Foundation—A non-profit organization, established by Kevin and Adam Pearce, dedicated to improving quality of life for people affected by traumatic brain injury.

http://www.LoveYourBrain.com/
See also https://www.facebook.com/LoveYourBrain-232366118918
info@LoveYourBrain.com

Adventures in Brain Trauma
Cavin Balaster, speaker and TBI survivor offering authentic experience, scientific research and candid wisdom about the process and strategies about healing from significant brain trauma
http://adventuresinbraininjury.com

National Institute of Neurological Disorders and Stroke (NINDS) - Offers information on all clinical trials occurring through the NIH. The webpage devoted to TBI can be found at:
http://www.ninds.nih.gov/disorders/tbi/tbi.htm

Family Caregiver Alliance/ National Center on Caregiving
http://www.caregiver.org

National Rehabilitation Information Center (NARIC)
http://www.naric.com

Centre for Neuro Skills – excellent reviews of TBI related research
http://www.NeuroSkills.com/resources/special-reports.php

National Institute on Disability and Rehabilitation Research (NIDRR)
U.S. Department of Education Office of Special Education and Rehabilitative Services
http://www.ed.gov/about/offices/list/osers/nidrr

Publicaciones en Español
Traumatismo Cerebral: Esperanza en la Investigación

One Flashlight, an organization promoting TBI awareness.
http://OneFlashlight.org

INTRODUCTION RESOURCES

"Dr. Dan Engle's "Full Spectrum Medicine" website.
http://www.FullSpectrumMedicine.com

The Crack in the Cosmic Egg by Joseph Chilton Pearce
Park Street Press; Revised edition (September 30, 2002)
ISBN: 978-0892819942

Exploring the Crack in the Cosmic Egg: Split Minds and Meta-Realities
by Joseph Chilton Pearce
Park Street Press; 6th Edition (February 15, 2014)
ISBN: 978-1620552544

For FAQs and more information about Chronic Traumatic Encephalopathy (CTE), check out the following links from the CTE Center, an independent academic research center located at Boston University School of Medicine:
http://www.bu.edu/cte/about/about-the-center/
http://www.bu.edu/cte/about/frequently-asked-questions/

The Lobotomist: A Maverick Medical Genius and His Tragic Quest to Rid the World of Mental Illness by Jack El-Hai
Wiley (February 9, 2007)
ISBN: 978-0470098301

The Human Brain Book by Rita Carter
DK (March 3, 2014)
ISBN: 978-1465416025

Brain: The Complete Mind: How It Develops, How It Works, and How to Keep It Sharp
by Michael S. Sweeney
National Geographic (November 17, 2009)
ISBN: 978-1426205477

CHAPTER 1 RESOURCES

FLOTATION REST THERAPY RESOURCES

"Where to Float"—An online, international collective of people who float
http://www.where-to-float.com/
Find a float center near you, buy or sell a used float tank, learn about float tanks for home or commercial use and much more.

Float Conference—Started in 2012, this annual conference brings together float center owners, float tank manufacturers, Flotation REST Therapy researchers and enthusiasts from all over the world.
http://FloatConference.com/

Floatation International LLC—Online purveyor of float pods, rooms and tanks
http://FloatationTanks.com/
contact@FloatationTanks.com
(941) 702-4763

True REST Float Spas—Dedicated float centers in Ohio, Arizona and California. Additional float center locations in other U.S. states coming soon.
http://TrueRest.com/
See also http://TrueRest.com/locations
info@TrueRest.com

Zero Gravity Institute—Dedicated float center in Austin, Texas.
http://ZeroGravityInstitute.com/
(512) 707-1191
float@ZeroGravityInstitute.com
2919 Manchaca Road Suite 105
Austin, TX, 78704

SELECTED FLOTATION PRODUCTS AND MANUFACTURERS:

The Float Pod
Manufactured by Float Pod Technologies LLC
http://www.FloatPod.com
(866) 295-8199
info@FloatPod.com
4440 S Rural Rd. Bldg F., Suite 111
Tempe, AZ 85282

Aqua Anima
manufactured by Floatingrest International AB
http://www.FloatingRest.com/
+46 70 715 76 63

Bergshyddebacken 5
S-187 76 TÄBY
Sweden

Aquason
+096 705 60 00
aquason.fl@gmail.com
Str. Gorodetsky, 11-well
metro Khreshchatyk
Ukraine

Elysium
Manufactured by Elysium Float Systems
+36 30 997 1235
info@ElysiumFloat.com
Kárpát utca 62-64
1133 Budapest
Hungary

Escape Pod
Manufactured by Umbra Heavy Industries, Inc.
http://www.EscapePodTank.com/
https://www.facebook.com/EscapePodFloatationTanks
(402) 480-5795
info@EscapePodTank.com

Evolution Float Pod
Manufactured by Superior Float Tanks
http://SuperiorFloatTanks.com/
(757) 966-6350
contact@SuperiorFloatTanks.com
431 W 25th St.
Norfolk, VA 23517

Float-es
Manufactured by San Juan Products, Inc.
http://www.FloatEpsomSalt.com/
(800) 535-7946
2302 Lasso Lane
Lakeland, FL 33801

Float Lab
http://FloatLab.com/
(310) 396-3336
sales@FloatLab.com

Float Spa
Manufactured by FloatSPA
http://FloatSpa.com/

Float Star
http://www.FloatStar.com/
0049 (0)176 76 177 660 (for Europe and bordering countries)
FloatingTank@hotmail.de (for Europe and bordering countries)
0064(0)6 9670 200 (for New Zealand, Australia and Asia)
info@FloatationTank.co.nz (for New Zealand, Australia and Asia)

i-sopod
Manufactured by Floatworks
http://www.i-sopod.com/
+44 (0)20 7357 0111 (for Europe)
(646) 500-8651 (for U.S.)

Oasis
Manufactured by Oasis Relaxation Systems
http://www.OasisRelaxation.com/
(619) 265-9391
info@OasisRelaxation.com
P.O. Box 15669
San Diego, CA 92175

Ocean Floatrooms
http://OceanFloatRooms.com/
+44 (0)1628 675 870
80-83 Long Lane
London EC1A 9ET

Samadhi
Samadhi Tank Company, Inc.
http://www.SamadhiTank.com/

https://www.facebook.com/SamadhiTankCompany
(530) 477-1319
Grass Valley, CA 95949

Zen Home Float Tank
Zen Float Co.
http://www.ZenFloatCo.com/
(801) 871-5140
1-855-ZEN-FLOAT (U.S. Only)
info@ZenFloatCo.com
4730 Riverside Drive
Salt Lake City, UT 84123

TBI RESOURCES:

The Neurometabolic Cascade of Concussion by C.C. Giza and D.A. Hovda. J Athl Train, 2001. 36(3): p. 228-235.

Posttraumatic Retrograde and Anterograde Amnesia: Pathophysiology and Implications in Grading and Safe Return to Play by R.C. Cantu. J Athl Train, 2001. 36(3): p. 244-248.

Predicting Neurocognitive and Behavioural Outcome After Early Brain Insult by V.A. Anderson, et al. Dev Med Child Neurol, 2014.

Overlap of Mild TBI and Mental Health Conditions in Returning OIF/OEF Service Members and Veterans by H.L. Lew, et al.. J Rehabil Res Dev, 2008.

SELECTED BOOKS by John C. Lilly, MD:

The Mind of the Dolphin: A Nonhuman Intelligence (Consciousness Classics) by John Cunningham Lilly, MD
Gateways Books & Tapes; Expanded edition (August 28, 2015)
ISBN: 978-0895561190

Programming and Metaprogramming in the Human Biocomputer: Theory and Experiments by Dr. John C. Lilly
Float On (May 8, 2014)
ISBN: 978-0692217894

Simulations of God: The Science of Belief by John C. Lilly, MD
Ronin Publishing; 2nd edition (August 21, 2012)
ISBN: 978-1579511579

Center of the Cyclone: Looking into Inner Space by John C. Lilly, MD
Ronin Publishing; First Trade Paper edition (June 5, 2007)
ISBN: 978-1579510381

The Deep Self: Consciousness Exploration in the Isolation Tank (Consciousness Classics) by John Cunningham Lilly, MD
Gateways Books & Tapes; 1 Reprint edition (May 28, 2006)
ISBN: 978-0895561169

The Quiet Center: Isolation and Spirit
by John C. Lilly, MD, Phillip Bailey Lilly, and Tom Robbins
Ronin Publishing (May 9, 2003)
ISBN: 978-1579510596

Tanks for the Memories: Floatation Tank Talks (Consciousness Classics) by John Cunningham Lilly, MD and E. J. Gold
Gateways Books & Tapes; 2nd edition (June 1, 1996)
ISBN: 978-0895560711

The Scientist: A Metaphysical Autobiography by John C. Lilly, MD
Ronin Publishing, Inc.; 3rd edition (October 23, 1996)
ISBN: 978-0914171720

John Lilly So Far. . . by Francis Jeffrey and John C. Lilly
Jeremy P. Tarcher, Inc.; 1st edition (February 1, 1991)
ISBN: 978-0874776133

The Dyadic Cyclone: the Autobiography of a Couple by John Lilly, MD and
Antonietta Lilly
Pocket Books (1977)

Lilly on Dolphins: Humans of the Sea by John C. Lilly
Anchor Books (1975)

Man and Dolphin: Adventures of a New Scientific Frontier by John C. Lilly
Doubleday & Company; 1st edition (1961)

Breathe2Relax—free app for iOS and Android devices, developed by the National Center for Telehealth and Technology
Available via Google Play, iTunes App Store and Amazon.com
"Breathe2Relax is a portable stress management tool which provides detailed information on the effects of stress on the body and instructions and practice exercises to help users learn the stress management skill called diaphragmatic breathing. Breathing exercises have been documented to decrease the body's 'fight-or-flight' (stress) response, and help with mood stabilization, anger control, and anxiety management. Breathe2Relax can be used as a stand-alone stress reduction tool, or can be used in tandem with clinical care directed by a healthcare worker."

LOW-LEVEL LASER (LIGHT) THERAPY (LLLT) RESOURCES

ColdLasers.org—Comprehensive site sells many different cold laser devices and includes buyers' guides, device specifications and tips on choosing a laser for at-home use
http://www.ColdLasers.org
(800) 388-0850
4450 Arapahoe Road Suite 100
Boulder, CO 80303

U.S. Food and Drug Administration
http://www.fda.gov/
Visit the "Medical Devices" section to determine whether a particular device has officially been "cleared" or "approved" for use by the FDA. Related, helpful links:
http://www.fda.gov/MedicalDevices/ResourcesforYou/Consumers/ucm142523.htm
http://www.fda.gov/MedicalDevices/ProductsandMedical Procedures/DeviceApprovalsandClearances/default.htm

SELECTED LLLT PRODUCTS AND MANUFACTURERS:

Aspen "Summit" and "Pinnacle" Series Laser Systems
Manufactured by Aspen Laser Systems
http://www.AspenLasers.com/
(877) 817-0365

info@AspenLasers.com
Dominion Towers
600 17th St #2800
Denver, CO 80202

LZ30p, LZ30x and LZ30z lasers
Manufactured by Avant Wellness Systems
http://www.lz30laser.com/
(949) 682-8268
sales@AvantWellness.com

PowerLaser PRO 1500
Manufactured by PowerMedic Lasers
http://PowerMedicLasers.com/
(608) 406-2020 (U.S.)
+45 5944 0832 (Europe)
S1609A Hughes Rd.
Westby, WI 54667

HYPERBARIC OXYGEN THERAPY (HBOT) RESOURCES

International Hyperbaric Medication Association
www.IHMA.org

Hyperbaric Medical Solutions
www.hmshbot.com

Scott Sherr, MD
Integrative Health Optimization Medical Doctor Specializing in HBOT
www.IntegrativeHBOT.com

The International Hyperbarics Association, Inc.—"Educational and charitable organization focusing on the needs of the hyperbaric community"
http://www.ihausa.org
(877) 442-8721
Email info@ihausa.org to find a hyperbaric treatment center near you.

SELECTED HBOT PRODUCTS AND MANUFACTURERS:

Portable hyperbaric chambers (23-, 28- and 40-inch-diameter models)
Manufactured by Healing Dives
http://www.HealingDives.com/
(888) 713-8700
+1 (818) 348-8700 (international)
info@HealingDives.com
4220 Lobos Road
Woodland Hills, CA 91364

Solace 210, Respiro 270, Vitaris 320, Quamvis 320 and Fortius 420
Manufactured by OxyHealth LLC
http://www.OxyHealth.com
(877) 789-0123
information@OxyHealth.com
10719 Norwalk Blvd.
Santa Fe Springs, CA 90670

Seal, Class 4 and Class 7 mild hyperbaric chambers
Newtowne Hyperbarics
http://www.NewtowneHyperbarics.com/
(410) 975-7414
sales@NewtowneHyperbarics.com
1106 Market St.
Pocomoke, MD 21851

SELECTED HBOT BOOKS:

Doc, I Want My Brain Back by Dan Greathouse
CreateSpace Independent Publishing Platform (November 22, 2013)
ISBN: 978-1493699070

The Hyperbaric Chamber: Science, Not Miracle by Nina Subbotina
CreateSpace Independent Publishing Platform (December 5, 2013)
ISBN: 978-1494361051

Hyperbaric Oxygen Therapy: The Ultimate Beginner's Guide to Understanding the Hyperbaric Chamber by Brad Durant

CreateSpace Independent Publishing Platform (March 5, 2014)
ISBN: 978-1507849644

Oxygen to the Rescue: Oxygen Therapies and How They Help Overcome Disease, Promote Repair, and Improve Overall Function by Pavel Yutsis, MD
Basic Health Publications; 1st edition (February 1, 2003)
ISBN: 978-1591200079

The Oxygen Revolution: Hyperbaric Oxygen Therapy: The New Treatment for Post Traumatic Stress Disorder (PTSD), Traumatic Brain Injury, Stroke, Autism and More by Paul G. Harch, MD and Virginia McCullough
Hatherleigh Press; Updated edition (October 26, 2010)
ISBN: 978-1578263264

PULSED ELECTROMAGNETIC FIELDS (PEMF) RESOURCES:

DrPawluk.com "Healing with Magnetic Field Energy"—Primer on choosing a PEMF system for at-home use
http://drpawluk.com/resources/buyers-guide/
Systems can also be rented or purchased via this site.

U.S. Food and Drug Administration
http://www.fda.gov/
Visit the "Medical Devices" section to determine whether a particular device has officially been "cleared" or "approved" for use by the FDA. Related, helpful links:
http://www.fda.gov/MedicalDevices/ResourcesforYou/Consumers/ucm142523.htm
http://www.fda.gov/MedicalDevices/ProductsandMedical Procedures/DeviceApprovalsandClearances/default.htm

SELECTED PEMF PRODUCTS AND MANUFACTURERS:

MAS Sport Multi and MAS Special Multi
Manufactured by MAS Magnetic Field Systems
http://MASMagnetics.com
+43 664 831 8477
fiona.zach@gmail.com
Gralla 61, Leibnitz, 8430
Leibnitz/Austria

iMRS Wellfit, iMRS Complete and iMRS Professional
Manufactured by Swiss Bionic Solutions
http://www.imrs.com/
See also http://www.imrs.com/en/system/imrs-systems.html and
www.SwissBionic.com
(954) 766 4153
us@SwissBionic.com
1200 NE. 7Th AVE. Suite 7
Fort Lauderdale, Florida 33304

Almag 01
Manufactured by ALMAGIA International
http://www.almagia.com/
(718) 930-5152
info@almagia.com
1775 East 18th Str, Suite 1E
Brooklyn, NY 11229

Bemer Classic Set and Bemer Pro-Set
Manufactured by Bemer
https://www.BemerGroup.com/
See also https://united-states.BemerGroup.com/en-US
(310) 295-9753
+423 399 39 99 (international)
info@BemerGroup.com

Curatron 2000 Ultra-Power 3D
Manufactured by Amjo Corp
http://www.curatron.com/
See also www.amjo.net
(513) 942-2770
(877) BUY-AMJO
support@amjo.net
P.O. Box 8304
West Chester, OH 45069

SELECTED PEMF BOOKS:

PEMF - The Fifth Element of Health: Learn Why Pulsed Electromagnetic Field (PEMF) Therapy Supercharges Your Health Like Nothing Else! by Bryant A. Meyers
BalboaPress (August 19, 2013)
ISBN: 978-1452579221

TRANSCRANIAL MAGNETIC STIMULATION (TMS) RESOURCES

Clinical TMS Society, Inc.—A membership organization for physicians, clinicians and TMS device industry professionals
http://www.ClinicalTMSSociety.org/
(877) 389-2333
c/o Shipman & Goodwin LLP
One Constitution Plaza, 14th Floor
Hartford, CT 06103-1919
Visit http://www.ClinicalTMSSociety.org/left/find-a-provider/ to find a TMS provider near you.

U.S. Food and Drug Administration
http://www.fda.gov/
Visit the "Medical Devices" section to determine whether a particular device has officially been "cleared" or "approved" for use by the FDA. Related, helpful links:
http://www.fda.gov/MedicalDevices/ResourcesforYou/Consumers/ucm142523.htm
http://www.fda.gov/MedicalDevices/ProductsandMedical Procedures/DeviceApprovalsandClearances/default.htm

SELECTED TMS DEVICE MANUFACTURERS:

Neurostar TMS Therapy
Manufactured by Neuronetics
https://neurostar.com/
See also http://www.neuronetics.com/
(877) 600-7555
info@neuronetics.com

3222 Phoenixville Pike
Malvern, PA 19355

Brainsway Deep TMS
Manufactured by Brainsway Ltd.
http://www.brainsway.com/us
(844) 386-7001 (U.S.)
+972-2-5813140 (international)
info@brainsway.com
2-98 Decker Blvd.
Bala Cynwyd, PA 19004

Magvita TMS Therapy
Manufactured by MagVenture A/S
http://www.MagVenture.com/
(888) 624-7764
infousa@MagVenture.com
303 Perimeter Center North, Suite 300
Atlanta, GA 30346

TRANSCRANIAL DIRECT CURRENT STIMULATION (tDCS) RESOURCES:

DIY tDCS—"Keeping Tabs [on] Transcranial Direct Current Stimulation"
http://www.diytdcs.com/
Instructables.com—"Build a Human Enhancement Device (Basic tDCS Supply)"
http://www.instructables.com/id/Build-a-Human-Enhancement-Device-Basic-tDCS-Suppl/

U.S. Food and Drug Administration
http://www.fda.gov/
Visit the "Medical Devices" section to determine whether a particular device has officially been "cleared" or "approved" for use by the FDA. Related, helpful links:
http://www.fda.gov/MedicalDevices/ResourcesforYou/Consumers/ucm142523.htm

http://www.fda.gov/MedicalDevices/ProductsandMedical
Procedures/DeviceApprovalsandClearances/default.htm

SELECTED tDCS PRODUCTS AND MANUFACTURERS:

The Brain Stimulator Basic tDCS Kit, The Brain Stimulator Advanced
tDCS Kit and The Brain Stimulator Deluxe tDCS Kit
Manufactured by Neurolectrics, Inc.
https://TheBrainStimulator.net/
See also https://www.facebook.com/TheBrainStimulator/
contact@TheBrainStimulator.net

The DC-Stimulator Plus
Manufactured by neuroConn
http://www.NeuroConn.de/
See also http://www.NeuroConn.de/dc-stimulator_plus_en/
+49 3677 689790 (international)
info@NeuroConn.de
Albert-Einstein-Straße 3
98693 Ilmenau Germany

The Brain Driver
Manufactured by the Brain Driver
https://TheBrainDriver.com/
(312) 685-1147
TheBrainDriver@gmail.com
564 W. Randolph Street
Chicago, IL 60661

The Soterix Medical 1×1
Manufactured by Soterix Medical Inc.
http://SoterixMedical.com/
(888) 990-8327
contact@SoterixMedical.com
160 Convent Ave.
New York, NY, 10031

Alpha-Stim (Microcurrent Electrical Therapy (MET) device)
Manufactured by Electromedical Products International, Inc.
http://www.alpha-stim.com/
(800) 367-7246
+(940) 328-0788 (international)
info@epii.com
2201 Garrett Morris Parkway
Mineral Wells, TX 76067-9034

CHAPTER 2 RESOURCES

HORMONE REPLACEMENT THERAPY (HRT) RESOURCES:

The American Association of Clinical Endocrinologists
https://www.aace.com
See also http://www.EmpowerYourHealth.org/ for patient resources
(904) 353-7878
245 Riverside Avenue Suite 200
Jacksonville, FL 32202
To find an endocrinologist near you visit https://www.aace.com/
resources/find-an-endocrinologist

Bioidentical Hormone Doctors—"Helping You Find Qualified
Bioidentical Hormone Doctors Nationwide"
http://www.BioidenticalHormoneDoctors.com/

ZRT Laboratories—Clinical Laboratory Improvement Amendments
(CLIA)-certified diagnostic laboratory that performs hormone and
wellness testing.
http://www.ZRTLab.com/
See also http://www.ZRTLab.com/patients/hormones-101 and
http://www.ZRTLab.com/patients-standard-tests
(866) 600-1636
info@ZRTLab.com
8605 SW Creekside Place
Beaverton, OR 97008

Dried Urine Test for Comprehensive Hormones (DUTCH)
Offered by Precision Analytical, a CLIA-certified diagnostic laboratory

http://DutchTest.com/
See also http://DutchTest.com/?q=catalog
(503) 687-2050
3138 NE Rivergate Street, Suite #301C
McMinnville, OR 97128

Assorted tests
Genova Diagnostics
https://www.gdx.net/
See also https://www.gdx.net/product/hormonal-health-hormone-test-serum and https://www.gdx.net/tests/alphabetical
(800) 522-4762
63 Zillicoa Street
Asheville, NC 28801

Assorted tests, including hormonal levels and metabolism
BioHealth Laboratory, Inc.
http://BioHealthLab.com/
See also http://BioHealthLab.com/test-menu/
(800) 570-2000
2216 Santa Monica Boulevard – Suite 102
Santa Monica, CA 90404

Sabre Sciences—"Products specifically designed to support the entire hormone system to enhance energy, adrenals, skin care, and libido."
http://www.SabreSciences.com/
(760) 448-2750
info@SabreSciences.com
2233 Faraday Ave # K
Carlsbad, CA 92008

SELECTED HRT BOOKS:

The Adrenal Reset Diet: Strategically Cycle Carbs and Proteins to Lose Weight, Balance Hormones, and Move from Stressed to Thriving by Alan Christianson, NMD
Harmony; 1st edition (December 30, 2014)
ISBN: 978-0804140539

The Hormone Cure: Reclaim Balance, Sleep and Sex Drive; Lose Weight; Feel Focused, Vital, and Energized Naturally with the Gottfried Protocol by Dr. Sara Gottfried
Scribner; Reprint edition (March 11, 2014)
ISBN: 978-1451666953

The Hormone Solution: Stay Younger Longer with Natural Hormone and Nutrition Therapies by Dr. Thierry Hertoghe
Harmony (August 20, 2002)
ISBN: 978-1400080854

SELECTED COGNITIVE REHABILITATION DEVICES AND MANUFACTURERS:

The Muse Brain Sensing Headband
Manufactured by InteraXon Inc.
http://www.ChooseMuse.com/
888-508-MUSE
CustomerCare@ChooseMuse.com
511 King St. W #303
Toronto, ON M5V 1K4
Canada

"Muse"—free app for iOS and Android devices, developed by InteraXon. To be used in conjunction with the Muse Brain Sensing Headband, the "Muse" app is available via Google Play, iTunes App Store and Amazon.com.
"Learn to meditate and improve your meditation practice with Muse: The Brain Sensing Headband. While you meditate Muse uses brain sensing technology to determine whether your mind is calm or active and translates those signals into guiding sounds that you select. Choose from soundscapes that include a beach, rainforest, a desert or event ambient music. When your mind is wandering the sounds intensify and when you're calm you'll hear peaceful sounds."

"Muse Monitor"—app for iOS and Android devices developed by James Clutterbuck. Available via Google Play and iTunes App Store.

"See what's really going on inside your head in real time! Muse Monitor is exclusively for use with "Muse: The Brain-Sensing Headband" from Interaxon. Get real time EEG brainwave data beautifully graphed, right on your phone or tablet. Split data by channel, into left brain/right brain, Front/Back, or even individual sensors."

Emotiv Insight, Emotiv EPOC and Emotiv EPOC+
Manufactured by Emotiv, Inc.
https://emotiv.com/
See also https://www.facebook.com/emotiv/
hello@emotiv.com
490 Post St. Suite 824
San Francisco, CA 94102

"Emotiv Insight"—free app for iOS and Android devices developed by Emotiv to be used with Emotiv Insight Brainwear. Available via Google Play and iTunes App Store.

"Helps improve brain fitness and promotes life-long brain health. Using this app, you can record your brain activity during everyday activities and learn to optimize your brain performance. Strengthen your focus, manage your stress levels, and learn ways to improve your brain fitness."

MindWave and MindWave Mobile EEG
manufactured by NeuroSky
http://neurosky.com/
See also https://www.facebook.com/NeuroSkyBCI
(408) 200-6675
support@NeuroSky.com
125 S Market St – #900
San Jose, CA 95113

"MindWave Mobile Tutorial"—free app for iOS and Android devices developed by NeuroSky to be used with the MindWave Mobile headset. Available via Google Play and iTunes App Store.

"Brainwave Visualizer"—free app for iOS and Android devices developed by NeuroSky to be used with the MindWave Mobile headset. Available via Google Play and iTunes App Store.

"The Brainwave Visualizer is a colorful, interactive application controlled by your brain, that shows you a graphical representation of your brain's activity. The Brainwave Visualizer includes the Brainwave Visualization, Brainwave Power Spectrum Graph, and the eSense Attention and Meditation meters."

FocusBand Mind Sensing Headset
manufactured by T 2 Green Pty Ltd.
http://www.ifocusband.com/
info@FocusBand.com

"FocusBand Brain Training"—free app for iOS and Android devices developed by T 2 Green Pty Ltd.
"The App's inbuilt Brain Wave Simulator allows you to familiarise yourself with all functions before purchasing the FocusBand Brain Training Headset."

Rift
Manufactured by Oculus VR, LLC
https://www.oculus.com/en-us/
(949) 502-2070
19800 MacArthur Boulevard, Suite 200
Irvine, CA 92612

Dynavision D2
Manufactured by Dynavision International LLC.
http://www.DynavisionInternational.com/
See also http://products.DynavisionInternational.com/products/d2
(513) 645 2503
info@DynavisionInternational.com
8800 Global Way
West Chester, OH. USA 45069

Interactive Rehabilitation and Exercise System (IREX)
Manufactured by GestureTek
http://www.GestureTekHealth.com/
See also http://www.GestureTekHealth.com/products-rehab-irex.php
(416) 340-9290
info@GestureTekHealth.com

317 Adelaide St. W, Suite 903
Toronto, ON M5V 1P9 Canada

PlayStation 4, PlayStation Camera and PlayStation Move motion controller
Manufactured by Sony Computer Entertainment, Inc.
https://www.PlayStation.com
See also https://www.PlayStation.com/en-us/explore/accessories/PlayStation-camera-ps4/ and https://www.PlayStation.com/en-us/explore/accessories/PlayStation-move/
2207 Bridgepointe Pkwy.
San Mateo, CA 94404

NEUROFEEDBACK RESOURCES

Biofeedback Certification International Alliance—Professional organization for biofeedback and neurofeedback practitioners
http://www.bcia.org/
720) 502-5829
info@bcia.org
5310 Ward Road, Suite 201
Arvada CO 80002
Visit http://certify.bcia.org/4dcgi/resctr/search.html to find a certified biofeedback provider near you. (Each provider listing includes designated certification type, such as "BCN" for those certified in neurofeedback or EEG biofeedback.)

International Society for Neurofeedback & Research—Professional organization for neurofeedback researchers, practitioners and industry
http://www.isnr.org/
See also http://www.isnr.org/#!visitor-landing/c12e3 for patient-focused resources
(703) 848-1994
office@isnr.net
1350 Beverly Road, Suite 115, PMB 114
McLean, VA 22101-3633

Bio-Medical Instruments—Online purveyor of biofeedback devices
and accessories
http://bio-medical.com/
(800) 521-4640
(586) 756-5070
sales@bio-medical.com
38875 Harper Ave.
Clinton Township, MI 48036

SELECTED NEUROFEEDBACK PRODUCTS AND MANUFACTURERS:

Nine levels of alpha brain state training and nine levels of theta brain
state training
Biocybernaut Institute
http://www.biocybernaut.com/
See also https://www.facebook.com/
Biocybernaut-Institute-134173223301707/
(250) 391-1237
info@biocybernaut.com
4431 Spellman Place
Victoria, British Columbia V9C 4C5
Canada

In-clinic, at-home and retreat-based neurofeedback training sessions
Brainworks
http://www.BrainWorksNeuroTherapy.com/
See also http://www.transformational-retreats.com/
(646) 583-1233 (U.S.)
(+44) 0207 193 4373 (international)
info@BrainWorksNT.com
2 John Street
London WC1N 2ES
United Kingdom

Discovery 24E, Discovery 20, Atlantis I, Atlantis II and other EEG
products and accessories
BrainMaster Technologies, Inc.

http://www.BrainMaster.com/
(440) 232-6000
info@brainm.com
195 Willis Street
Bedford, OH 44146

SELECTED NEUROFEEDBACK BOOKS:

Conquering Concussion: Healing TBI Symptoms with Neurofeedback and without Drugs by Mary Lee Esty
Round Earth Publishing (September 15, 2014)
ISBN: 978-0965342506

The Neurofeedback Solution: How to Treat Autism, ADHD, Anxiety, Brain Injury, Stroke, PTSD, and More by Stephen Larsen
Healing Arts Press (March 26, 2012)
ISBN: 978-1594773662

ACUPUNCTURE RESOURCES:

American Association of Acupuncture and Oriental Medicine—U.S.-based membership organization of acupuncture and Oriental medicine (AOM) practitioners and supporters
http://www.aaaomOnline.org/
(866) 455-7999
P.O. Box 96503 #44114
Washington, DC 20090-6503
Visit http://www.aaaomOnline.org/search/custom.asp?id=320 to find a practitioner near you.

National Certification Commission for Acupuncture and Oriental Medicine
http://www.nccaom.org/
See also http://www.nccaom.org/consumers/
(904) 598-1005
76 South Laura Street, Suite 1290
Jacksonville, FL, 32202
Visit http://mx.nccaom.org/FindAPractitioner.aspx to find a certified acupuncturist.

Acutrials - Acupuncture review database of available research
Visit http://acutrials.ocom.edu/

STEM CELL THERAPY RESOURCES:

The International Society for Stem Cell Research—
http://www.isscr.org/
See http://www.CloserLookAtStemCells.org/ for patient resources
(224) 592-5700
info@isscr.org
5215 Old Orchard Road, Suite 270
Skokie, IL 60077 USA

Harvard Stem Cell Institute (HSCI)—"Focused on bringing stem cell-based treatments to patients as quickly as possible"
http://hsci.harvard.edu/
(617) 496-4050
hsci@harvard.edu
Bauer Building, Administrative Suite
7 Divinity Avenue
Cambridge, MA 02138

The Institute for Stem Cell Biology and Regenerative Medicine
http://StemCell.stanford.edu/
(650) 736-8325
StemCellInstitute@med.stanford.edu
265 Campus Drive, 3rd Floor
Stanford, CA 94305
Matt Cook, MD
BioReset Medical
Los Gatos, CA
(650) 204-3858
www.BiroResetMedical.com

U.S. National Institutes of Health ClinicalTrials.gov—Searchable database of ongoing clinical trials.
www.ClinicalTrials.gov
(Enter "stem cell" AND "traumatic brain injury" in the trial search box to find ongoing clinical trials which may be recruiting new patients.)
See also http://www.CenterWatch.com/clinical-trials/listings/

PHARMACEUTICAL NOOTROPICS RESOURCES

"Limitless Mindset"—Nootropics-related podcast, blog, resources, product reviews and more
http://www.LimitlessMindset.com/
See also http://www.LimitlessMindset.com/mind-power-products/
1008-pharmaceutical-grade-nootropics.html
(720) 924-1872
info@LimitlessMindset.com

SELECTED PHARMACEUTICAL NOOTROPIC PRODUCTS:

Cerebrolysin
Nootropic EU—Online retailer that sells assorted nootropics including
Cerebrolysin
http://nootropic.eu/
(+44) 7428 036 621
CerebroPeptide@gmail.com
54 Southcroft Road
London SW17 9TR

United Kingdom
Modafinil
ModUP.net—Online retailer that sells the generic modafinil known as
"Modvigil"
https://www.modup.net/
support@modup.net

Piracetam and Aniracetam
Powder City—Online retailer that sells assorted nootropics including
Piracetam and Aniracetam
http://www.PowderCity.com/
See also http://www.PowderCity.com/products/aniracetam and
http://www.PowderCity.com/products/piracetam-benefits
(717) 745-4795
support@cs.PowderCity.com

CHAPTER 3 RESOURCES

NOOTROPICS RESOURCES

Physica Energetics—"An internationally renowned professional, family owned, natural remedy company"
http://www.PhysicaEnergetics.com/
(800) 404-4163
480 Sovereign Rd. Unit 7
London Ontario N6M 1A4
Canada

Apex Energetics—"Advanced Nutritional & Bioenergetic Products & Services"
http://www.ApexEnergetics.com/
(800) 736-4381
info@ApexEnergetics.com
16592 Hale Ave.
Irvine, CA 92606

Pure Encapsulations—Hypo-allergenic nutritional supplements
http://www.PureEncapsulations.com/
(800) 753-2277
490 Boston Post Road
Sudbury, MA 01776

Thorne Research, Inc.
https://www.thorne.com/
See also https://www.thorne.com/products/neurological-support
(800) 228-1966
info@thorne.com
P.O. Box 25
Dover, ID 83825

Standard Process—supplier of "whole food nutrient" supplements
https://www.StandardProcess.com/
(800) 558-8740
info@StandardProcess.com

1200 W. Royal Lee Dr.
Palmyra, WI 53156

Onnit Labs, LLC
https://www.onnit.com/
(855) ONNIT-99
info@onnit.com
4401 Freidrich Ln. Suite 302
Austin, TX 78744

Biotics Research NW, Inc.
http://www.BioticsNW.com/
See also http://www.BioticsResearch.com/
(360) 438-3600
biotics@BioticsNW.com
6977 Littlerock Rd. SW
Tumwater, WA 98512

Neuro-Hacker Collective — Research body and blog posts on peak cognitive performance.
Nootropic: Qualia
https://www.NeuroHacker.com

Liquid glutathione
Key Compounding Pharmacy
www.KeyCompounding.com/
(206) 878-3900
(800) 878-1322
530 S 336th St.
Federal Way, WA 98003

CHAPTER 4 RESOURCES

SLEEP-RELATED RESOURCES

National Sleep Foundation
www.SleepFoundation.org

See also https://sleep.org/ and https://www.facebook.com/
NationalSleepFoundation
(703) 243-1697
nsf@SleepFoundation.org
1010 N. Glebe Road, Suite 420
Arlington, VA 22201 USA
Visit https://SleepFoundation.org/find-sleep-professional to find a
sleep professional.

American Academy of Sleep Medicine—U.S.-based professional organization dedicated to the medical subspecialty of sleep medicine.
http://www.aasmnet.org/
See also http://www.SleepEducation.org/
(630) 737-9700
2510 North Frontage Road
Darien, IL 60561
Visit http://www.SleepEducation.org/find-a-facility to find a sleep
center near you.

SELECTED SLEEP AID PRODUCTS AND MANUFACTURERS:

Valerian, chamomile, hops, passion flower, and many other herbs
Bulk Herb Store—Online retailer that sells dried and powdered herbs
and herb mixes in bulk
http://www.BulkHerbStore.com/
(877) 278-4257
info@BulkHerbStore.com
38 3rd Ave. East
Lobelville, TN 37097

Kava kava
KV Naturals, Inc.—Online retailer that sells powdered kava root, as
well as kava capsules and tinctures
https://www.kava.com/
(716) 989-5577
shop@kava.com
770 Sycamore Ave, 122-493
Vista, CA 92083

Magnesium supplements
Drugstore.com—Online retailer that sells magnesium, melatonin and many other types of supplements and vitamins
http://www.DrugStore.com/
(800) 378-4786
(425) 372-4401
411 108th Ave NE, Suite 1600
Bellevue, WA 98004

Spoonk acupressure pillow and mat sets
Manufactured by Spoonk
http://www.SpoonkSpace.com/
See also https://www.facebook.com/SpoonkSpace/
(888) 583.2880
info@SpoonkSpace.com

SELECTED SLEEP-RELATED BOOKS:

Sleep Smarter: 21 Proven Tips to Sleep Your Way To a Better Body, Better Health and Bigger Success by Shawn Stevenson
Model House Publishing (May 22, 2014)
ISBN: 978-0984574520

The Insomnia Workbook: A Comprehensive Guide to Getting the Sleep You Need by Stephanie Silberman
New Harbinger Publications; 1st edition (June 1, 2009)
ISBN: 978-1572246355

Say Good Night to Insomnia: The Six-Week, Drug-Free Program Developed At Harvard Medical School by Gregg D. Jacobs
Holt Paperbacks; 1st edition (September 15, 2009)
ISBN: 978-0805089585

The Harvard Medical School Guide to a Good Night's Sleep (Harvard Medical School Guides) by Lawrence Epstein and Steven Mardon
McGraw-Hill Education; 1st edition (October 16, 2006)
ISBN: 978-0071467438

HELIOTHERAPY RESOURCES

Center for Environmental Therapeutics U.S./CAN—"An independent, non-profit professional organization dedicated to education and research on the new environmental therapies. We offer a variety of services, including background information, self-assessment questionnaires, and environmental therapy products."
http://www.cet.org/
(646) 395-8241
337 West 20th Street, Suite 4M
New York NY 10011

Vitamin D Council
http://www.VitaminDCouncil.org/
See https://www.VitaminDCouncil.org/about-vitamin-d/testing-for-vitamin-d/ for information and sources for in-home vitamin D test kits
(805) 439-1075
info@VitaminDCouncil.org
1241 Johnson Ave. #134
San Luis Obispo, CA 93401

SELECTED HELIOTHERAPY PRODUCTS AND MANUFACTURERS:

The Day-Light Classic, The Day-Light Classic Plus and The Day-Light Sky (10,000-lux, white light therapy devices)
Manufactured by Carex Health Brands Inc.
http://www.carex.com/products/95/Bright-Light-Therapy/
See also https://www.facebook.com/CarexHealthBrands
(800) 526-8051
customerservice@carex.com

GoLITE BLU Energy Light (natural blue light)
Manufactured by Philips
http://www.usa.philips.com/c-p/HF3332_60/golite-blu-energy-light
(866) 832-4361
3000 Minuteman Rd.
Andover, MA 01810

Per2 LED Daylight Lamp (simulates natural daylight rhythm from dusk to dawn) and SunTouch Plus (10,000-lux and includes negative ion generator)
Manufactured by Nature Bright
https://www.NatureBright.com/
(949) 625-4900
(800) 622-0231
19200 Von Karman Ave, Suite 350
Irvine, California 92612

UVB Midband Ultraviolet Lamp (provides UVB only)
Manufactured by Rayminder Engineered Lighting
http://www.rayminder.org/
info@rayminder.org

Vitamin D3 10,000 IU Liquid
Manufactured by DaVinci Laboratories of Vermont
http://www.DaVinciLabs.com/
(800) 325-1776
20 New England Dr. Suite 10
Essex Junction, VT 05452
Phone: (800) 325-1776 • Fax: (802

Superior Source Vitamin D Extra Strength MicroLingual Tablets (10,000 IU)
Manufactured by Continental Vitamin Company
http://SuperiorSourceVitamins.com/
See also http://SuperiorSourceVitamins.com/microlingual-tablets/a-d-k-vitamins/
(800) 421.6175
information@SuperiorSource1.com
4510 S. Boyle Ave.
Los Angeles, CA 90058

Free blue light reduction software
F.lux—"Software to warm up your computer display at night, to match your indoor lighting."
https://JustGetFlux.com/
See also https://www.facebook.com/JustGetFlux
support@JustGetFlux.com

SELECTED HELIOTHERAPY BOOKS:

Reset Your Inner Clock: The Drug-Free Way to Your Best-Ever Sleep, Mood, and Energy by Michael Terman, PhD and Ian McMahan, PhD
Avery; Reprint edition (October 29, 2013)
ISBN: 978-1583335345

SEX-RELATED RESOURCES

American Association of Sexuality Educators, Counselors and Therapists (AASECT)—A not-for-profit, professional organization including sexuality educators, counselors, therapists, and others.
https://www.aasect.org/
(202) 449-1099
info@aasect.org
1444 I Street, NW, Suite 700
Washington, DC 20005
Visit https://www.aasect.org/referral-directory to find a sexuality therapist or counselor near you.

International Professional Surrogates Association—"Non-profit organization dedicated to advancing the science, art and availability of Surrogate Partner Therapy"
http://www.SurrogateTherapy.org/
See also http://www.SurrogateTherapy.org/contact-us/referral-contact/
(413) 247-4722
3679 Motor Avenue, Suite 205
Los Angeles, CA 90034

SELECTED SEXUAL DYSFUNCTION/THERAPY PRODUCTS AND MANUFACTURERS:

Maca powder
Navitas Naturals—Online retailer that sells powdered maca, maca cashews and other superfoods
http://NavitasNaturals.com/
888-645-4282
info@NavitasNaturals.com

SELECTED SEXUAL DYSFUNCTION/THERAPY BOOKS:

Sex Made Simple: Clinical Strategies for Sexual Issues in Therapy by Barry McCarthy
PESI Publishing & Media (June 15, 2015)
ISBN: 978-1559570275

Sexual Healing: The Complete Guide to Overcoming Common Sexual Problems by Barbara Keesling, PhD
Hunter House; 3rd edition (February 3, 2006)
ISBN: 978-0897934657

MUSIC THERAPY RESOURCES:

Integrated Listening Systems
Visit - http://IntegratedListening.com/about/

Neurologic Music Therapy - The Center for Biomedical Research in Music at Colorado State University
Visit - http://cbrm.ColoState.edu/

EARTHING-RELATED RESOURCES:

Earthing Institute Inc.—Research, advisories, earthing FAQs, videos and more
http://www.EarthingInstitute.net/
(760) 325-0151
367 South Cahuilla Road
Palm Springs, CA 92262

National Electrical Contractors Association
http://www.necanet.org/
(301) 657-3110
3 Bethesda Metro Center, Suite 1100
Bethesda, MD 20814
Visit http://www.necanet.org/find-a-contractor to find a qualified electrical contractor near you.

SELECTED EARTHING-RELATED PRODUCTS AND
MANUFACTURERS:

Earthing universal grounding mats, throws and pads, pillows, sheet sets,
accessories and other earthing products
Earthing.com—Manufacturer and online retailer
https://www.earthing.com/
(888) 223-8454
72320 Manufacturing Rd,
Thousand Palms, CA 92276

Minimalist earthing shoes
Manufactured by Earth Runners
http://www.EarthRunners.com/
See also http://www.EarthRunners.com/pages/earthing-shoes
(408) 564-1966
EarthRunner1987@gmail.com
1229 Hecker Pass Road
Watsonville, California 95076

Earthing footwear, sheets and bedding
The Earthing Store—Online retailer
http://www.TheEarthingStore.com/
(855) 273-2181
info@TheBrownBear.ca

SELECTED EARTHING-RELATED BOOKS:

Earthing: The Most Important Health Discovery Ever! by Clinton Ober
Basic Health Publications; 2nd edition (March 15, 2014)
ISBN: 978-1591203742

*Grounding Therapy: Nature's Most POWERFUL Natural Health Secret Redis-
covered* by James Edgar
Wyeland Publishing; Kindle Edition (August 29, 2014)

HORTICULTURE THERAPY RESOURCES:

American Horticultural Therapy Association
http://ahta.org

Media review article with listing of farms owned and operated by veterans
http://HealthImpactNews.com/2011/war-vets-turn-to-organic-farming-for-mental-health-instead-of-drugs/

HT program in Bryn Mawr Rehabilitation Hospital
http://www.MainLineHealth.org/rehab/services/horticultural-therapy

CHAPTER 5 RESOURCES

Academy of Certified Brain Injury Specialists
http://www.biausa.org/acbis
(703) 761-0750 ext. 631
acbis@biausa.org
c/o Brain Injury Association of America
1608 Spring Hill Road, Suite 110
Vienna, VA 22182

Onnit Academy and DeFranco's Gym
http://www.onnit.com
1-855-ONNIT-99
4401 Freidrich Ln.
Suite 302
Austin, TX 78744

YMCA
http://www.ymca.net/
See also http://www.ymca.net/find-your-y/ to find your local YMCA
(800) 872-9622 (U.S.)
(312) 977-0031 (International)
fulfillment@ymca.net
101 N Wacker Drive
Chicago, IL 60606

Gym and Fitness Clubs.com—Includes a gym finder for U.S. and Canada, diet and fitness resources and more
http://www.GymsAndFitnessClubs.com/
See also http://www.GymsAndFitnessClubs.com/gyms-by-location/
531 Main Street #902
El Segundo, CA 90245

ExerciseFriends.com—Free site to "connect people all over the [U.S.] who want to meet new people, achieve their health goals, and get out and exercise." Enter your zip code and preferred activity to find potential exercise partners nearby.
http://ExerciseFriends.com/
support@ExerciseFriends.com

FitLink—Find a workout partner, personal trainer or other fitness professional. Site also includes free workout plans and other resources.
http://www.FitLink.com/
See also http://www.FitLink.com/workout-partners and
http://www.FitLink.com/personal-trainers
(646) 652.6574
info@FitLink.com

"SportsBuddy"—Free app for iOS devices developed by Buddy Tech, LLC. Available via iTunes App Store.
"The world's first smart-matching app that connects you to sports partners at your level and in your area. From tennis buddies, to running buddies, to yoga buddies, to gym buddies... we've got you covered."
https://www.GetSportsBuddy.com/

"Fitspur"—Free app for iOS devices developed by Goquest Media Ventures Private Limited. Available via iTunes App Store.
"Find your activity partners, pair up with them, enjoy your favorite sport and most importantly stay motivated throughout the course of it."
http://fitspur.com/

"SwollMates"—Free app for iOS devices developed by Apptreneur LLC. Available via iTunes App Store.
"Connecting with your perfect fitness partner has never been easier. Match, meet and get fit! Browse through tons of people within your customized search filters to connect with others."

"Workout Plan"—Free fitness schedule and journal app for iOS devices developed by Matcha Labs. Available via iTunes App Store.
http://GetWorkoutPlan.com/

Onnit Academy—Diet and fitness information, resources, podcasts and more
https://www.onnit.com/academy/
(855) ONNIT-99
info@onnit.com
4401 Freidrich Ln. Suite 302
Austin, TX 78744

BALANCE AND BODYWEIGHT TRAINING RESOURCES:

"Bodyweight Workout" and "MMA Spartan System 3.0 Free"—Free apps for Android devices developed by Arsutech. Available via Google Play. "Spartan bodyweight" workout routines for beginners and athletes. http://www.GorillaSoft.me.pn/
"MMA Spartan Workouts & Exercises"—Free app for iOS devices developed by Arslan Hajdarevic. Available via iTunes App Store.
Balance and wobble boards, resistance bands and tubing, rebounders, jump ropes and much more
Perform Better!—Online retailer specializing in functional training, rehab and sports performance
http://www.PerformBetter.com/
(888) 556-7464
PerformBetter@PerformBetter.com
1600 Division Rd.
West Warwick, RI 02893

Butter NUB Balance Board, Flow Balance Board w/Rock, Zone Balance Pro Board w/Rocks and others
Manufactured by Vew-Do
https://www.VewDo.com/
See also https://www.VewDo.com/Where-To-Buy-Vew-Do-Balance-Boards_ep_89-1.html
(802) 362-2893
254 Airport Rd.
Manchester Center, VT 05255

SI Balance Board
Manufactured by SI Boards
http://www.Si-Boards.com

See also https://www.onnit.com/Si-Board/
(714) 809-5109
PO Box 61272
Irvine, CA 92602

Slackline kits, hardware, webbing, accessories
Balance Community, LLC—Online retailer
http://www.BalanceCommunity.com/
(818) 527-5225
info@BalanceCommunity.com
PO Box 601
Germantown, MD 20875

SELECTED BALANCE AND BODYWEIGHT TRAINING BOOKS:

You Are Your Own Gym: The Bible of Bodyweight Exercises by Mark Lauren
Ballantine Books; Reprint edition (January 4, 2011)
ISBN: 978-0345528582

100 No-Equipment Workouts by Neila Rey
New Line Publishing (November 6, 2013)
ISBN: 978-1844819805

Bodyweight Strength Training Anatomy by Bret Contreras
Human Kinetics; 2nd edition (September 6, 2013)
ISBN: 978-1450429290

YOGA RESOURCES:

Resources for Yoga Instructors

- Yoga Teacher Central — http://YogaTeacherCentral.com/free-teaching-tools/our-bookshelf/
- Yoga Teacher Resource — http://TeachingYoga.net
- Teach Asana — http://www.TeachAsana.com
- International Association of Yoga Teachers — http://www.iayt.org
- British Wheel of Yoga — http://www.bwy.org.uk
- International Yoga Teachers Association — http://iyta.org.au

Resources for Yoga Students
- Yoga Basics — http://www.YogaBasics.com/practice/yoga-for-beginners/

- *The Yoga Bible* by Christina Brown, 2003.
  ISBN: 9781841811925

- *Yoga Anatomy* by Leslie Kaminoff, 2007.
  ISBN: 978-1450400244

- *The Key Muscles of Yoga: Scientific Keys Series, Vol. 1,* by Ray Long, 2009.
  ISBN: 978-1607432382

- *The Key Poses of Yoga: Scientific Keys Series, Vol. 2,* by Ray Long, 2009.
  ISBN: 978-1607432395

QI GONG RELATED RESOURCES:

Master Zhongxian Wu – lineage holder of multiple Qi Gong schools. Visit - http://www.MasterWu.net/

MEDITATION RESOURCES:

"Stop, Breathe & Think!"—free app for iOS and Android devices developed by Tools for Peace. Available via Google Play and iTunes App Store. "Become more mindful and compassionate using our Meditation Guide. Check in daily, track your progress, and feel the calm."
http://StopBreatheThink.org/

HeartMath Institute—"A nonprofit research and education organization offering prevention and intervention strategies for improved emotional health, decision-making [and] learning skills."
https://www.HeartMath.org/
(800) 711-6221
info@HeartMath.org
http://www.HeartMath.com/emwave-technology/ and
http://www.HeartMath.com/InnerBalance/
14700 West Park Ave.
Boulder Creek, California 95006

Herbert Benson, MD and the Relaxation Response
http://www.RelaxationResponse.org/

SELECTED MEDITATION BOOKS:

Presence Process: A Journey Into Present Moment Awareness by Michael Brown
Namaste Publishing (June 22, 2010)
ISBN: 978-1897238462

The Miracle of Mindfulness: An Introduction to the Practice of Meditation by
Thich Nhat Hanh
Beacon Press; 1st edition (May 1, 1999)
ISBN: 978-0807012390

Meditation for Beginners by Jack Cornfield
Sounds True; 1st edition (August 1, 2008)
ISBN: 978-1591799429

INVERSION THERAPY RESOURCES:

Inversion USA—Online retailer of inversion tables, gravity boots and
racks
http://www.InversionUSA.com/
(877) 843-2424
CustomerService@inversionusa.com

SELECTED INVERSION THERAPY PRODUCTS AND
MANUFACTURERS:

EP 560 Ltd. Inversion Table, EP 960 Ltd. Inversion Table and
accessories
Manufactured by Teeter Hang Ups
http://TeeterTV.com/
(800) 847-0143
info@teeter-inversion.com
9902 162nd Street Ct E
Puyallup, WA 98375

Ironman Gravity 4000 Inversion Table, Ironman High Capacity Gravity 3000 Inversion Table and others
Manufactured by Ironman Fitness
https://www.IronmanFitness.com/
https://www.IronmanFitness.com/products/Inversion+Tables/
(626) 810-2100
(844) 641-7922

SELECTED INVERSION THERAPY BOOKS:

Inversion Therapy: Relieve lower back and sciatica pain, improve posture, and revolutionize your health by Mia Campbell
Green Pony Press, Inc. (February 12, 2014)
ISBN: 978-0615971285

FAITH AND PERSEVERANCE RESOURCES:

"TBI Hope & Inspiration" Facebook Group—Founded by brain injury survivor and author David A. Grant. "Here, TBI stands for 'To Be Inspired!'"
https://www.facebook.com/TBIHopeAndInspiration
(See also *TBI Hope & Inspiration Magazine*—A free, all-digital publication that supports the brain injury/concussion community at http://www.TBIHopeAndInspiration.com/subscribe.htm)

"Traumatic Brain Injury Healing & Recovery Support Group" Facebook Group—A closed forum for brain injury survivors, their caregivers and loved ones. "Please feel free to post questions, advice, resources and your feelings on this life changing and challenging journey."
https://www.facebook.com/groups/186712754690242/

"Life After Brain Injury—Friendship, Support, and Laughter" Facebook Group—Closed forum for brain injury survivors, their caregivers and relatives. "This group can be used for networking with other survivors, friendship, and supporting your fellow brain injury survivor. Please feel free to share factual information regarding brain injury and ways for brain injury survivors to find support."
https://www.facebook.com/groups/LifeAfterBrainInjury/

"Brain Injury Help, News, and Support" Facebook Group—A closed forum and Brain Injury Network survivor advocacy group. With the permission of the survivor, close family members and friends may join; however, "Medical providers and certain other service providers are not eligible for this group even if they meet the other criteria."
https://www.facebook.com/groups/brain.injury.help.news.and.support.community/

"Brain Injury Survivors' Worldwide Community" Facebook Group—An open group also affiliated with the Brain Injury Network.
https://www.facebook.com/brain.injury.survivors.worldwide.community

VolunteerMatch—Provides volunteer information, listings and search options for local and remote volunteer opportunities
http://www.VolunteerMatch.org/
(415) 241-6868
support@VolunteerMatch.org
550 Montgomery Street, 8th Floor
San Francisco, CA 94111

All for Good—Affiliated with Points of Light, All for Good provides volunteer information, listings and search options for local and remote volunteer opportunities
http://www.AllForGood.org/
See also http://www.PointsOfLight.org/
support@AllForGood.org

Mental Health America—"Community-based nonprofit dedicated to addressing the needs of those living with mental illness"
http://www.MentalHealthAmerica.net/
See also http://www.MentalHealthAmerica.net/finding-help and http://www.MentalHealthAmerica.net/find-support-groups
(703) 838-7553
2000 N. Beauregard Street, 6th Floor
Alexandria, VA 22311

GoodTherapy.org—"Helping people find therapists. Advocating for ethical therapy."

http://www.GoodTherapy.org/
(888) 563-2112 ext. 1
2103 Harrison Ave. NW #2-347
Olympia, WA 98502
Visit http://www.GoodTherapy.org/find-therapist.html to search for a therapist near you.

Help Finding a Therapist: 1-800-THERAPIST (1-800-843-7274)

"Talkspace"—Online counseling and therapy app for iOS and Android devices developed by Groop Internet Platform Inc. Available via Google Play and iTunes App Store. "For only $25 per week (paid monthly), Talkspace members gain unlimited access to a licensed therapist." See also http://www.talkspace.com/

BrainLine.org—Comprehensive information and resources about preventing, treating and living with TBI. Includes webcasts, an e-newsletter and much more.
http://www.BrainLine.org
sSee also http://www.BrainLine.org/resources/index.php and
http://www.BrainLine.org/landing_pages/Family.html
(703) 998-2020
info@BrainLine.org
2775 South Quincy Street
Arlington, VA 22206

CHAPTER 6 RESOURCES

Epi-paleo Rx: The Prescription for Disease Reversal and Optimal Health by Dr. Jack Kruse
Optimized Life PLC; 1st edition (March 20, 2013)
ISBN: 978-0989057738

The Better Brain Book: The Best Tool for Improving Memory and Sharpness and Preventing Aging of the Brain by David Perlmutter
Riverhead Books; reprint edition (August 2, 2005)
ISBN: 978-1594480935

Primal Body, Primal Mind: Beyond the Paleo Diet for Total Health and a Longer Life by Nora T. Gedgaudas
Healing Arts Press; 2nd edition (May 27, 2011)
ISBN: 978-1594774133
The 4 Hour Body by Timothy Ferriss
Harmony Books; 1st edition 2010
ISBN: 978-0307463630

Seeds, sprouters, kits and supplies, plus free sprouting instructions and resources
Sprout People—Online retailer of organic seed and food-grade, seed-sprouting equipment
https://SproutPeople.org
(877) 777-6887
170 Mendell St.
San Francisco, CA 94124

Beyond Organic Beef—"Exclusively Grassfed Beef"
http://BeyondOrganicBeef.com/
(541) 805-1124
info@BeyondOrganicBeef.com
1782 S. Main St.
Union, OR 97883

Clean: The Revolutionary Program to Restore the Body's Natural Ability to Heal Itself by Alejandro Junger
HarperOne; 2nd updated edition (April 17, 2012)
ISBN: 978-0062201669

The Second Brain: A Groundbreaking New Understanding of Nervous Disorders of the Stomach and Intestine
by Michael Gershon
Harper Perennial (November 17, 1999)
ISBN: 978-0060930721

Brain Maker: The Power of Gut Microbes to Heal and Protect Your Brain—for Life by Dr. David Perlmutter with Kristin Loberg
Little, Brown and Company; 1st edition (April 28, 2015)
ISBN: 978-0316380102

Local Harvest—Find locally grown produce near you. Site includes search tools to help you locate farmers' markets, family farms, Community Supported Agriculture (CSA) programs, food co-ops and farm stands throughout the U.S.
http://www.LocalHarvest.org/
See also http://www.LocalHarvest.org/csa/ and http://www.LocalHarvest.org/farmers-markets/
(831) 515-5602
contact@LocalHarvest.org
P.O. Box 1292
Santa Cruz, CA 95061

Chia protein powder
Distributed by Foods Alive
http://www.FoodsAlive.com/
See also http://www.FoodsAlive.com/Chia-Protein-Powder-Organic-8-oz-p/0043.htm
(260) 488-4497
300 Industrial Dr., Suite C; P.O. Box 210
Angola, IN 46703

Pea protein powder and rice protein powder
Distributed by Growing Naturals, LLC
http://GrowingNaturals.com/
See also http://store.GrowingNaturals.com/pea-proteins/ and http://store.GrowingNaturals.com/rice-proteins/
(888) 572-5827
info@GrowingNaturals.com
12049 W Jefferson Blvd.
Culver City, CA 90230

The Dolce Whey—whey protein isolate
Distributed by Onnit Labs, LLC
https://www.onnit.com
See also https://www.onnit.com/dolce-whey/
(855) ONNIT-99
info@onnit.com
4401 Freidrich Ln. Suite 302
Austin, TX 78744

Intermittent Fasting: Everything You Need to Know About Intermittent Fasting For Beginner to Expert - Build Lean Muscle and Change Your Life by James Sinclair
Amazon Digital Services, Inc.; Kindle edition (November 15, 2015)

The Fast Diet: Lose Weight, Stay Healthy, and Live Longer with the Simple Secret of Intermittent Fasting by Michael Mosley
Atria Books; revised, updated edition (January 6, 2015)
ISBN: 978-1501102011

Blood testing for Omega 6:3 ratios
Quest Diagnostics
http://www.QuestDiagnostics.com/home.html
See also http://www.QuestDiagnostics.com/home/contact.html#locations
(866) 697-8378

GENETIC PROFILE TESTING FOR NUTRIGENOMICS AND PROVIDERS:

23andMe—CLIA certified lab

https://www.23andMe.com/
See also https://www.23andMe.com/howitworks/ and
https://www.facebook.com/23andMe/
(800) 239-5230
899 W Evelyn Ave.
Mountain View, CA 94041

Holistic Health International (Dr. Amy Yasko)
http://www.HolisticHealth.com/
See also http://www.DrAmyYasko.com/ and
http://www.HolisticHealth.com/
800-768-8744
info@HolisticHealth.com
279 Walkers Mills Rd.
Bethel, ME 04217

Know your Genetics
https://www.KnowYourGenetics.com/

MTHFR.net—"Your Expert Resource on MTHFR Gene Mutations"
http://mthfr.net/
See also https://www.facebook.com/DrBenjaminLynch/

NeuroSenory Centers of America—"Focused on the diagnosis and treatment of Neuroimmune disorders."
http://www.DrKendalStewart.com/
(512) 338-9840
info@DrKendalStewart.com
11719 Bee Caves Rd. #204
Austin, TX 78738

KETOGENIC DIET RESOURCES:

Ketogenic Diet Mistakes You Need to Know by Sara Givens
Amazon Digital Services, Inc.; Kindle edition (April 26, 2015)

The Ketogenic Cookbook: Nutritious Low-Carb, High-Fat Paleo Meals to Heal Your Body by Jimmy Moore
Victory Belt Publishing; 1st edition (July 28, 2015)
ISBN: 978-1628600780

OILY FISH RESOURCES:

Krill oil (DHA and EPA supplement)
Distributed by Onnit Labs, LLC
https://www.onnit.com
See also https://www.onnit.com/krill-oil/
(855) ONNIT-99
info@onnit.com
4401 Freidrich Ln. Suite 302
Austin, TX 78744

COCONUT OIL RESOURCES:

Organic Extra Virgin Coconut Oil Softgel Capsules
Distributed by Paradise's Blend
http://www.ParadisesBlend.com/
See also http://www.ParadisesBlend.com/products/organic-coconut-oil-capsules
(206) 552-8449
cs@ParadisesBlend.com
2926 South Steele St., Suite 500
Tacoma, WA 98409

TURMERIC RESOURCES:

Turmeric Curcumin Extract w/Bioperine Capsules
Distributed by BioGanix, Ltd.
http://www.BioGanix.com/
BioGanix Ltd.
(281) 402-6747
support@BioGanix.com
10685-B Hazelhurst Dr. # 15634
Houston, TX 77043

EGG YOLKS AND LECITHIN RESOURCES:

Local Harvest—Find locally grown produce and fresh eggs near you. Site includes search tools to help you locate farmers' markets, family farms, Community Supported Agriculture (CSA) programs, food co-ops and farm stands throughout the U.S.
http://www.LocalHarvest.org/
See also http://www.LocalHarvest.org/csa/ and http://www.LocalHarvest.org/farmers-markets/
(831) 515-5602
contact@LocalHarvest.org
P.O. Box 1292
Santa Cruz, CA 95061

U.S. Department of Agriculture (USDA) Local Food Directories—Find a local Community Supported Agriculture (CSA) program, farmers' market, on-farm market or other food hub with free, online search tools from the USDA's Agricultural Marketing Service.
http://www.USDALocalFoodDirectories.com/
(202) 720-2791
1400 Independence Ave., S.W.
Washington, DC 20250

Sunflower-derived lecithin in liquid, powder and capsule forms
Distributed by LEKITHOS Inc.
https://www.MySunflowerLecithin.com/
(888) 938-5188
info@lekithos.com

Non-GMO, soy-derived lecithin powder
Distributed by HealthForce Nutritionals
https://HealthForce.com
See also https://HealthForce.com/longevity-immunity/non-gmo-lecithin-powder
(800) 357-2717

Soy-derived and sunflower-derived lecithin in softgel capsules, liquid, powder and granulated forms
Distributed by Piping Rock Health Products
http://www.PipingRock.com
See also http://www.PipingRock.com/lecithin
(800) 544-1925
customerservice@PipingRock.com
2120 Smithtown Ave
Ronkonkoma, NY 11779

CHAPTER 7 RESOURCES

SUGAR-RELATED RESOURCES:

All-natural sugar alternatives, including glycine, stevia, monk fruit, erythritol and xylitol
Swanson Health Products—Online retailer

http://www.SwansonVitamins.com/
See also http://www.SwansonVitamins.com/food-beverage-sugar-substitutes
(800) 824-4491
customercare@SwansonVitamins.com
P.O. Box 2803
Fargo, ND 58108-2803

SELECTED SUGAR-RELATED BOOKS:

JJ Virgin's Sugar Impact Diet: Drop 7 Hidden Sugars, Lose Up to 10 Pounds in Just 2 Weeks by J.J. Virgin
Grand Central Life & Style; 1st edition (November 4, 2014)
ISBN: 978-1455577842

JJ Virgin's Sugar Impact Diet Cookbook: 150 Low-Sugar Recipes to Help You Lose Up to 10 Pounds in Just 2 Weeks by J.J. Virgin
Grand Central Life & Style; 1st edition (May 26, 2015)
ISBN: 978-1455577873

Grain Brain: The Surprising Truth about Wheat, Carbs, and Sugar—Your Brain's Silent Killers
by David Perlmutter with Kristin Loberg
Little, Brown and Company; 1st edition (September 17, 2013)
ISBN: 978-0316234801

The Blood Sugar Solution: The Ultra Healthy Program for Losing Weight, Preventing Disease, and Feeling Great Now! by Mark Hyman
Little, Brown and Company; reprint edition (December 30, 2014)
ISBN: 978-0316127363

The Blood Sugar Solution 10-Day Detox Diet Cookbook: More than 150 Recipes to Help You Lose Weight and Stay Healthy for Life by Mark Hyman
Little, Brown and Company; 1st edition (March 10, 2015)
ISBN: 978-0316338813

OBESITY-RELATED RESOURCES:

"Fitter Fitness Calculator & Weight Tracker"—free app for iOS devices developed by MigoApps, LLC. Available via iTunes App Store. Includes weight tracking tools and calulators for Body Mass Index, Body Fat Percentage, Basal Metabolic Rate and more.

"BMI Calculator Weight Tracker"—free app for Android devices developed by Appovo. Available via Google Play. "With BMI Calculator you can calculate your Body Mass Index, Waist-to-Height Ratio, Body Fat Percentage and Calorie Consumption (BMR + PAL) to find your ideal weight based on age and gender. It can also be used to find your healthy weight if you want to lose weight or are on diet."

FitLink—Online BMI calculator
http://www.fitlink.com/bmi-calculator
(646) 652.6574
info@FitLink.com

DoctorFinders—Free, U.S.-based search for specific procedures, including DXA body scans.
http://DoctorFinders.com/dexa.php
(480) 704-4716
SalesLoop@DoctorFinders.com

Body Spec—Provider of DXA body scans with locations in northern and southern California.
https://www.body-spec.com/
See also https://www.body-spec.com/scan-me
310-601-8184
support@body-spec.com
2148 Federal Ave, Suite C
Los Angeles, CA 90025

DexaFit LLC—Provider of DXA body scans with locations in Chicago, San Francisco, Atlanta, Tampa and others.
http://www.DexaFit.com/
3727 North Broadway Street
Chicago, IL 60613

Overeaters Anonymous
http://www.oa.org/
See also https://www.oa.org/membersgroups/find-a-meeting/
(505) 891-2664
P.O. Box 44020
Rio Rancho, New Mexico 87174-4020

SELECTED FASTING-RELATED BOOKS:

Intermittent Fasting: Everything You Need to Know About Intermittent Fasting For Beginner to Expert - Build Lean Muscle and Change Your Life by James Sinclair
Amazon Digital Services, Inc.; Kindle edition (November 15, 2015)

The Fast Diet: Lose Weight, Stay Healthy, and Live Longer with the Simple Secret of Intermittent Fasting by Michael Mosley
Atria Books; revised, updated edition (January 6, 2015)
ISBN: 978-1501102011

ALCOHOL ABSTINENCE PROGRAMS AND RESOURCES:

Being True to You — An empowerment based recovery coaching program for healing from addiction
http://www.beingtruetoyou.com
650-690-2088
coaching@beingtruetoyou.com

The Traumatic Brain Injury Network—A substance abuse treatment program for individuals who have sustained a traumatic brain injury (TBI)
http://www.TBI-Network.org/
(614) 685-8511
3300 Morehouse Medical Plaza Pavilion
2050 Kenny Road
Columbus, OH 43221
Alcoholics Anonymous
http://www.aa.org/
(212) 870-3400

P.O. Box 459, Grand Central Station
New York, NY 10163
Be Sober Hotline: (800) BE-SOBER (1-800-237-6237)

Secular Organizations for Sobriety (SOS)—non-religious, member-driven support program for "anyone sincerely seeking sobriety from alcohol addiction, drug addiction and compulsive eating."
http://www.SOSSobriety.org/
See also http://www.SOSSobriety.org/meetings.html
(323) 666-4295
sos@cfiwest.org
4773 Hollywood Blvd.
Los Angeles, CA 90027

SMART Recovery—"the leading self-empowering addiction recovery support group. Our participants learn tools for addiction recovery based on the latest scientific research and participate in a world-wide community which includes free, self-empowering, science-based mutual help groups."
http://www.SmartRecovery.org/
(866) 951-5357
7304 Mentor Avenue Suite F
Mentor, OH 44060

Women For Sobriety—"A non-profit organization dedicated to helping women overcome alcoholism and other addictions."
http://www.WomenForSobriety.org/
(215) 536-8026
contact@WomenForSobriety.org
P.O. Box 618
Quakertown, PA 18951

Dual Recovery Anonymous—"An independent, nonprofessional, Twelve Step, self-help membership organization for people with a dual diagnosis." (Members with a "dual diagnosis" deal with chemical dependence and psychiatric conditions.)
(913) 991-2703
draws@DRAOnline.org

See also http://DRAOnline.QWKNetLLC.com/meetings.html
P.O. Box 8107
Prairie Village, Kansas 66208

Substance Abuse and Mental Health Services Administration (SAM-HSA)—Site includes a Behavioral Health Treatment Services Locator tool for those seeking substance abuse/addiction or mental health service in the U.S.
http://www.samhsa.gov/
See also https://FindTreatment.samhsa.gov/
(800) 487-4889
1 Choke Cherry Road
Rockville, MD 20857

"Step Away"—free app for iOS devices developed by Here and Now Systems LLC. Available via iTunes App Store. "Step Away offers alcohol addiction help when friends, family, therapists or groups may not be available or immediately present. Step Away provides strategies and reminders to help you overcome alcohol addiction during high risk times."

"Quit Drinking with Andrew Johnson"—app for Android devices developed by HiveBrain Software. Available via Google Play. "Designed to help listeners relax and overcome the emotional and physical cravings for alcohol. Whether you are wanting to stop drinking altogether or regain control and cut down, this app will start to help you break those negative habits that lead to reaching for a drink." (See also "Stop Drinking with Andrew Johnson"—app for iOS devices developed by Michael Schneider. Available via iTunes App Store.)

CHAPTER 8 RESOURCES

TBI ASSESSMENT TOOLS

Sport Concussion Assessment Tool – 3rd edition
http://bjsm.bmj.com/content/47/5/259.full.pdf

Sport Concussion Recognition Tool (SCRT)—Free, downloadable PDF assessment tool, including visible clues and signs and symptoms of suspected concussion.
Available from ParachuteCanada.org
http://horizon.ParachuteCanada.org/wp-content/uploads/2014/10/Pocket-Concussion-Recognition-Tool2013.pdf
(647) 776-5100
info@ParachuteCanada.org
150 Eglinton Ave East Suite 300
Toronto, Ontario M4P 1E8
Canada

Sports Concussion Assessment Tool, 3rd edition (SCAT3)—This free, downloadable PDF assessment tool was the result of the Third International Commission on Concussion in Sports in Zurich, 2008.
Available from *The British Journal of Sports Medicine*
http://bjsm.bmj.com/content/47/5/259.full.pdf
+ 44 (0) 207 111 1105
bjsm@bmj.com
Tavistock Square
London, WC1H 9JR
UK

Sports Concussion Assessment Tool for children ages five to 12, 3rd edition (Child-SCAT3)—This free, downloadable PDF assessment tool was the result of the Third International Commission on Concussion in Sports in Zurich, 2008.
Available from *The British Journal of Sports Medicine*
http://bjsm.bmj.com/content/47/5/263.full.pdf
+ 44 (0) 207 111 1105
bjsm@bmj.com
Tavistock Square
London, WC1H 9JR
UK

Brain Network Activation (BNA) testing
Developed by ElMindA Ltd.
http://ElMindA.com/
See also http://ElMindA.com/the-bna-platform/

(224) 888-0060 (U.S.)
972-9-951-6476 (International)
16 Haminhara St.
Herzliya 46586
Israel

Athletico Physical Therapy—Brain Network Activation (BNA) testing available in five Illinois-based locations, including Athletico Aurora Eola, Midtown Athletic Club, Athletico Lagrange Park, Athletico Niles and Athletico Orland Park North
http://www.athletico.com/
See also http://www.athletico.com/locations/
(630) 575-6200
(877) ATHLETI
concussion@athletico.com

Single Photon Emission Computer Tomography (SPECT)
Performed at Amen Clinics, Dr. Daniel G. Amen
http://www.AmenClinics.com/
See also http://www.AmenClinics.com/locations/ and http://www.AmenClinics.com/about-us/spect-frequently-asked-questions/
(866) 260-8227

Immediate Post-Concussion Assessment and Cognitive Testing (ImPACT)
ImPACT Applications, Inc.
https://www.ImpactTest.com
See also www.ImpactTest.com/find_care_provider
(877) 646-7991
info@ImpactTest.com
2000 Technology Drive, Suite 150
Pittsburgh, PA 15219

COGNISON test
Developed by Neuronetrix
http://www.neuronetrix.com/
See also http://neuronetrix.com/cognision-i-26.html
(502) 410-0219

info@neuronetrix.com
1044 E Chestnut St
Louisville KY 40204

Videonystagmography (VNG)
Carrick Institute of Clinical Neuroscience and Rehabilitation
http://CarrickInstitute.com/
See also http://CarrickInstitute.com/become-a-patient/
(321) 868-6464
info@CarrickInstitute.com
203-8941 Lake Drive
Cape Canaveral, FL 32920

CHAPTER 9 RESOURCES

"PUTTING IT ALL TOGETHER" RESOURCES

"T2 Mood Tracker"—free app for iOS and Android devices developed by the National Center for Telehealth & Technology. Available via Google Play and iTunes App Store.

"Allows users to monitor their moods on six pre-loaded scales (anxiety, stress, depression, brain injury, post-traumatic stress, general well-being). Custom scales can also be built. Users rate their moods by swiping a small bar to the left or to the right. The ratings are displayed on graphs to help users track their moods over time. Notes can be recorded to document daily events, medication changes and treatments that may be associated with mood changes, providing accurate information to help health care providers make treatment decisions."

"How Are You"—app for iOS and Android devices developed by Quantum Lab Co. Available via Google Play and iTunes App Store. "Easy tool for mood tracking in the form of a personal journal. Developed to help people who suffer from depression, anxiety, stress, bipolar disorder, mood swings and OCD."

Miscellaneous Resources

Nutrient Power: Heal Your Biochemistry and Heal Your Brain by William Walsh
Skyhorse Publishing; 1st revised, updated edition (May 6, 2014)
ISBN: 978-1626361287

Why Isn't My Brain Working?: A Revolutionary Understanding of Brain Decline and Effective Strategies to Recover Your Brain's Health by Dr. Datis Kharrazian
Elephant Press; 1st edition (May 1, 2013)
ISBN: 978-0985690434

Change Your Brain, Change Your Life: The Breakthrough Program for Conquering Anxiety, Depression, Obsessiveness, Lack of Focus, Anger, and Memory Problems by Daniel G. Amen, MD
Harmony; revised, expanded edition (November 3, 2015)
ISBN: 978-1101904640

National Alliance on Mental Illness
http://www.nami.org/
See also http://www.nami.org/Find-Support and http://www.nami.org/Learn-More/Mental-Health-Conditions/Related-Conditions/Dual-Diagnosis
(703) 524-7600
3803 N. Fairfax Drive, Suite 100
Arlington, VA 22203

National Institute of Mental Health
http://www.nimh.nih.gov/
(866) 615-6464
nimhinfo@nih.gov
6001 Executive Boulevard, Room 6200, MSC 9663
Bethesda, MD 20892-9663

Anxiety and Depression Association of America Support Groups—"National nonprofit organization dedicated to the prevention, treatment, and cure of anxiety and mood disorders, OCD, and PTSD and to improving the lives of all people who suffer from them through education, practice, and research."

http://www.adaa.org/
See also http://www.adaa.org/SupportGroups
(240) 485-1001
8701 Georgia Ave., Suite #412
Silver Spring, MD 20910

Depression and Bipolar Support Alliance (DBSA)
http://www.DBSAlliance.org/
See also http://www.DBSAlliance.org/site/PageServer?pagename=
peer_support_group_locator
(800) 826-3632
55 E. Jackson Blvd, Suite 490
Chicago, Illinois 60604

REFERENCES

1. Zaloshnja E, Miller T, Langlois J, Selassie A. Prevalence of Long-Term Disability From Traumatic Brain Injury in the Civilian Population of the United States, 2005. *Journal of Head Trauma Rehabilitation.* 2008;23(6):394-400. doi:10.1097/01.htr.0000341435.52004.ac.

2. Coronado VG, McGuire LC, Sarmiento K, et al. Trends in Traumatic Brain Injury in the U.S. and the public health response: 1995-2009. *J Safety Res.* 2012;43(4):299-307.

3. Rates of TBI-related Emergency Department Visits, Hospitalizations, and Deaths — United States, 2001–2010. (2014, February 24). Retrieved June 9, 2015, from http://www.cdc.gov/traumaticbraininjury/data/rates.html

4. Taylor C, Greenspan A, Xu L, Kresnow M. Comparability of National Estimates for Traumatic Brain Injury-Related Medical Encounters. *Journal of Head Trauma Rehabilitation.* 2015;30(3):150-159. doi:10.1097/htr.0000000000000105.

5. Coronado VG, Haileyesus T, Cheng TA, et al. Trends in Sports- and Recreation-Related Traumatic Brain Injuries Treated in US Emergency Departments: The National Electronic Injury Surveillance System-All Injury Program (NEISS-AIP) 2001-2012. J Head Trauma Rehabil. 2015;30(3):185-97.

6. Coronado VG, Haileyesus T, Cheng TA, et al. Trends in Sports- and Recreation-Related Traumatic Brain Injuries Treated in US Emergency Departments: The National Electronic Injury Surveillance System-All Injury Program (NEISS-AIP) 2001-2012. J Head Trauma Rehabil. 2015;30(3):185-97.

7. The CDC, NIH, DoD, and VA Leadership Panel. Report to Congress on Traumatic Brain Injury in the United States: Understanding the Public Health Problem among Current and Former Military Personnel. Centers for Disease Control and Prevention (CDC), the National Institutes of Health (NIH), the Department of Defense (DoD), and the Department of Veterans Affairs (VA). 2013.

8. The CDC, NIH, DoD, and VA Leadership Panel. Report to Congress on Traumatic Brain Injury in the United States: Understanding the Public

Health Problem among Current and Former Military Personnel. Centers for Disease Control and Prevention (CDC), the National Institutes of Health (NIH), the Department of Defense (DoD), and the Department of Veterans Affairs (VA). 2013.

9. National Institute of Neurological Disorders and Stroke. Traumatic brain injury: hope through research. Bethesda (MD): National Institutes of Health; 2002 Feb. NIH Publication No.: 02-158.

10. Plassman BL, Havlik RJ, Steffens DC, et al. Documented head injury in early adulthood and risk of Alzheimer's disease and other dementias. *Neurology*. 2000;55(8):1158–1166.

11. Silver J, McAllister T, Yudofsky S. *Textbook Of Traumatic Brain Injury, Second Edition*. Washington, D.C.: American Psychiatric Publishing; 2011.

12. Silver J, McAllister T, Yudofsky S. *Textbook Of Traumatic Brain Injury, Second Edition*. Washington, D.C.: American Psychiatric Publishing; 2011.

13. Finkelstein E, Corso P, Miller T. *The Incidence And Economic Burden Of Injuries In The United States*. Oxford: Oxford University Press; 2006.

14. Cuthbert J, Harrison-Felix C, Corrigan J, Bell J, Haarbauer-Krupa J, Miller A. Unemployment in the United States After Traumatic Brain Injury for Working-Age Individuals. *Journal of Head Trauma Rehabilitation*. 2015;30(3):160-174. doi:10.1097/htr.0000000000000090.

15. Schwarzbold, M., Diaz, A., Martins, E. T., Rufino, A., Amante, L. N., Thais, M. E., … Walz, R. (2008). Psychiatric disorders and traumatic brain injury. *Neuropsychiatric Disease and Treatment*, *4*(4), 797–816.

16. Horner, M. D., Ferguson, P. L., Selassie, A. W., Labbate, L. a, Kniele, K., & Corrigan, J. D. (2005). Patterns of alcohol use 1 year after traumatic brain injury: a population-based, epidemiological study. *Journal of the International Neuropsychological Society : JINS*, *11*(3), 322–30. http://doi.org/10.1017/S135561770505037X

17. Kshettry V, Mindea S, Batjer H. The management of cranial injuries in antiquity and beyond. *Neurosurgical FOCUS*. 2007;23(1):1-8. doi:10.3171/foc-07/07/e8.

18. Finger S, Clower WT: Victor Horsley on "Trephining in Pre- historic Times." Neurosurgery 48:911–918, 2001.

19. Gross, C. G. (2009). *A hole in the head : more tales in the history of neuroscience*. Cambridge, Mass.: MIT Press.

20. Kshettry V, Mindea S, Batjer H. The management of cranial injuries in antiquity and beyond. *Neurosurgical FOCUS*. 2007;23(1):1-8. doi:10.3171/foc-07/07/e8.

21. Faria M. Violence, mental illness, and the brain - A brief history of psychosurgery: Part 1 - From trephination to lobotomy. *Surg Neurol Int.* 2013;4(1):49. doi:10.4103/2152-7806.110146.

22. Robison RA, Taghva A, Liu CY, Apuzzo ML. Surgery of the mind, mood and conscious state: an idea in evolution. *World Neurosurg.* 2012;77:662–86.

23. Laskowski, R., Creed, J., & Raghupathi, R. (2015). Pathophysiology of Mild TBI: Implications for Altered Signaling Pathways –PubMed - NCBI. In F. Kobeissy (Ed.), *Brain Neurotrauma: Molecular, Neuropsychological and Rehabilitation Aspects.* Boca Raton (FL): CRC Press. Retrieved from http://www.ncbi.nlm.nih.gov/pubmed/26269903

24. Kim, E., Lauterbach, E. C., Reeve, A., Arciniegas, D. B., Coburn, K. L., Mendez, M. F., … Coffey, E. C. (2007). Neuropsychiatric complications of traumatic brain injury: a critical review of the literature (a report by the ANPA Committee on Research). *The Journal of Neuropsychiatry and Clinical Neurosciences, 19*(2), 106–27. http://doi.org/10.1176/jnp.2007.19.2.106

25. Horner, M. D., Ferguson, P. L., Selassie, A. W., Labbate, L. a, Kniele, K., & Corrigan, J. D. (2005). Patterns of alcohol use 1 year after traumatic brain injury: a population-based, epidemiological study. *Journal of the International Neuropsychological Society : JINS, 11*(3), 322–30. http://doi.org/10.1017/S135561770505037X

26. Nolan, S. (2005). Traumatic brain injury: a review. *Critical Care Nursing Quarterly, 28*(2), 188–94. Retrieved from http://www.ncbi.nlm.nih.gov/pubmed/15875448

27. Himanen L, Portin R, Isoniemi H, Helenius H, et al. Longitudinal cognitive changes in traumatic brain injury: a 30-year follow-up study. *Neurology* 2006;66(2):187-92.

28. Plassman BL, Havlik RJ, Steffens DC, et al. Documented head injury in early adulthood and risk of Alzheimer's disease and other dementias. *Neurology.* 2000;55(8):1158–1166.

29. Farrer L. Effects of Age, Sex, and Ethnicity on the Association Between Apolipoprotein E Genotype and Alzheimer Disease. *JAMA.* 1997;278(16):1349. doi:10.1001/jama.1997.03550160069041.

30. Mahley R, Weisgraber K, Huang Y. Apolipoprotein E4: A causative factor and therapeutic target in neuropathology, including Alzheimer's disease. Proceedings of the National Academy of Sciences. 2006;103(15):5644-5651. doi:10.1073/pnas.0600549103.

31. Caselli, R J. Age-related memory decline and apolipoprotein. *Discovery Medicine.* 2009;8(41):47.

32. Mayeux R, Ottman R, Maestre G et al. Synergistic Effects of Traumatic Head Injury and Apolipoprotein-epsilon4 in Patients With Alzheimer's Disease. *Neurology*. 1995;45(3):555-557. doi:10.1212/wnl.45.3.555.

33. Stoller, K. P. (2015). All the right moves: the need for the timely use of hyperbaric oxygen therapy for treating TBI/CTE/PTSD. *Medical Gas Research*, 5(1), 7. http://doi.org/10.1186/s13618-015-0028-0

34. Addington, C. P., Roussas, A., Dutta, D., & Stabenfeldt, S. E. (2015). Endogenous repair signaling after brain injury and complementary bioengineering approaches to enhance neural regeneration. *Biomarker Insights*, 10(Suppl 1), 43–60. http://doi.org/10.4137/BMI.S20062

35. Perman, S. M., Goyal, M., Neumar, R. W., Topjian, A. A., & Gaieski, D. F. (2014). Clinical applications of targeted temperature management. *Chest*, 145(2), 386–93. http://doi.org/10.1378/chest.12-3025

36. Pietrzak, E., Pullman, S., & McGuire, A. (2014). Using Virtual Reality and Videogames for Traumatic Brain Injury Rehabilitation: A Structured Literature Review. *Games for Health Journal*, 3(4), 202–14. http://doi.org/10.1089/g4h.2014.0013

37. Morries, L. D., Cassano, P., & Henderson, T. A. (2015). Treatments for traumatic brain injury with emphasis on transcranial near infrared laser phototherapy. *Neuropsychiatric Disease and Treatment*, 11, 2159–75. http://doi.org/10.2147/NDT.S65809

38. Addington, C. P., Roussas, A., Dutta, D., & Stabenfeldt, S. E. (2015). Endogenous repair signaling after brain injury and complementary bioengineering approaches to enhance neural regeneration. *Biomarker Insights*, 10(Suppl 1), 43–60. http://doi.org/10.4137/BMI.S20062

39. Giza, C.C. and Hovda, D.A. The Neurometabolic Cascade of Concussion. *Journal of Athletic Training*. 2001;36(3):228-235.

40. van Dierendonck D, Te Nijenhuis J. Flotation restricted environmental stimulation therapy (REST) as a stress-management tool: A meta-analysis. *Psychology & Health*. 2005;20(3):405-412. doi:10.1080/0887044041233133 7093.

41. Turner J, Fine T. Effects of relaxation associated with brief restricted environmental stimulation therapy (REST) on plasma cortisol, ACTH, and LH. *Biofeedback and Self-Regulation*. 1983;8(1):115-126. doi:10.1007/bf01000542.

42. Fine, T.H., Mills, D. and Turner, J.W. Jr. (1993). Differential effects of wet and dry flotation REST on EEG frequency and amplitude. In A.F. Barabasz and M. Barabasz (Eds.), Clinical and experimental restricted

environmental stimulation: New developments and perspectives (pp. 206-213). New York: Springer-Verlag.

43. Hashmi J, Huang Y, Osmani B, Sharma S, Naeser M, Hamblin M. Role of Low-Level Laser Therapy in Neurorehabilitation. PM&R. 2010;2(12):S292-S305. doi:10.1016/j.pmrj.2010.10.013.

44. Whelan, H. T., Smits Jr, R. L., Buchman, E. V., Whelan, N. T., Turner, S. G., Margolis, D. A., ... & Caviness, J. Effect of NASA light emitting diode irradiation on wound healing. *Journal of Clinical Laser Medicine & Surgery. 2001;*19(6), 305-314.

45. Xuan W, Vatansever F, Huang L, Hamblin M. Transcranial low-level laser therapy enhances learning, memory, and neuroprogenitor cells after traumatic brain injury in mice. *J Biomed Opt.* 2014;19(10):108003. doi:10.1117/1.jbo.19.10.108003.

46. Xuan W, Vatansever F, Huang L et al. Transcranial Low-Level Laser Therapy Improves Neurological Performance in Traumatic Brain Injury in Mice: Effect of Treatment Repetition Regimen. PLoS ONE. 2013;8(1):e53454. doi:10.1371/journal.pone.0053454.

47. Hashmi J, Huang Y, Osmani B, Sharma S, Naeser M, Hamblin M. Role of Low-Level Laser Therapy in Neurorehabilitation. *PM&R.* 2010;2(12):S292-S305. doi:10.1016/j.pmrj.2010.10.013.

48. Naeser M, Saltmarche A, Krengel M, Hamblin M, Knight J. Improved Cognitive Function After Transcranial, Light-Emitting Diode Treatments in Chronic, Traumatic Brain Injury: Two Case Reports. *Photomedicine and Laser Surgery.* 2011;29(5):351-358. doi:10.1089/pho.2010.2814.

49. Naeser M, Saltmarche A, Krengel M, Hamblin M, Knight J. Improved Cognitive Function After Transcranial, Light-Emitting Diode Treatments in Chronic, Traumatic Brain Injury: Two Case Reports. *Photomedicine and Laser Surgery.* 2011;29(5):351-358. doi:10.1089/pho.2010.2814.

50. Fda.gov. Illuminating the Hazards of Powerful Laser Products. 2015. Available at: http://www.fda.gov/ForConsumers/ConsumerUpdates/ucm166649.htm. Accessed July 6, 2015.

51. Los Angeles Times online. The Healthy Skeptic: What it means to be "FDA approved" or "FDA registered". 2001. Available at: http://articles.latimes.com/2010/mar/01/health/la-he-0301-skeptic-20100301. Accessed July 8, 2015.

52. Stoller K. All the right moves: the need for the timely use of hyperbaric oxygen therapy for treating TBI/CTE/PTSD. *Medical Gas Research.* 2015.

Available at: http://www.medicalgasresearch.com/content/pdf/s13618-015-0028-0.pdf. Accessed July 1, 2015.

53. FDA Consumer Health Information. Hyperbaric Oxygen Therapy: Don't Be Misled. August 2013. Available at: http://www.fda.gov/downloads/forconsumers/consumerupdates/ucm366015.pdf. Accessed July 1, 2015.

54. Rossignol D, Rossignol L, Smith S et al. Hyperbaric treatment for children with autism: a multicenter, randomized, double-blind, controlled trial. *BMC Pediatrics*. 2009;9(1):21. doi:10.1186/1471-2431-9-21.

55. Harch PG, Andrews SR, Fogarty EF, Amen D, Pezzullo JC, Lucarini J, et al. A phase I study of low-pressure hyperbaric oxygen therapy for blast-induced post-concussion syndrome and post-traumatic stress disorder. *J Neurotrauma*. 2012;29(1):168–85.

56. Harch PG, Andrews SR, Fogarty EF, Amen D, Pezzullo JC, Lucarini J, et al. A phase I study of low-pressure hyperbaric oxygen therapy for blast-induced post-concussion syndrome and post-traumatic stress disorder. *J Neurotrauma*. 2012;29(1):168–85.

57. Wikipedia. Hyperbaric medicine. 2015. Available at: https://en.wikipedia.org/wiki/Hyperbaric_medicine. Accessed July 2, 2015.

58. Markov M. Pulsed electromagnetic field therapy history, state of the art and future. *Environmentalist*. 2007;27(4):465-475. doi:10.1007/s10669-007-9128-2.

59. Markov M. *Electromagnetic Fields In Biology And Medicine*. CRC Press; 2015.

60. Markov M. Pulsed electromagnetic field therapy history, state of the art and future. *Environmentalist*. 2007;27(4):465-475. doi:10.1007/s10669-007-9128-2.

61. Goodwin, Thomas J. *Physiological and molecular genetic effects of time-varying electromagnetic fields on human neuronal cells*. National Aeronautics and Space Administration, Lyndon B. Johnson Space Center, 2003.

62. Rasouli J, Lekhraj R, White N et al. Attenuation of interleukin-1beta by pulsed electromagnetic fields after traumatic brain injury. *Neuroscience Letters*. 2012;519(1):4-8. doi:10.1016/j.neulet.2012.03.089.

63. Shiozaki T, Hayakata T, Tasaki O et al. Cerebrospinal fluid concentrations of anti-inflammatory mediators in early-phase severe traumatic brain injury. *Shock*. 2005;23(5):406-410. doi:10.1097/01.shk.0000161385.62758.24.

64. Holmin S, Mathiesen T. Intracerebral administration of interleukin-1β and induction of inflammation, apoptosis, and vasogenic edema. *Journal of Neurosurgery*. 2000;92(1):108-120. doi:10.3171/jns.2000.92.1.0108.

65. B.W. McColl, N.J. Rothwell, S.M. Allan, Systemic inflammation alters the kinetics of cerebrovascular tight junction disruption after experimental stroke in mice, *Journal of Neuroscience.* 2008;(28):9451–9462.

66. Rasouli J, Lekhraj R, White N et al. Attenuation of interleukin-1beta by pulsed electromagnetic fields after traumatic brain injury. *Neuroscience Letters.* 2012;519(1):4-8. doi:10.1016/j.neulet.2012.03.089.

67. Dr. Pawluk. PEMF Contraindications - Dr. Pawluk. 2015. Available at: http://drpawluk.com/education/contraindications/. Accessed July 9, 2015.

68. Dr. Pawluk. PEMF Contraindications - Dr. Pawluk. 2015. Available at: http://drpawluk.com/education/contraindications/. Accessed July 9, 2015.

69. Dr. Pawluk. PEMF Contraindications - Dr. Pawluk. 2015. Available at: http://drpawluk.com/education/contraindications/. Accessed July 9, 2015.

70. Nahas Z. Handbook of Transcranial Magnetic Stimulation. *J Psychiatry Neurosci.* 2013;28(5):373–375.

71. Pascual-Leone A. *Handbook Of Transcranial Magnetic Stimulation.* London: Arnold; 2002.

72. Herrold A, Kletzel S, Harton B, Chambers R, Jordan N, Pape T. Transcranial magnetic stimulation: potential treatment for cooccurring alcohol, traumatic brain injury and posttraumatic stress disorders. *Neural Regeneration Research.* 2014;9(19):1712. doi:10.4103/1673-5374.143408.

73. Koski L, Kolivakis T, Yu C, Chen J, Delaney S, Ptito A. Noninvasive Brain Stimulation for Persistent Postconcussion Symptoms in Mild Traumatic Brain Injury. *Journal of Neurotrauma.* 2015;32(1):38-44. doi:10.1089/neu.2014.3449.

74. Coffman B, Clark V, Parasuraman R. Battery powered thought: Enhancement of attention, learning, and memory in healthy adults using transcranial direct current stimulation. *NeuroImage.* 2014;85:895-908. doi:10.1016/j.neuroimage.2013.07.083.

75. You D, Kim D, Chun M, Jung S, Park S. Cathodal transcranial direct current stimulation of the right Wernicke's area improves comprehension in subacute stroke patients. *Brain and Language.* 2011;119(1):1-5. doi:10.1016/j.bandl.2011.05.002.

76. Hesse S, Waldner A, Mehrholz J, Tomelleri C, Pohl M, Werner C. Combined Transcranial Direct Current Stimulation and Robot Assisted Arm Training in Subacute Stroke Patients: An Exploratory, Randomized

Multicenter Trial. *Neurorehabilitation and Neural Repair.* 2011;25(9):838-846. doi:10.1177/1545968311413906.

77. Fregni F, Li S, Zaninotto A, Santana Neville I, Paiva W, Nunn D. Clinical utility of brain stimulation modalities following traumatic brain injury: current evidence. *NDT.* 2015:1573. doi:10.2147/ndt.s65816.

78. Kang E, Kim D, Paik N. Transcranial direct current stimulation of the left prefrontal cortex improves attention in patients with traumatic brain injury: A pilot study. *J Rehabil Med.* 2012;44(4):346-350. doi:10.2340/16501977-0947.

79. Schneider H. Prevalence of anterior pituitary insufficiency 3 and 12 months after traumatic brain injury. *European Journal of Endocrinology.* 2006;154(2):259-265. doi:10.1530/eje.1.02071.

80. Bondanelli M, De Marinis L, Ambrosio M et al. Occurrence of Pituitary Dysfunction following Traumatic Brain Injury. *Journal of Neurotrauma.* 2004;21(6):685-696. doi:10.1089/0897715041269713.

81. Schneider H, Kreitschmann-Andermahr I, Ghigo E, Stalla G, Agha A. Hypothalamopituitary Dysfunction Following Traumatic Brain Injury and Aneurysmal Subarachnoid Hemorrhage. *JAMA.* 2007;298(12):1429. doi:10.1001/jama.298.12.1429.

82. Schneider H, Kreitschmann-Andermahr I, Ghigo E, Stalla G, Agha A. Hypothalamopituitary Dysfunction Following Traumatic Brain Injury and Aneurysmal Subarachnoid Hemorrhage. *JAMA.* 2007;298(12):1429. doi:10.1001/jama.298.12.1429.

83. Zihl J, Almeida O. Neuropsychology of Neuroendocrine Dysregulation after Traumatic Brain Injury. *Journal of Clinical Medicine.* 2015;4(5):1051-1062. doi:10.3390/jcm4051051.

84. Prinz, P.N.; Scanlan, J.N.; Vitaliano, P.P.; Moe, K.E.; Borson, S.; Toivola, B.; Merriam, G.R.; Larsen, L.H.; Reed, H.L. Thyroid hormones: Positive relationships with cognition in healthy, euthyroid older men. *J. Gerontol. A Biol. Sci. Med. Sci.* 1999, *54*, M111–M116.

85. Rivas, M.; Naranjo, J.R. Thyroid hormones, learning and memory. *Genes Brain Behav.* 2007, *1*, 40–44.

86. Zihl J, Almeida O. Neuropsychology of Neuroendocrine Dysregulation after Traumatic Brain Injury. *Journal of Clinical Medicine.* 2015;4(5):1051-1062. doi:10.3390/jcm4051051.

87. Samuels, M.H. Cognitive function in untreated hypothyroidism and hyperthyroidism. *Curr. Opin. Endocrinol. Diabetes Obes.* 2008, *15*, 429–433.

88. Zihl J, Almeida O. Neuropsychology of Neuroendocrine Dysregulation after Traumatic Brain Injury. *Journal of Clinical Medicine*. 2015;4(5):1051-1062. doi:10.3390/jcm4051051.

89. Zihl J, Almeida O. Neuropsychology of Neuroendocrine Dysregulation after Traumatic Brain Injury. *Journal of Clinical Medicine*. 2015;4(5):1051-1062. doi:10.3390/jcm4051051.

90. León-Carrión, J.; Leal-Cerro, A.; Murillo Cabezas, F.; Madrazo Atutxa, A.; García Gomez, G.; Flores A.; Rincón Ferrari, M.D.; Domínguez-Morales, M. Cognitive deterioration due to GH deficiency in patients with traumatic brain injury: A preliminary report. *Brain Injury* 2007, *21*, 871–875.

91. High, E.M.; Briones-Galang, M.; Clark, J.A.; Gilkison, C.; Mossberg, K.A., Zgaljardic, D.J.; Masel, B.E.; Urban, R.J. Effect of growthhormone therapy on cognition after traumatic brain injury. *J. Neurotrauma* 2010, *27*, 1565–1575.

92. Moreau, O.K.; Cortel-Rudelli, C.; Yollin, E.; Merlen, E.; Daveluy, W.; Rousseaux, M. Growth replacement therapy in patients with   traumatic brain injury. *J. Neurotrauma* 2013, *30*, 998–1006.

93. Reimunde, P.; Quintana, A.; Castanon, B.; Casteleiro, N.; Vilarnovo, Z.; Otero, A.; Devesa, A.; Otero-Cepeda, X.L.; Devesa, J. Effects of growth hormone (GH) replacement and cognitive rehabilitation in patients with cognitive disorders after traumatic brain injury. *Brain Injury* 2011, *25*, 65–73.

94. Muse: The Brain Sensing Headband Tech Spec Sheet. 2015.

95. Gesturetekhealth.com. GestureTek Health - Products - IREX: Interactive Rehabilitation & Exercise Systems. 2015. Available at: http://www.gesturetekhealth.com/products-rehab-irex.php. Accessed June 30, 2015.

96. Selzer M, Clarke S, Cohen L, Kwakkel G, Miller R. *Textbook Of Neural Repair And Rehabilitation*. Cambridge: Cambridge University Press; 2014.

97. Kim B, Chun M, Kim L, Park J. Effect of Virtual Reality on Cognition in Stroke Patients. *Ann Rehabil Med*. 2011;35(4):450. doi:10.5535/arm.2011.35.4.450.

98. Mirelman A, Patritti B, Bonato P, Deutsch J. Effects of virtual reality training on gait biomechanics of individuals post-stroke. *Gait & Posture*. 2010;31(4):433-437. doi:10.1016/j.gaitpost.2010.01.016.

99. Selzer M, Clarke S, Cohen L, Kwakkel G, Miller R. *Textbook Of Neural Repair And Rehabilitation*. Cambridge: Cambridge University Press; 2014.

100. Stanney K, Mourant R, Kennedy R. Human Factors Issues in Virtual Environments: A Review of the Literature. *Presence: Teleoperators and Virtual Environments*. 1998;7(4):327-351. doi:10.1162/105474698565767.

101. Nield D. How Oculus Rift works: Everything you need to know about the VR sensation. *Wareable*. 2015. Available at: http://www.wareable.com/oculus-rift/how-oculus-rift-works. Accessed June 30, 2015.

102. Klavora P, Warren M. Rehabilitation of Visuomotor Skills in Poststroke Patients Using the Dynavision Apparatus. *Perceptual and Motor Skills*. 1998;86(1):23-30. doi:10.2466/pms.1998.86.1.23.

103. Klavora P, Gaskovski P, Martin K et al. The Effects of Dynavision Rehabilitation on Behind-the-Wheel Driving Ability and Selected Psychomotor Abilities of Persons After Stroke. *American Journal of Occupational Therapy*. 1995;49(6):534-542. doi:10.5014/ajot.49.6.534.

104. Dynavisioninternational.com. Experience the Proven Power of Dynavision!. 2015. Available at: http://dynavisioninternational.com/. Accessed June 25, 2015.

105. Hardt J. Alpha EEG Feedback: Closer Parallel with Zen than with Yoga. *Biocybernaut Institute*. 2015. Available at: http://www.biocybernaut.com/wp-content/uploads/2013/12/ScienceArticle_AlpEEGFee.pdf. Accessed July 17, 2015.

106. Leon-Carrion J, Martin-Rodriguez J, Damas-Lopez J, Barroso y Martin J, Dominguez-Morales M. Delta–alpha ratio correlates with level of recovery after neurorehabilitation in patients with acquired brain injury. *Clinical Neurophysiology*. 2009;120(6):1039-1045. doi:10.1016/j.clinph.2009.01.021.

107. Niedermeyer E. Cerebrovascular disorders and EEG. In: Niedermeyer E, Lopes da Silva F, editors. Electroencephalography: basic principles, clinical applications and related fields. 5th ed. Philadelphia: Lippincott Williams & Wilkins; 2005;339–62.

108. Leon-Carrion J, Martin-Rodriguez J, Damas-Lopez J, Barroso y Martin J, Dominguez-Morales M. Delta–alpha ratio correlates with level of recovery after neurorehabilitation in patients with acquired brain injury. *Clinical Neurophysiology*. 2009;120(6):1039-1045. doi:10.1016/j.clinph.2009.01.021.

109. Goldman R, Stern J, Engel J, Cohen M. Simultaneous EEG and fMRI of the alpha rhythm. *NeuroReport*. 2002;13(18):2487-2492. doi:10.1097/00001756-200212200-00022.

110. Tornero D, Wattananit S, Gronning Madsen M et al. Human induced pluripotent stem cell-derived cortical neurons integrate in stroke-injured cortex and improve functional recovery. *Brain.* 2013;136(12):3561-3577. doi:10.1093/brain/awt278.

111. Takahashi K, Tanabe K, Ohnuki M et al. Induction of Pluripotent Stem Cells from Adult Human Fibroblasts by Defined Factors. *Cell.* 2007;131(5):861-872. doi:10.1016/j.cell.2007.11.019.

112. Yu J, Vodyanik M, Smuga-Otto K et al. Induced Pluripotent Stem Cell Lines Derived from Human Somatic Cells. *Science.* 2007;318(5858):1917-1920. doi:10.1126/science.1151526.

113. Bao S, Tang F, Li X et al. Epigenetic reversion of post-implantation epiblast to pluripotent embryonic stem cells. *Nature.* 2009;461(7268):1292-1295. doi:10.1038/nature08534.

114. Espuny-Camacho I, Michelsen K, Gall D et al. Pyramidal Neurons Derived from Human Pluripotent Stem Cells Integrate Efficiently into Mouse Brain Circuits In Vivo. *Neuron.* 2013;77(3):440-456. doi:10.1016/j.neuron.2012.12.011.

115. Chen H, Qian K, Chen W et al. Human-derived neural progenitors functionally replace astrocytes in adult mice. *Journal of Clinical Investigation.* 2015;125(3):1033-1042. doi:10.1172/jci69097.

116. Tian C, Wang X, Wang X et al. Autologous Bone Marrow Mesenchymal Stem Cell Therapy in the Subacute Stage of Traumatic Brain Injury by Lumbar Puncture. *Experimental and Clinical Transplantation.* 2013;11(2):176-181. doi:10.6002/ect.2012.0053.

117. Lakkis F, Billiar T. Molecular analysis of transplant rejection: marching onward. *Journal of Experimental Medicine* 2013;210(11):2147-2149. doi:10.1084/jem.20131810.

118. Tan Y, Ooi S, Wang L. Immunogenicity and Tumorigenicity of Pluripotent Stem Cells and their Derivatives: Genetic and Epigenetic P e r - spectives. *CSCR.* 2013;9(1):63-72. doi:10.2174/1574888x113086660068.

119. Clinicalcenter.nih.gov. NIH Clinical Center: FAQ About Clinical Studies. 2014. Available at: http://clinicalcenter.nih.gov/participate/faqaboutcs.shtml. Accessed November 4, 2015.

120. Novacellsinstitute.com. Discover stem cell treatments for Neurologic Diseases, NCIM. Available at: http://www.novacellsinstitute.com/neurologic-diseases.html. Accessed November 4, 2015.

121. Lin, Yuan-Chi, Acupuncture for Pain Management, Springer New York, 2014. Page 4.

122. Zhou, Jia, Acupuncture anesthesia for open heart surgery in contemporary China. International Journal of Cardiology, July 2011, Volume 150, Issue 1, 12-16.

123. Robert L. Koffman, "Downrange Acupuncture", Medical Acupuncture. 2011, 23, 215-218.

124. Williams T, Mueller K, Cornwall MW. Effect of acupuncture-point stimulation on diastolic blood pressure in hypertensive subjects. Phys Ther 1991;71:523-9.

125. Ohsawa H, Yamaguchi S, Ishimaru H, et al. Neural mechanism of pupillary dilation elicited by electro-acupuncture stimulation in anesthetized rats. J Auton Nerv Syst 1997;64:101-6.

126. Hsu CC, Weng CS, Liu TS, et al. Effects of electrical acupuncture on acupoint BL15 evaluated in terms of heart rate variability, pulse rate variability and skin conductance response. Am J Chin Med 2006;34:23-36.

127. Huang W, Kutner N, Bliwise D. A systematic review of the effects of acupuncture in treating insomnia. *Sleep Med Rev* 2009;13:73-104.

128. Wei Huang, M.D., Ph.D., Nancy Kutner, Ph.D., Donald L. Bliwise, Ph.D, Autonomic Activation in Insomnia: The Case for Acupuncture. *Journal of Clinical Sleep Medicine*, Vol. 7, No. 1, 2011: 96.

129. Malykh A, Sadaie M. Piracetam and Piracetam-Like Drugs. *Drugs*. 2010;70(3):287-312. doi:10.2165/11319230-000000000-00000.

130. Giurgea C. The 'nootropic' approach to the pharmacology of the integrative activity of the brain. *Cond Reflex* 1973 Apr-Jun; 8 (2): 108-15.

131. Zhang Y, Chopp M, Meng Y et al. Cerebrolysin improves cognitive performance in rats after mild traumatic brain injury. *Journal of Neurosurgery*. 2015;122(4):843-855. doi:10.3171/2014.11.jns14271.

132. Sharma H, Zimmermann-Meinzingen S, Johanson C. Cerebrolysin reduces blood-cerebrospinal fluid barrier permeability change, brain pathology, and functional deficits following traumatic brain injury in the rat. *Annals of the New York Academy of Sciences*. 2010;1199(1):125-137. doi:10.1111/j.1749-6632.2009.05329.x.

133. Zhang Y, Chopp M, Meng Y et al. Improvement in functional recovery with administration of Cerebrolysin after experimental closed head injury. *Journal of Neurosurgery*. 2013;118(6):1343-1355. doi:10.3171/2013.3.jns122061.

134. Muresanu D, Ciurea A, Gorgan R et al. A Retrospective, Multi-Center Cohort Study Evaluating the Severity- Related Effects of Cerebrolysin Treatment on Clinical Outcomes in Traumatic Brain Injury. *CNS &*

Neurological Disorders - Drug Targets. 2015;14(5):587-599. doi:10.2174/18 715273146661150430162531.

135. Onose G, Mureșanu D F, Ciurea A V, et al. Neuroprotective and consequent neurorehabilitative clinical outcomes, in patients treated with the pleiotropic drug cerebrolysin. *Journal of medicine and life.* 2009;2(4):350.

136. Chen C, Wei S, Tsaia S, Chen X, Cho D. Cerebrolysin enhances cognitive recovery of mild traumatic brain injury patients: double blind, placebo-controlled, randomized study. *British Journal of Neurosurgery.* 2013;27(6):803-807. doi:10.3109/02688697.2013.793287.

137. Formichi P, Radi E, Battisti C, Di Maio G, Muresanu D, Federico A. Cerebrolysin administration reduces oxidative stress-induced apoptosis in limphocytes from healthy individuals. *J Cell Mol Med.* 2012;16(11):2840-2843. doi:10.1111/j.1582-4934.2012.01615.x.

138. Álvarez X A, Lombardi V R M, Corzo L, et al. *Oral Cerebrolysin enhances brain alpha activity and improves cognitive performance in elderly control subjects.* Springer Vienna;2000;315-328.

139. Thome J, Doppler E. Safety profile of Cerebrolysin: clinical experience from dementia and stroke trials. *Drugs of today.* 2012;48: 63-69.

140. Drugscase.net. Cerebrolysin - Memory problems Without Prescription! Buy Cerebrolysin Online!. Available at: http://www.drugscase.net/memory-problems/cerebrolysin.html. Accessed November 17, 2015.

141. Battleday R, Brem A. Modafinil for cognitive neuroenhancement in healthy non-sleep-deprived subjects: A systematic review. *European Neuropsychopharmacology.* 2015. doi:10.1016/j.euroneuro.2015.07.028.

142. Sahakian B, Morein-Zamir S. Professor's little helper. *Nature.* 2007;450(7173):1157-1159.

143. Maher B. Poll results: look who's doping. *Nature.* 2008;452(7188):674-675. doi:10.1038/452674a.

144. Talsky A, Pacione L R, Shaw T, et al. Pharmacological interventions for traumatic brain injury. *British Columbia Medical Journal.* 2010;53(1):1.

145. Elovic E. Use of Provigil for Underarousal Following TBI. *Journal of Head Trauma Rehabilitation.* 2000;15(4):1068-1071. doi:10.1097/00001199-200008000-00009.

146. Teitelman E. Off-label uses of Modafinil. *Am J Psychiatry* 2001;158:1341.

147. Raminder, K. Approved and Investigational Uses of Modafinil: An Evidence-Based Review. *Drugs.* 2008;68(13):1803-1839.

148. Wikipedia. Modafinil. Available at: https://en.wikipedia.org/wiki/Modafinil#Legal_status. Accessed November 17, 2015.

149. Malykh A, Sadaie M. Piracetam and Piracetam-Like Drugs. *Drugs.* 2010;70(3):287-312. doi:10.2165/11319230-000000000-00000.

150. Zavadenko N, Guzilova L. Sequelae of Closed Craniocerebral Trauma and the Efficacy of Piracetam in Its Treatment in Adolescents. *Neurosci Behav Physi.* 2009;39(4):323-328. doi:10.1007/s11055-009-9146-2.

151. Waegemans T, Wilsher CR, Danniau A, et al. Clinical efficacy of piracetam in cognitive impairment: a meta-analysis. *Dement Geriatr Cogn Disord.* 2002;13(4):217-24.

152. Zavadenko N, Guzilova L. Sequelae of Closed Craniocerebral Trauma and the Efficacy of Piracetam in Its Treatment in Adolescents. *Neurosci Behav Physi.* 2009;39(4):323-328. doi:10.1007/s11055-009-9146-2.

153. Ovanesov K B, Shikina I B, Arushanian E B, et al. Effect of pyracetam on the color discriminative function of retina in patients with craniocerebral trauma. *Eksperimental'naia i klinicheskaia farmakologiia.* 2002;66(4):6-8.

154. Zhang S. Effect of piracetam on the cognitive performance of patients undergoing coronary bypass surgery: A meta-analysis. *Experimental and Therapeutic Medicine.* 2013. doi:10.3892/etm.2013.1425.

155. Batysheva TT, Bagir LV, Kostenko EV, et al. Experience of the out-patient use of memotropil in the treatment of cognitive disorders in patients with chronic progressive cerebrovascular disorders. *Neurosci Behav Physiol.* 2009;39(2):193-7.

156. Waegemans T, Wilsher CR, Danniau A, et al. Clinical efficacy of piracetam in cognitive impairment: a meta-analysis. *Dement Geriatr Cogn Disord.* 2002;13(4):217-24.

157. Wikipedia. Piracetam. Available at: https://en.wikipedia.org/wiki/Piracetam#Approval_and_usage. Accessed November 17, 2015.

158. Nootriment - Supplement Reviews and Healthy Ideas. How Short is Aniracetam's Half Life? 2014. Available at: http://nootriment.com/aniracetam-half-life/. Accessed November 17, 2015.

159. Baranova A, Whiting M, Hamm R. Delayed, Post-Injury Treatment with Aniracetam Improves Cognitive Performance after Traumatic Brain Injury in Rats. *Journal of Neurotrauma.* 2006;23(8):1233-1240. doi:10.1089/neu.2006.23.1233.

160. Canonico V, Forgione L, Paoletti C, et al. Efficacy and tolerance of aniracetam in elderly patients with primary or secondary mental deterioration. *Rivista di neurologia.* 1990;61(3):92-96.

161. Senin U, Abate G, Fieschi C, et al. Aniracetam (Ro 13- 5057) in the treatment of senile dementia of Alzheimer type (SDAT): results of a

placebo controlled multicentre clinical study. *Eur Neuropsychopharmacol*. 1991;1(4):511-7.

162. Nakamura K, Shirane M, Koshikawa N. Site-specific activation of dopamine and serotonin transmission by aniracetam in the mesocortico-limbic pathway of rats. *Brain Research*. 2001;897(1-2):82-92. doi:10.1016/s0006-8993(01)02096-0.

163. Nootriment - Supplement Reviews and Healthy Ideas. Is Aniracetam Legal Where You Live? 2014. Available at: http://nootriment.com/is-aniracetam-legal/. Accessed November 17, 2015.

164. Altern Med Rev 2007 Sep; 12(3):207-27.

165. McCann JC, Ames BN. Is docosahexaenoic acid, an n-3 long-chain polyunsaturated fatty acid, required for development of normal brain function? An overview of evidence from cognitive and behavioral tests in humans and animals. Am J Clin Nutr 2005;82:281-295.

166. Altern Med Rev 2007 Sep; 12(3): 221.

167. Journal of the Clinical Psychiatry 2006;67:1954–1967

168. Crook T, Petne W. Wells C, Massari DC. Effects of phosphatidylserine in Alzheimer's disease, Psychopharmacol Bull 1992:28:61-6.

169. Baumeister J, Barthel T, Geiss KR, Weiss M. Influence of phosphatidylserine on cognitive performance and cortical activity after induced stress. Nutr Neurosci. 2008;11:103–110.

170. Montelenne P, Beinat L. Tanzillo C, et al. Effects of phosphatidylserine on the neuroendocrine response to physical stress in humans. Neuroendocrinology, 1990;52:243-248.

171. Fahey TD, Pearl MS. The hormonal and perceptive effects of phosphatidylserine administration during two weeks of resistive exercise-induced overtraining. Biol Sport 1998; 15:135-144

172. Fioravanti M, Yanagi M. Cytidinediphosphocholine (CDP-choline) for cognitive and behavioural disturbances associated with chronic cerebral disorders in the elderly. Cochrane Database Syst. Rev. 2,CD000269 (2005).

173. Altern Med Rev 2007 Sep; 12(3):224.

174. Ghezzi P. Role of glutathione in immunity and inflammation in the lung. Int J Gen Med. 2011;4:105–113.

175. Sido B, Braunstein J, Breitkreutz R, Herfarth C, Meuer SC. Thiol-mediated redox regulation of intestinal lamina propria T lymphocytes. J Exp Med. 2000;192(6):907–912.

176. Oliver JM, Albertini DF, Berlin RD. Effects of glutathione-oxidizing agents on microtubule assembly and microtubule-dependent surface properties of human neutrophils. J Cell Biol. 1976;71(3):921–932.

177. Chen, Swanson, "Astrocytes and Brain Injury", Journal of Cerebral Blood Flow & Metabolism 2003, 23:137–149

178. Drukarch, B., Schepens, E., Stoof, J.C., Langeveld, C.H. Anethole dithiolethione prevents oxidative damage in glutathione depleted astrocytes. Eur. J. Pharmacol. 1997: 329, 259-262.

179. Wade, L.A., Brady, H.M. "Cysteine and cystine transport at the blood brain barrier." J. Neurochem. 1981, 37, 730-734.

180. Rice, M.E., Russo-Menna, I. Differential compartimentalization of brain ascorbate and glutathione between neurons and glia.Neuroscience, 1998, 82, 1213-1223.

181. Wilson, J.X. Antioxidant defense of the brain: a role for astrocytes. Can. J. Physiol. Pharmacol. 1997, 75, 1149-1163.

182. Greenblatt, J, Grossman, K. Lithium: The Untold Story of the Magic Mineral That Charges Cell Phones and Preserves Memory. Townsend Letter. October 2015, pg 63-67.

183. Shorter, Edward. "The History of Lithium Therapy." *Bipolar disorders* 11.0 2 (2009): 4–9

184. Mauer S, Vergne D, Ghaemi NS. Standard and trace-dose lithium: a systematic review of dementia prevention and other behavioral benefits. Aust N Z J Psychiatry. 2014;48(9):809–818.

185. Farah R et al. "Lithium's gene expression profile, a cDNA microarray study." Cellular and Molecular Neurobiology. April 2013, Volume 33, Issue 3, pp 411-420

186. M. Kikuchi, S. Kashii, Y. Honda, Y. Tamura, K. Kaneda, and A. Akaike, "Protective effects of methylcobalamin, a vitamin B12 analog, against glutamate-induced neurotoxicity in retinal cell culture," Investigative Ophthalmology and Visual Science, vol. 38, no. 5, pp. 848–854, 1997.

187. Katayama, Y M.D., Ph.D., Becker, D M.D.., et al. Massive increases in extracellular potassium and the indiscriminate release of glutamate following concussive brain injury Journal of neurosurgery. February 2010, Vol. 112, No. 2, Pages 889-900.

188. X. Kong, X. Sun, and J. Zhang, "The protective role of Mecobalamin following optic nerve crush in adult rats," *Yan Ke Xue Bao*, vol. 20, no. 3, pp. 171–177, 2004.

189. A. Pfohl-Leszkowicz, G. Keith, and G. Dirheimer, "Effect of cobalamin derivatives on in vitro enzymatic DNA methylation: methylcobalamin can act as a methyl donor," *Biochemistry*, vol. 30, no. 32, pp. 8045–8051, 1991.

190. Packer L, Witt EH, Tritschler HJ. Alpha-lipoic acid as a biological anti-oxidant. Free Rad Biol Med 1995;19:227–50.

191. Rosenburg HR, Culik R. Effects of α–lipoic acid on vitamin C and vitamin E deficiencies. *Arch Biochem Biophys* 1959;80:86-93.

192. Scholich H, Murphy ME, Sies H. Antioxidant activity of dihydrolipoate against microsomal lipid peroxidation and its dependence on α– tocopherol. *Biochem Biophys Acta* 1989;1001:256-261.

193. Busse E, Zimmer G, Schopohl B, et al. Influence of alpha–lipoic acid on intracellular glutathione in vitro and in vivo. *Arzneimittel-Forschung* 1992;42:829-831.

194. Kagan V, Serbinova E, Packer L. Antioxidant effects of ubiquinones in microsomes and mitochondria are mediated by tocopherol recycling. *Biochem Biophys Res Comm* 1990;169:851-857.

195. Bertoni-Freddari C, Fattoretti P, Casoli T, et al. Morphological adaptive response of the synaptic junctional zones in the human dentate gyrus during aging and alzheimer's disease. *Brain Res* 1990;517:69-75.

196. Bertoni-Freddari C, Fattoretti, P, Casoli T, et al. Dynamic morphology of the synaptic junctional areas during aging: the effect of chronic ace-tyl-L-carnitine administration. *Brain Res* 1994;656:359-366.

197. Bonavita E. Study of the efficacy and tolerability of L-acetylcarnitine therapy in the senile brain. *Int J Clin Pharmacol Ther Tox* 1986;24:511-516.

198. DiGiacomo C, Latteri F, Fichera C, et al. Effect of acetyl-L-carnitine on lipid peroxidation and xanthine oxidase activity in rat skeletal muscle. *Neurochem Res* 1993;18:1157-1162.

199. Fernandez E, Pallini R, Gangitano C, et al. Effects of L-carnitine, L-ace-tylcarnitine and gangliosides on the regeneration of the transected sciat-ic nerve in rats. *Neurological Res* 1989;11:57-62.

200. Mathias J, Alvaro P. Prevalence of sleep disturbances, disorders, and problems following traumatic brain injury: A meta-analysis.   *Sleep Medicine*. 2012;13(7):898-905. doi:10.1016/j.sleep.2012.04.006.

201. Beetar J, Guilmette T, Sparadeo F. Sleep and pain complaints in symp-tomatic traumatic brain injury and neurologic populations. *Archives of Physical Medicine and Rehabilitation*. 1996;77(12):1298-1302. doi:10.1016/s0003-9993(96)90196-3.

202. Dikmen S, McLean A, Temkin N. Neuropsychological and psychosocial consequences of minor head injury. *Journal of Neurology, Neurosurgery & Psychiatry.* 1986;49(11):1227-1232. doi:10.1136/jnnp.49.11.1227.

203. Gilbert K, Kark S, Gehrman P, Bogdanova Y. Sleep disturbances, TBI and PTSD: Implications for treatment and recovery. *Clinical Psychology Review.* 2015;40:195-212. doi:10.1016/j.cpr.2015.05.008.

204. Gilbert K, Kark S, Gehrman P, Bogdanova Y. Sleep disturbances, TBI and PTSD: Implications for treatment and recovery. *Clinical Psychology Review.* 2015;40:195-212. doi:10.1016/j.cpr.2015.05.008.

205. Gilbert K, Kark S, Gehrman P, Bogdanova Y. Sleep disturbances, TBI and PTSD: Implications for treatment and recovery. *Clinical Psychology Review.* 2015;40:195-212. doi:10.1016/j.cpr.2015.05.008.

206. Kemp S, Biswas R, Neumann V, Coughlan A. The value of melatonin for sleep disorders occurring post-head injury: a pilot RCT. *Brain Inj.* 2004;18(9):911-919. doi:10.1080/02699050410001671892.

207. Naseem, M. and Parvez, S. Role of Melatonin in traumatic brain injury and spinal cord injury. Scientific World Journal 2014;2014:586270. doi: 10.1155/2014/586270. Epub 2014 Dec 21.

208. Rao, V. et al. Does acute TBI-related sleep disturbance predict subsequent neuropsychiatric disturbance? Brain Inj. 2014;28(1):20-6.doi: 10.3109/02699052.2013.847210.

209. Lin, L. et al. Melatonin in Alzheimer's Disease. Int J Mol Sci. 2013 Jul 12;14(7):14575-93. doi: 10.3390/ijms140714575.

210. Classen, HG. Magnesium orotate—experimental and clinical evidence. Rom J Intern Med. 2004;42(3):491-501.

211. Slutsky, Inna et al. Enhancement of learning and memory by elevating brain magnesium. Neuron. 2010 Jan 28; 65(2):165-177.

212. Nutrition and Traumatic Brain Injury: Improving Acute and Subacute Outcomes in Military Personnel. 2011. The National Academies Press. Chapter 12 Magnesium. pg 157.

213. Holick M. F. Sunlight and vitamin D for bone health and prevention of autoimmune diseases, cancers, and cardiovascular disease. *The American Journal of Clinical Nutrition.* 2004;80(6):1678S-1688S.

214. Baggerly C, Cuomo R, French C et al. Sunlight and Vitamin D: Necessary for Public Health. *Journal of the American College of Nutrition.* 2015;34(4):359-365. doi:10.1080/07315724.2015.1039866.

215. Garcion E, Wion-Barbot N, Montero-Menei C, Berger F, Wion D. New clues about vitamin D functions in the nervous system. *Trends*

in Endocrinology & Metabolism. 2002;13(3):100-105. doi:10.1016/s1043-2760(01)00547-1.

216. Holick M. F. Sunlight and vitamin D for bone health and prevention of autoimmune diseases, cancers, and cardiovascular disease. *The American Journal of Clinical Nutrition.* 2004;80(6):1678S-1688S.

217. Archer M.D. D. Vitamin D Deficiency and Depression. *Psychology Today.* 2015. Available at: https://www.psychologytoday.com/blog/reading-between-the-headlines/201307/vitamin-d-deficiency-and-depression. Accessed July 30, 2015.

218. Baggerly C, Cuomo R, French C et al. Sunlight and Vitamin D: Necessary for Public Health. *Journal of the American College of Nutrition.* 2015;34(4):359-365. doi:10.1080/07315724.2015.1039866.

219. Skincancer.org. Facts about Sunburn and Skin Cancer - SkinCancer.org. 2015. Available at: http://www.skincancer.org/prevention/sunburn/facts-about-sunburn-and-skin-cancer. Accessed July 30, 2015.

220. Holick M. F. Sunlight and vitamin D for bone health and prevention of autoimmune diseases, cancers, and cardiovascular disease. *The American Journal of Clinical Nutrition.* 2004;80(6):1678S-1688S.

221. Baggerly C, Cuomo R, French C et al. Sunlight and Vitamin D: Necessary for Public Health. *Journal of the American College of Nutrition.* 2015;34(4):359-365. doi:10.1080/07315724.2015.1039866.

222. Holick M. F. Sunlight and vitamin D for bone health and prevention of autoimmune diseases, cancers, and cardiovascular disease. *The American Journal of Clinical Nutrition.* 2004;80(6):1678S-1688S.

223. Lam R, Levitt A, Levitan R et al. The Can-SAD Study: A Randomized Controlled Trial of the Effectiveness of Light Therapy and Fluoxetine in Patients With Winter Seasonal Affective Disorder. *American Journal of Psychiatry.* 2006;163(5):805-812. doi:10.1176/ajp.2006.163.5.805.

224. Flory R, Ametepe J, Bowers B. A randomized, placebo-controlled trial of bright light and high-density negative air ions for treatment of Seasonal Affective Disorder. *Psychiatry Research.* 2010;177(1-2):101-108. doi:10.1016/j.psychres.2008.08.011.

225. Goel N, Terman M, Su Terman J, Macchi M, Stewart J. Controlled trial of bright light and negative air ions for chronic depression. *Psychological Medicine.* 2005;35(7):945-955. doi:10.1017/s0033291705005027.

226. Ponsford J. Sexual changes associated with traumatic brain injury. *Neuropsychological Rehabilitation.* 2003;13(1-2):275-289. doi:10.1080/09602010244000363.

227. Wylie K. *ABC Of Sexual Health*. Hoboken: Wiley; 2015.

228. Lennington J B, Yang Z, Conover J C. Neural stem cells and the regulation of adult neurogenesis. *Reprod Biol Endocrinol*, 2003;1(1):99-105.

229. Dvorsky G. 10 Reasons Why Oxytocin Is The Most Amazing Molecule In The World. *io9*. 2015. Available at: http://io9.com/5925206/10-reasons-why-oxytocin-is-the-most-amazing-molecule-in-the-world. Accessed July 28, 2015.

230. Borland S. Revealed: What goes on in a woman's brain when she has an orgasm. *Mail Online*. 2010. Available at: http://www.dailymail.co.uk/news/article-1327489/What-goes-womans-brain-orgasm.html. Accessed July 27, 2015.

231. Shin B, Lee M, Yang E, Lim H, Ernst E. Maca (L. meyenii) for improving sexual function: a systematic review. *BMC Complementary and Alternative Medicine*. 2010;10(1):44. doi:10.1186/1472-6882-10-44.

232. Dording C, Schettler P, Dalton E et al. A Double-Blind Placebo-Controlled Trial of Maca Root as Treatment for Antidepressant Induced Sexual Dysfunction in Women. *Evidence-Based Complementary and Alternative Medicine*. 2015;2015:1-9. doi:10.1155/2015/949036.

233. Daniel J. Levitin, This Is Your Brain On Music The Science of a Human Obsession, pages 8-9.

234. Doidge M.D., Norman, The Brain's Way of Healing. Viking Penguin, New York. Chapter 14.

235. Sacks, Oliver, "The Power of Music". http://dx.doi.org/10.1093/brain/awl234 2528-2532 First published online: 25 September 2006

236. Vestibulocochlear nerve, cranial nerve VIII, codes for both hearing and vestibular sensory input.

237. Doidge M.D., Norman, The Brain's Way of Healing. Viking Penguin, New York. Chapter 8, 241.

238. Fritz J, Elhiliali M, Shamma S (2005b) Active listening: task-dependent plasticity of receptive fields in primary auditory cortex. Hear Res 206:159–176.

239. Khalfa S, Bella SD, Roy M, Peretz I, Lupein SJ. Effects of relaxing music on salivary cortisol level after psychological stress. Ann N Y Acad Sci (2003) 999:374–6.

240. Blood AJ, Zatorre RJ. Intensely pleasurable responses to music correlate with activity in brain regions implicated in reward and emotion. Proc Natl Acad Sci U S A (2001) 98:11818–2310.

241. Peretz I. The nature of music from a biological perspective. Cognition (2006) 100:1–32.

242. H. Hummelsheim, "Rationales for improving motor function," Current Opinion in Neurology 12 (1999): 697–701.

243. A. Pascual Leone, "The brain that plays music and is changed by it," Annals of the New York Academy of Sciences 930 (2001): 315-329.

244. Fukui H, Toyoshima K. Music facilitate the neurogenesis, regeneration and repair of neuron. Med Hypotheses (2008) 71:765–9.

245. Thaut MH. Neurologic music therapy in sensorimotor rehabilitation. In: Thaut MH, editor. , editor. Rhythm, Music and the Brain. New York: Routledge; Taylor and Francis group; (2005). p. 137–64.

246. M. I. Posner and B. Patoine, "How arts training improves attention and cognition," Cerebrum (2009): http://dana.org/news/cerebrum/detail.aspx?id=23206.

247. G. Schlaug, "Music, musicians, and brain plasticity," in S. Hallam, I. Cross, and M. H. Thaut, eds., The Oxford Handbook of Music Psychology (Oxford: Oxford University Press, 2008), 197–208.

248. Thaut MH. Neurologic music therapy in speech and language rehabilitation. In: Thaut MH, editor. , editor. Rhythm, Music and the Brain. New York: Routledge; Taylor and Francis group; (2005). p. 165–78.

249. Sacks, Oliver. Musicophilia: Tales of Music and the Brain. New York: Alfred A. Knopf, 2007. pg 236-238.

250. Sacks, Oliver. Musicophilia: Tales of Music and the Brain. New York: Alfred A. Knopf, 2007. pg xii, preface.

251. M. H. Thaut, G. C. McIntosh, and R. R. Rice, "Rhythmic facilitation of gait training in hemiparetic stroke rehabilitation," Journal of Neurological Sciences 151 (1997): 207–212.

252. M. H. Thaut, A. K. Leins, R. R. Rice, et al., "Rhythmic auditory stimulation improves gait more than NDT/Bobath training in near ambulatory patients early post stroke: A single blind randomized control trial," Neurorehabilitation and Neural Repair 21 (2007): 455–459.

253. Verghese,J, et. al. "Leisure Activities and the Risk of Dementia in the Elderly" N Engl J Med 2003; 348:2508-2516.

254. M. H. Thaut, J. C. Gardiner, D. Holmberg, et al., "Neurologic music therapy improves executive function and emotional adjustment in traumatic brain injury rehabilitation," Annals of the New York Academy of Sciences 1169 (2009): 406–416.

255. Brown S, Martinez MJ, Parsons LM. Passive music listening spontaneously engages limbic and paralimbic systems.

256. M. H. Thaut, D. A. Peterson, and G. C. McIntosh, "Temporal entrainment of cognitive functions: Musical mnemonics induce brain plasticity and oscillatory synchrony in neural networks underlying memory," Annals of the New York Academy of Sciences 1060 (2005): 243–254.

257. Missal, Mouraux, Nozaradan, and Peretz, "Tagging the Neuronal Entrainment to Beat and Meter." The Journal of Neuroscience, July 13, 2011 • 31(28):10234 –10240.

258. Doidge M.D., Norman, The Brain's Way of Healing. Viking Penguin, New York. Chapter 14.

259. Bower J, Catroppa C, Grocke D, Shoemark H. Music therapy for early cognitive rehabilitation post-childhood TBI: an intrinsic mixed methods case study. Dev Neurorehabil (2013).

260. P. Belin, P. Van Eeckhout, M. Zilbovicius, et al., "Recovery from non-fluent aphasia after melodic intonation therapy," Neurology 47 (1996): 1504–1511.

261. Chevalier G, Sinatra S, Oschman J, Sokal K, Sokal P. Earthing: Health Implications of Reconnecting the Human Body to the Earth's Surface Electrons. *Journal of Environmental and Public Health*. 2012;2012:1-8. doi:10.1155/2012/291541.

262. Chevalier G. Changes in pulse rate, respiratory rate, blood oxygenation, perfusion index, skin conductance, and their variability induced during and after grounding human subjects for 40 minutes. *Journal of Alternative and Complementary Medicine*. 2010;16(1):1–7.

263. G. Chevalier, K. Mori, and J. L. Oschman, "The effect of Earthing (grounding) on human physiology," *European Biology and Bioelectromagnetics*, vol. 2, no. 1, pp. 600–621, 2006.

264. Chevalier G, Sinatra S, Oschman J, Sokal K, Sokal P. Earthing: Health Implications of Reconnecting the Human Body to the Earth's Surface Electrons. *Journal of Environmental and Public Health*. 2012;2012:1-8. doi:10.1155/2012/291541.

265. Oschman J. Charge transfer in the living matrix. *Journal of Bodywork and Movement Therapies*. 2009;13(3):215-228. doi:10.1016/j.jbmt.2008.06.005.

266. Chevalier G, Sinatra S, Oschman J, Sokal K, Sokal P. Earthing: Health Implications of Reconnecting the Human Body to the Earth's Surface Electrons. *Journal of Environmental and Public Health*. 2012;2012:1-8. doi:10.1155/2012/291541.

267. Chevalier G, Sinatra S, Oschman J, Delany R. Earthing (Grounding) the Human Body Reduces Blood Viscosity—a Major Factor in Cardiovascular Disease. *The Journal of Alternative and Complementary Medicine.* 2013;19(2):102-110. doi:10.1089/acm.2011.0820.

268. Chevalier G, Sinatra S, Oschman J, Sokal K, Sokal P. Earthing: Health Implications of Reconnecting the Human Body to the Earth's Surface Electrons. *Journal of Environmental and Public Health.* 2012;2012:1-8. doi:10.1155/2012/291541.

269. Ghaly M, Teplitz D. The Biologic Effects of Grounding the Human Body During Sleep as Measured by Cortisol Levels and Subjective Reporting of Sleep, Pain, and Stress. *J Altern Complement Med.* 2004;10(5):767-776. doi:10.1089/1075553042476696.

270. Sokol M. Failures in Outlet Testing Exposed. *Ecmwebcom.* 2013. Available at: http://ecmweb.com/contractor/failures-outlet testing-exposed. Accessed August 11, 2015.

271. Drijkoningen D, Caeyenberghs K, Leunissen I et al. Training-induced improvements in postural control are accompanied by alterations in cerebellar white matter in brain injured patients. *NeuroImage: Clinical.* 2015;7:240-251. doi:10.1016/j.nicl.2014.12.006.

272. Peters D, Jain S, Liuzzo D et al. Individuals With Chronic Traumatic Brain Injury Improve Walking Speed and Mobility With Intensive Mobility Training. *Archives of Physical Medicine and Rehabilitation.* 2014;95(8):1454-1460. doi:10.1016/j.apmr.2014.04.006.

273. Black JE, Isaacs KR, Anderson BJ, Alcantara AA, Greenough WT. Learning causes synaptogenesis, whereas motor activity causes angiogenesis in cerebellar cortex of adult rats. Proc Natl Acad Sci U S A. 1990;87:5568–5572.

274. Rhyu IJ, Boklewski J, Ferguson B, et al. Exercise training associated with increased cortical vascularization in adult female cynomologus monkeys. Abstr Soc Neurosci. 2003;920.

275. Cotman CW, Berchtold NC. Exercise: a behavioral intervention to enhance brain health and plasticity. Trends Neurosci. 2002;25: 295–301.

276. van Praag H, Christie BR, Sejnowski TJ, Gage FH. Running enhances neurogenesis, learning, and long-term potentiation in mice. Proc Natl Acad Sci U S A. 1999;96:13427–13431.

277. Chin L, Keyser R, Dsurney J, Chan L. Improved Cognitive Performance Following Aerobic Exercise Training in People With Traumatic Brain

Injury. *Archives of Physical Medicine and Rehabilitation.* 2015;96(4):754-759. doi:10.1016/j.apmr.2014.11.009.

278. Raz N. Regional Brain Changes in Aging Healthy Adults: General Trends, Individual Differences and Modifiers. *Cerebral Cortex.* 2005;15(11):1676-1689. doi:10.1093/cercor/bhi044.

279. Erickson K, Voss M, Prakash R et al. Exercise training increases size of hippocampus and improves memory. *Proceedings of the National Academy of Sciences.* 2011;108(7):3017-3022. doi:10.1073/pnas.1015950108.

280. M.Merzenich and R.Decharms, "Neural Representations, Experience and Change," *The Mind-Brain Continuum,* ed. R. Llinas and P.S. Church land (Cambridge, MA: MIT Press, 1996), pg 77. Reported in Move Into Life, Anat Baniel, 2009, pg 267.

281. To look further into the work of Michael Merzenich, see N. Doidge, 2007, *The Brain That Changes Itself,* Chapter 3.

282. M. Jueptner, K.M. Stephan, C.D. Frith, D.J. Brooks, R.S.Frackowiak, and R.E. Passingham, 1997, "Anatomy of Motor Learning: I. Frontal Cortex and Attention to Action," *Journal of Neurophysiology* 77(3):1313-1324.

283. Xerri C1, Merzenich MM, Peterson BE, Jenkins W, "Plasticity of primary somatosensory cortex paralleling sensorimotor skill recovery from stroke in adult monkeys", J Neurophysiol. 1998 Apr;79(4):2119-48.

284. Doidge, N. "The Brain's Way of Healing". Scribe Books, London. 2015, Chapter 5.

285. Robbins, Jim, *A Symphony in the Brain,* 1999. pg 49.

286. Doidge, N. "The Brain's Way of Healing". Scribe Books, London. 2015, Chapter 3.

287. Llinas, Rudolfo R. *I of the Vortex: From Neurons to Self.* Mass Inst of Technology, 2001. pg 134-170.

288. Rosenthal JZ, Grosswald S, Ross R, Rosenthal N: Effects of transcendental meditation in veterans of Operation Enduring Freedom and Operation Iraqi Freedom with posttraumatic stress disorder: a pilot study. Mil Med 2011; 176(6): 626 –30.

289. BarnesVernon A.RiggJohn L.WilliamsJennifer J.. (2013) Clinical Case Series: Treatment of PTSD With Transcendental Meditation in Active Duty Military Personnel. Military Medicine 178:7, e836-e840.

290. Rosenthal JZ, Grosswald S, Ross R, Rosenthal N: Effects of transcendental meditation in veterans of Operation Enduring Freedom and Oper- ation Iraqi Freedom with posttraumatic stress disorder: a pilot study. Mil Med 2011; 176(6): 626 –30.

291. JW Hoffman, H Benson, PA Arns, GL Stainbrook, GL Landsberg, JB Young, A Gill, "Reduced sympathetic nervous system responsivity associated with the relaxation response", Science 8. January 1982: Vol. 215 no. 4529 pp. 190-192.

292. Mattson, A.J., Levin, H.S., "Frontal lobe dys- function following closed head injury. A review of the literature." J. Nerv. Ment. 1990: Dis. 178, 282–291.

293. Lazar SW, Kerr CE, Wasserman RH, et al. Meditation experience is associated with increased cortical thickness. *Neuroreport.* 2005;16(17):1893-1897.

294. Kabat-Zinn, J. (2005). Wherever you go, there you are : mindfulness meditation in everyday life. New York: Hyperion.

295. Grossman, P., Niemann, L., Schmidt, S., & Walach, H. (2004). Mindfulness-based stress reduction and health benefits. A meta analysis. Journal Psychosomatic Research,57(1), 35-43.

296. Davidson, R. J., Kabat-Zinn, J., Schumacher, J., Rosenkranz, M., Muller, D., Santorelli, S. F., Urbanowski, F., Harrington, A., Bonus, K., & Sheridan, J. F. (2003). Alterations in brain and immune function produced by mindfulness meditation.[see comment]. Psychosomatic Medicine, 65(4), 564-570.

297. Miller, G. E., Cohen, S., Pressman, S., Barkin, A., Rabin, B. S., & Treanor, J. J. (2004). Psychological stress and antibody response to influenza vaccination: when is the critical period for stress, and how does it get inside the body? Psychosomatic Medicine, 66(2), 215-223.

298. Orme-Johnson DW, Walton KG: All approaches of preventing or revers-ing effects of stress are not the same. Am J Health Promot 1998; 12(5): 297– 9.

299. The Relaxation Response, Herbert Benson, C. 1975, pg 12-13.

300. Goldman R M, Tarr R S, Pinchuk B G, Kappler R E. The effects of oscillating inversion on systemic blood pressure, pulse, intraocular pressure, and central retinal arterial pressure. *The Physician and Sportsmedicine.* 1985;13(3):93-96.

301. Prasad K M, Gregson B A, Hargreaves G, Byrnes T, Winburn P, Mendelow A D. Inversion therapy in patients with pure single level lumbar discogenic disease: a pilot randomized trial. *Disability and Rehabilitation.* 2012;*34*(17):1473-1480.

302. DiMatteo M. Social Support and Patient Adherence to Medical Treatment: A Meta-Analysis. *Health Psychology.* 2004;23(2):207 218. doi:10.1037/0278-6133.23.2.207.

303. DiMatteo M. Social Support and Patient Adherence to Medical Treatment: A Meta-Analysis. *Health Psychology.* 2004;23(2):207 218. doi:10.1037/0278-6133.23.2.207.

304. DiMatteo M. Social Support and Patient Adherence to Medical Treatment: A Meta-Analysis. *Health Psychology.* 2004;23(2):207 218. doi:10.1037/0278-6133.23.2.207.

305. Ellison L, Morrison H. Low Serum Cholesterol Concentration and Risk of Suicide. *Epidemiology.* 2001;12(2):168-172. doi:10.1097/00001648-200103000-00007.

306. Stafstrom, Carl and Rho, Jong. The ketogenic diet as a treatment paradigm for diverse neurological disorders. *Frontiers in Pharmacology.* 2012;3:59. doi:10.3389/fphar.2012.00059.

307. Mady M, Kossoff E, McGregor A, Wheless J, Pyzik P, Freeman J. The Ketogenic Diet: Adolescents Can Do It, Too. *Epilepsia.* 2003;44(6):847-851. doi:10.1046/j.1528-1157.2003.57002.x.

308. El-Mallakh R, Paskitti M. The ketogenic diet may have mood-stabilizing properties. *Medical Hypotheses.* 2001;57(6):724-726. doi:10.1054/mehy.2001.1446.

309. Evangeliou A, Vlachonikolis I, Mihailidou H, et al. Application of a Ketogenic Diet in Children With Autistic Behavior: Pilot Study. *Journal of Child Neurology.* 2003;18(2):113-118. doi:10.1177/08830738030180020501.

310. Roberts RO, Roberts LA, Geda YE, et al. Relative Intake of Macronutrients Impacts Risk of Mild Cognitive Impairment or dementia. *Journal of Alzheimer's disease : JAD.* 2012;32(2):329-339. doi:10.3233/JAD-2012-120862.

311. Farooqui AA, Horrocks LA, Farooqui T. Modulation of inflammation in brain: A matter of fat. J Neurochem. 2007;101:577–99.

312. Wu A, Ying Z, Gomez-Pinilla F. Dietary Omega-3 Fatty Acids Normalize BDNF Levels, Reduce Oxidative Damage, and Counteract Learning Disability after Traumatic Brain Injury in Rats. *Journal of Neurotrauma.* 2004;21(10):1457-1467. doi:10.1089/neu.2004.21.1457.

313. Wu A, Ying Z, Gomez-Pinilla F. Dietary Omega-3 Fatty Acids Normalize BDNF Levels, Reduce Oxidative Damage, and Counteract Learning Disability after Traumatic Brain Injury in Rats. *Journal of Neurotrauma.* 2004;21(10):1457-1467. doi:10.1089/neu.2004.21.1457.

314. Bailes J, Mills J. Docosahexaenoic Acid Reduces Traumatic Axonal Injury in a Rodent Head Injury Model. *Journal of Neurotrauma.* 2010;27(9):1617-1624. doi:10.1089/neu.2009.1239.

315. Mills J, Hadley K, Bailes J. Dietary Supplementation With the Omega-3 Fatty Acid Docosahexaenoic Acid in Traumatic Brain Injury. *Neurosurgery.* 2011;68(2):474-481. doi:10.1227/neu.0b013e3181ff692b.

316. Haast RAM, Kiliaan AJ. Impact of fatty acids on brain circulation, structure and function. *Prostaglandins, Leukotrienes and Essential Fatty Acids (PLEFA).* 2015;92:3-14.

317. Muldoon M, Ryan C, Sheu L, Yao J, Conklin S, Manuck S. Serum Phospholipid Docosahexaenonic Acid Is Associated with Cognitive Functioning during Middle Adulthood. *Journal of Nutrition.* 2010;140(4):848-853. doi:10.3945/jn.109.119578.

318. Yurko-Mauro K, McCarthy D, Rom D et al. Beneficial effects of docosahexaenoic acid on cognition in age-related cognitive decline. *Alzheimer's & Dementia.* 2010;6(6):456-464. doi:10.1016/j.jalz.2010.01.013.

319. van Gelder B M, Tijhuis M, Kalmijn S, et al. Fish consumption, n–3 fatty acids, and subsequent 5-y cognitive decline in elderly men: the Zutphen Elderly Study. *The American journal of clinical nutrition.* 2007;85:1142–7.

320. Scudder B C, Chasar LC, Wentz DA, Bauch NJ, et al. Mercury in fish, bed sediment, and water from streams across the United States, 1998–2005: U.S. Geological Survey *Scientific Investigations Report 2009–5109.* 2009:1-76.

321. Nevin K, Rajamohan T. Beneficial effects of virgin coconut oil on lipid parameters and in vitro LDL oxidation. *Clinical Biochemistry.* 2004;37(9):830-835. doi:10.1016/j.clinbiochem.2004.04.010.

322. Cahill G F, Veech R L. Ketoacids? Good medicine? *Transactions of the american clinical and climatological association.* 2003;114:149.

323. Dreon D M, Fernstrom H A, Campos H, Blanche P, et al. Change in dietary saturated fat intake is correlated with change in mass of large low-density-lipoprotein particles in men. *The American journal of clinical nutrition.* 1998;67(5):828-836.

324. Morris M, Tangney C. Dietary fat composition and dementia risk. *Neurobiology of Aging.* 2014;35:S59-S64. doi:10.1016/j.neurobiolaging.2014.03.038.

325. Nafar F, Mearow K M. Coconut oil attenuates the effects of amyloid-β on cortical neurons in vitro. *Journal of Alzheimer's disease.* 2013;39(2):233-237.

326. Fernando W, Martins I, Goozee K, et al. The role of dietary coconut for the prevention and treatment of Alzheimer's disease: potential

mechanisms of action. *British Journal of Nutrition*. 2015;114(01):1-14. doi:10.1017/s0007114515001452.

327. Holly L, Blaskiewicz D, Wu A, et al. Dietary therapy to promote neuroprotection in chronic spinal cord injury. *Journal of Neurosurgery: Spine*. 2012;17(2):134-140. doi:10.3171/2012.5.spine1216.

328. Yeap S, Beh B, Ali N, et al. Antistress and antioxidant effects of virgin coconut oil in vivo. *Experimental and Therapeutic Medicine*. 2014. doi:10.3892/etm.2014.2045.

329. DebMandal M, Mandal S. Coconut (Cocos nucifera L.: Arecaceae): In health promotion and disease prevention. *Asian Pacific Journal of Tropical Medicine*. 2011;4(3):241-247. doi:10.1016/s1995-7645(11)60078-3.

330. Bayir H, Kagan V, Tyurina Y, et al. Assessment of Antioxidant Reserves and Oxidative Stress in Cerebrospinal Fluid after Severe Traumatic Brain Injury in Infants and Children. *Pediatr Res*. 2002;51(5):571-578. doi:10.1203/00006450-200205000-00005.

331. Ng T, Chiam P, Lee T, Chua H, Lim L, Kua E. Curry Consumption and Cognitive Function in the Elderly. *American Journal of Epidemiology*. 2006;164(9):898-906. doi:10.1093/aje/kwj267.

332. Mamtani R, Mamtani R. Ayurveda and Yoga in Cardiovascular Diseases. *Cardiology in Review*. 2005;13(3):155-162. doi:10.1097/01.crd.0000128730.31658.36.

333. Schraufstätter E, Bernt H. Antibacterial Action of Curcumin and Related Compounds. *Nature*. 1949;164(4167):456-457. doi:10.1038/164456a0.

334. Singh A, Sidhu G, Deepa T, Maheshwari R. Curcumin inhibits the proliferation and cell cycle progression of human umbilical vein endothelial cell. *Cancer Letters*. 1996;107(1):109-115. doi:10.1016/0304-3835(96)04357-1.

335. Sharma O. Antioxidant activity of curcumin and related compounds. *Biochemical Pharmacology*. 1976;25(15):1811-1812. doi:10.1016/0006-2952(76)90421-4.

336. DeWitt D, Prough D. Blast-Induced Brain Injury and Posttraumatic Hypotension and Hypoxemia. *Journal of Neurotrauma*. 2009;26(6):877-887. doi:10.1089/neu.2007.0439.

337. Weber J, Slemmer J, Shacka J, Sweeney M. Antioxidants and Free Radical Scavengers for the Treatment Of Stroke, Traumatic Brain Injury and Aging. *CMC*. 2008;15(4):404-414. doi:10.2174/092986708783497337.

338. Srimal R, Dhawan B. Pharmacology of diferuloyl methane (curcumin), a non-steroidal anti-inflammatory agent. *Journal of Pharmacy and Pharmacology*. 1973;25(6):447-452. doi:10.1111/j.2042-7158.1973.tb09131.x.

339. Zhu H, Bian C, Yuan J et al. Curcumin attenuates acute inflammatory injury by inhibiting the TLR4/MyD88/NF-κB signaling pathway in experimental traumatic brain injury. *Journal of Neuroinflammation*. 2014;11(1):59. doi:10.1186/1742-2094-11-59.

340. Yuan J, Zou M, Xiang X et al. Curcumin improves neural function after spinal cord injury by the joint inhibition of the intracellular and extracellular components of glial scar. *Journal of Surgical Research*. 2015;195(1):235-245. doi:10.1016/j.jss.2014.12.055.

341. Bhutani M, Bishnoi M, Kulkarni S. Anti-depressant like effect of curcumin and its combination with piperine in unpredictable chronic stress-induced behavioral, biochemical and neurochemical changes. *Pharmacology Biochemistry and Behavior*. 2009;92(1):39-43. doi:10.1016/j.pbb.2008.10.007.

342. Hurley L, Akinfiresoye L, Nwulia E, Kamiya A, et al. Antidepressant-like effects of curcumin in WKY rat model of depression is associated with an increase in hippocampal BDNF. *Behavioural Brain Research*. 2013;239:27-30. doi:10.1016/j.bbr.2012.10.049.

343. Kulkarni S, Bhutani M, Bishnoi M. Antidepressant activity of curcumin: involvement of serotonin and dopamine system. *Psychopharmacology*. 2008;201(3):435-442. doi:10.1007/s00213-008-1300-y.

344. Tsai H, Lin H, Lu Y, Chen Y, Mahady G. A Review of Potential Harmful Interactions between Anticoagulant/Antiplatelet Agents and Chinese Herbal Medicines. *PLoS ONE*. 2013;8(5):e64255. doi:10.1371/journal.pone.0064255.

345. Somasundaram S, Edmund N A, Moore D T, Small G W, et al. Dietary Curcumin Inhibits Chemotherapy-Induced Apoptosis in Models of Human Breast Cancer. *Cancer Research*. 2002;*62*(13):3868-3875.

346. Bohn T. Dietary factors affecting polyphenol bioavailability. *Nutr Rev*. 2014;72(7):429-452. doi:10.1111/nure.12114.

347. Shoba G, Joy D, Joseph T, Majeed M, Rajendran R, Srinivas P. Influence of Piperine on the Pharmacokinetics of Curcumin in Animals and Human Volunteers. *Planta Med*. 1998;64(04):353-356. doi:10.1055/s-2006-957450.

348. Hani U, Shivakumar H. Solubility Enhancement and Delivery Systems of Curcumin a Herbal Medicine: A Review. *Current Drug Delivery*. 2014;11(6):792-804. doi:10.2174/1567201811666140825130003.

349. Fda.gov. 2013. Available at: http://www.fda.gov/downloads/Food/IngredientsPackagingLabeling/GRAS/NoticeInventory/UCM346902.

350. Nath S. Spicy Approach to Cancer Treatment. *JNCI Journal of the National Cancer Institute*. 2011;103(24):1817-1818. doi:10.1093/jnci/djr526.

351. Lao C D, Ruffin M T, Normolle D, Heath D D, et al. Dose Escalation of a Curcuminoid Formulation. *BMC Complementary and Alternative Medicine*. 2006;6(1):10.

352. Ndb.nal.usda.gov. Show Foods. Available at: http://ndb.nal.usda.gov/ndb/foods/show/112. Accessed November 24, 2015.

353. Lichtenstein A. Diet and Lifestyle Recommendations Revision 2006: A Scientific Statement From the American Heart Association Nutrition Committee. *Circulation*. 2006;114(1):82-96. doi:10.1161/circulationaha.106.176158.

354. Berger S, Raman G, Vishwanathan R, Jacques P, Johnson E. Dietary cholesterol and cardiovascular disease: a systematic review and meta-analysis. *American Journal of Clinical Nutrition*. 2015;102(2):276-294. doi:10.3945/ajcn.114.100305.

355. Gao S, Jin Y, Hall K et al. Selenium Level and Cognitive Function in Rural Elderly Chinese. *American Journal of Epidemiology*. 2007;165(8):955-965. doi:10.1093/aje/kwk073.

356. Gómez-Pinilla F. Brain foods: the effects of nutrients on brain function. *Nature Reviews Neuroscience*. 2008;9(7):568-578. doi:10.1038/nrn2421.

357. Ribaya-Mercado J, Blumberg J. Lutein and Zeaxanthin and Their Potential Roles in Disease Prevention. *Journal of the American College of Nutrition*. 2004;23(sup6):567S-587S. doi:10.1080/07315724.2004.10719427.

358. Fernandez M. Dietary cholesterol provided by eggs and plasma lipoproteins in healthy populations. *Current Opinion in Clinical Nutrition and Metabolic Care*. 2006;9(1):8-12. doi:10.1097/01.mco.0000171152.51034.bf.

359. Johnson E. A possible role for lutein and zeaxanthin in cognitive function in the elderly. *American Journal of Clinical Nutrition*. 2012;96(5):1161S-1165S. doi:10.3945/ajcn.112.034611.

360. Vishwanathan R, Iannaccone A, Scott T et al. Macular pigment optical density is related to cognitive function in older people. *Age and Ageing*. 2014;43(2):271-275. doi:10.1093/ageing/aft210.

361. McCann J, Hudes M, Ames B. An overview of evidence for a causal relationship between dietary availability of choline during development and cognitive function in offspring. *Neuroscience & Biobehavioral Reviews*. 2006;30(5):696-712. doi:10.1016/j.neubiorev.2005.12.003.

362. Gómez-Pinilla F. Brain foods: the effects of nutrients on brain function. *Nature Reviews Neuroscience*. 2008;9(7):568-578. doi:10.1038/nrn2421.

363. Poly C, Massaro J, Seshadri S et al. The relation of dietary choline to cognitive performance and white-matter hyperintensity in the Framingham Offspring Cohort1,2. *American Journal of Clinical Nutrition.* 2011;94(6):1584-1591. doi:10.3945/ajcn.110.008938.

364. Ushistory.org. Fire Department. 2015. Available at: http://www.ushistory.org/franklin/philadelphia/fire.htm. Accessed September 11, 2015.

365. Cohen J, Cottrell S. An overview of concussion protocols across professional sports leagues. *LawInSport.* 2015. Available at: http://www.lawinsport.com/features/item/an-overview-of-concussion-protocols-across-professional-sports-leagues.

366. Cohen J, Cottrell S. An overview of concussion protocols across professional sports leagues. *LawInSport.* 2015. Available at: http://www.lawinsport.com/features/item/an-overview-of-concussion-protocols-across-professional-sports-leagues.

367. Cohen J, Cottrell S. An overview of concussion protocols across professional sports leagues. *LawInSport.* 2015. Available at: http://www.lawinsport.com/features/item/an-overview-of-concussion-protocols-across-professional-sports-leagues.

368. Guskiewicz K, Marshall S, Bailes J, et al. Association between Recurrent Concussion and Late-Life Cognitive Impairment in Retired Professional Football Players. *Neurosurgery.* 2005:719-726. doi:10.1227/01.neu.0000175725.75780.dd.

369. Breslow J. 76 of 79 Deceased NFL Players Found to Have Brain Disease – Concussion Watch - FRONTLINE. *FRONTLINE.* 2015. Available at: http://www.pbs.org/wgbh/pages/frontline/sports/concussion-watch/76-of-79-deceased-nfl-players-found-to-have-brain-disease/.

370. Schwarz A. Dave Duerson Found to Have the Brain Trauma He Suspected. *Nytimescom.* 2011. Available at: http://www.nytimes.com/2011/05/03/sports/football/03duerson.html.

371. Hutchison M, Lawrence D, Cusimano M, Schweizer T. Head Trauma in Mixed Martial Arts. *The American Journal of Sports Medicine.* 2014;42(6):1352-1358. doi:10.1177/0363546514526151.

372. Lustig R, Schmidt L, Brindis C. Public health: The toxic truth about sugar. *Nature.* 2012;482(7383):27-29. doi:10.1038/482027a.

373. Ferdman R. Where people around the world eat the most sugar and fat. *Washington Post.* 2015. Available at: http://www.washingtonpost.com/news/wonkblog/wp/2015/02/05/where-people-around-the-world-eat-the-most-sugar-and-fat/.

374. Lustig R, Schmidt L, Brindis C. Public health: The toxic truth about sugar. *Nature*. 2012;482(7383):27-29. doi:10.1038/482027a.

375. Cohen R. Ngm.nationalgeographic.com. Sugar. 2013. Available at: http://ngm.nationalgeographic.com/2013/08/sugar/cohen-text. Accessed September 17, 2015.

376. Cohen R. Ngm.nationalgeographic.com. Sugar. 2015. Available at: http://ngm.nationalgeographic.com/2013/08/sugar/cohen-text. Accessed September 17, 2015.

377. Lustig R, Schmidt L, Brindis C. Public health: The toxic truth about sugar. *Nature*. 2012;482(7383):27-29. doi:10.1038/482027a.

378. Chen J. Your Brain on Sugar. *Marie Claire*. 2012;(7):101-101.

379. Kerti L, Witte V, Winkler A, et al. "Higher glucose levels associated with lower memory and reduced hippocampal microstructure." Neurology. 2013;81(20):1746-1752.

380. Schoenthaler, S J. Diet and crime: An empirical examination of the value of nutrition in the control and treatment of incarcerated juvenile offenders. *International Journal of Biosocial Research*. 1983;4(1): 25-39.

381. The Huffington Post. Ask JJ: Natural Sweetener Alternatives. 2015. Available at: http://www.huffingtonpost.com/jj-virgin/ask-jjnatural-sweetener-_b_6497816.html. Accessed September 17, 2015.

382. Cardello, H. M. A. B., Da Silva, M. A. P. A., & Damasio, M. H. Measurement of the relative sweetness of stevia extract, aspartame and cyclamate/saccharin blend as compared to sucrose at different concentrations. *Plant Foods for Human Nutrition*. 1999;54(2):119-129.

383. The Huffington Post. Ask JJ: Natural Sweetener Alternatives. 2015. Available at: http://www.huffingtonpost.com/jj-virgin/ask-jjnatural-sweetener-_b_6497816.html. Accessed September 17, 2015.

384. Roussell D, Roussell D. Ask the Diet Doctor: Monk Fruit. *Shape Magazine*. 2013. Available at: http://www.shape.com/healthyeating/diet-tips/ask-diet-doctor-monk-fruit. Accessed September 30, 2015.

385. The Huffington Post. Ask JJ: Natural Sweetener Alternatives. 2015. Available at: http://www.huffingtonpost.com/jj-virgin/ask-jjnatural-sweetener-_b_6497816.html. Accessed September 17, 2015.

386. Wikipedia. Xylitol. 2015. Available at: https://en.wikipedia.org/wiki/Xylitol. Accessed September 30, 2015.

387. Ishikawa M, Miyashita M, Kawashima Y, Nakamura T, Saitou N, Modderman J. Effects of Oral Administration of Erythritol on Patients with

Diabetes. *Regulatory Toxicology and Pharmacology*. 1996;24(2):S303-S308. doi:10.1006/rtph.1996.0112.

388. Wikipedia. Erythritol. 2015. Available at: https://en.wikipedia.org/wiki/Erythritol. Accessed September 30, 2015.

389. Cdc.gov. FastStats. 2015. Available at: http://www.cdc.gov/nchs/fastats/obesity-overweight.htm. Accessed October 15, 2015.

390. Ogden C, Carroll M, Kit B, Flegal K. Prevalence of Childhood and Adult Obesity in the United States, 2011-2012. *JAMA*. 2014;311(8):806. doi:10.1001/jama.2014.732.

391. (US) N. Section 1: Overweight and Obesity as Public Health Problems in America. *Office of the Surgeon General (US)*. 2001. Available at: http://www.ncbi.nlm.nih.gov/books/NBK44210/. Accessed October 15, 2015.

392. Brown C, Neville A, Rhee P, Salim A, Velmahos G, Demetriades D. The Impact of Obesity on the Outcomes of 1,153 Critically Injured Blunt Trauma Patients. *The Journal of Trauma: Injury, Infection, and Critical Care*. 2005:1048-1051. doi:10.1097/01.ta.0000189047.65630.c5.

393. Pannacciulli N, Del Parigi A, Chen K, Le D, Reiman E, Tataranni P. Brain abnormalities in human obesity: A voxel-based morphometric study. *NeuroImage*. 2006;31(4):1419-1425. doi:10.1016/j.neuroimage.2006.01.047.

394. Mattson M, Duan W, Chan S et al. Neuroprotective and neurorestorative signal transduction mechanisms in brain aging: modification by genes, diet and behavior. *Neurobiology of Aging*. 2002;23(5):695-705. doi:10.1016/s0197-4580(02)00025-8.

395. Naderali E, Ratcliffe S, Dale M. Review: Obesity and Alzheimer's Disease: A Link Between Body Weight and Cognitive Function in Old Age. *American Journal of Alzheimer's Disease and Other Dementias*. 2009;24(6):445-449. doi:10.1177/1533317509348208.

396. Xu W, Atti A, Gatz M, Pedersen N, Johansson B, Fratiglioni L. Midlife overweight and obesity increase late-life dementia risk: A population-based twin study. *Neurology*. 2011;76(18):1568-1574. doi:10.1212/wnl.0b013e3182190d09.

397. Gustafson D, Rothenberg E, Blennow K, Steen B, Skoog I. An 18-Year Follow-up of Overweight and Risk of Alzheimer Disease. *Arch Intern Med*. 2003;163(13):1524. doi:10.1001/archinte.163.13.1524.

398. Naderali E, Ratcliffe S, Dale M. Review: Obesity and Alzheimer's Disease: A Link Between Body Weight and Cognitive Function in Old Age. *American Journal of Alzheimer's Disease and Other Dementias*. 2009;24(6):445-449. doi:10.1177/1533317509348208.

399. Halagappa V, Guo Z, Pearson M et al. Intermittent fasting and caloric restriction ameliorate age-related behavioral deficits in the triple-transgenic mouse model of Alzheimer's disease. *Neurobiology of Disease.* 2007;26(1):212-220. doi:10.1016/j.nbd.2006.12.019.

400. Johnson J, Summer W, Cutler R et al. Alternate day calorie restriction improves clinical findings and reduces markers of oxidative stress and inflammation in overweight adults with moderate asthma. *Free Radical Biology and Medicine.* 2007;42(5):665-674. doi:10.1016/j.freeradbiomed.2006.12.005.

401. Young E. Deprive yourself: the real benefits of fasting. *New Scientist.* 2012;216(2891):46-49. doi:10.1016/s0262-4079(12)62960-1.

402. Martin B, Mattson M, Maudsley S. Caloric restriction and intermittent fasting: Two potential diets for successful brain aging. *Ageing Research Reviews.* 2006;5(3):332-353. doi:10.1016/j.arr.2006.04.002.

403. Freeman S. Alcohol Kills Brain Cells. *HowStuffWorks.* 2015. Available at: http://science.howstuffworks.com/life/inside-themind/human-brain/10-brain-myths9.htm. Accessed October 1, 2015.

404. Jorge R E, Starkstein S E, Arndt S, et al. Alcohol misuse and mood disorders following traumatic brain injury. *Archives of General Psychiatry.* 2005;*62*(7):742-749.

405. Rapp, P.E., et al., Traumatic brain injury detection using electrophysiological methods. Front Hum Neurosci, 2015. 9: p. 11.6.

406. ElMindA. BNA™ Basics - ElMindA. 2015. Available at: http://elminda.com/bna-basics/. Accessed November 13, 2015.

407. Impacttest.com. About ImPACT | ImPACT Testing & Computerized Neurocognitive Assessment Tools. 2015. Available at: https://www.impacttest.com/about/. Accessed November 15, 2015.

408. Mucha, Anne et al. A brief vestibular ocular motor screening (VOMS) assessment to evaluate concussions. *Am J of Sports Med,* 2014 Oct: 42 (10) 2479-2486.

409. http://kingdevicktest.com/for-concussions/research-and-publications/

CPSIA information can be obtained
at www.ICGtesting.com
Printed in the USA
LVOW04s1210310817
547041LV00003B/5/P